Cortical Mechanisms of Vision

The advent of sensors capable of localizing portions of the brain involved in specific computations, has provided significant insights into normal visual information processing and specific neurological conditions. Aided by devices such as fMRI, researchers are now able to construct highly detailed models of how the brain processes specific patterns of visual information. This book brings together some of the strongest thinkers in this field, to explore cortical visual information processing and its underlying mechanisms. It is a great resource for vision researchers with both biological and computational backgrounds, and is an essential guide for graduate students just starting out in the field.

MICHAEL JENKIN is Professor of Computer Science and Engineering at York University, Ontario, Canada. His research interests include perception and guidance for autonomous robotic systems, and the development and analysis of virtual reality systems. In 2005 he was the recipient of the CIPPRS/ACTIRF award for research excellence and service to the Canadian Computer and Robot Vision research community.

LAURENCE HARRIS is Chair of the Department of Psychology, and a member of the Centre for Vision Research at York University in Toronto. He received his Ph.D. from Cambridge University and was a lecturer in Physiology at the University of Wales until going to Canada in 1990. He is interested in how information coming through different senses is combined to determine orientation and self motion perception and to localize events in space and time and how these perceptions may be altered in unusual environments such as the microgravity of space or by clinical conditions such as Parkinson's syndrome.

CORTICAL MECHANISMS OF VISION

Edited by

MICHAEL R. M. JENKIN

York University,
Toronto, Ontario, Canada

LAURENCE R. HARRIS

York University,
Toronto, Ontario, Canada

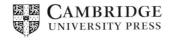

CAMBRIDGE
UNIVERSITY PRESS

CAMBRIDGE UNIVERSITY PRESS
Cambridge, New York, Melbourne, Madrid, Cape Town, Singapore, São Paulo, Delhi

Cambridge University Press
The Edinburgh Building, Cambridge CB2 8RU, UK

Published in the United States of America by Cambridge University Press, New York

www.cambridge.org
Information on this title: www.cambridge.org/9780521889612

First published 2009

Printed in the United Kingdom at the University Press, Cambridge

A catalog record for this publication is available from the British Library

Library of Congress Cataloging in Publication data

ISBN 978-0-521-88961-2 hardback

All material contained within the CD-ROM is protected by copyright and other intellectual property laws. The customer acquires only the right to use the CD-ROM and does not acquire any other rights, express or implied, unless these are stated explicitly in a separate licence.

To the extent permitted by applicable law, Cambridge University Press is not liable for direct damages or loss of any kind resulting from the use of this product or from errors or faults contained in it, and in every case Cambridge University Press's liability shall be limited to the amount actually paid by the customer for the product.

The CD-ROM that accompanies this book contains color imagery and other material associated with various chapters and the York Vision Conference. The CD-ROM is presented in HTML format, and is viewable with any standard browser (e.g. Netscape Navigator or Microsoft Internet Explorer). To view the CD-ROM, point your browser at the file **index.htm** on the CD-ROM.

Contents

Contributors

Galia Avidan
Department of Psychology
Ben Gurion University of the Negev
POB 653
Beer Sheva 84105, Israel

Raymundo Báez-Mendoza
Department of Physiology,
Development and Neuroscience
University of Cambridge
Cambridge, CB2 3DY, UK

Marlene Behrmann
Department of Psychology
Carnegie Mellon University
Pittsburgh, PA 15213, USA

James W. Bisley
Department of Neurobiology
David Geffin School of Medicine
P. O. Box 951763
Los Angeles, CA 90025, USA

Sandra E. Black
Department of Medicine
Sunnybrook Health Sciences Centre
2075 Bayview Ave.
Toronto, Ontario M4N 3M5, Canada

Annabelle Blangero
Espace et Action
16 avenue du doyen Lépine
69500, Bron, Rhone-Alpes, France

J. Douglas Crawford
Centre for Vision Research and Depart-
ment of Psychology
York University
4700 Keele St.
Toronto, Ontario M3J 1P3, Canada

Joseph F. X. DeSouza
Department of Psychology
York University
4700 Keele St.
Toronto, Ontario M3J 1P3, Canada

Marc J. Dubin
University of Rochester Medical Center
601 Elmwood Ave.
Rochester, NY 14642-0673, USA

Charles J. Duffy
University of Rochester Medical Center
601 Elmwood Ave.
Rochester, NY 14642-0673, USA

Mazyar Fallah
School of Kinesiology and Health Science
York University
4700 Keele St.
Toronto, Ontario M3J 1P3, Canada

Florin D. Feloiu
Department of Physiotherapy
McMaster University
1280 Main St. W.
Hamilton, Ontario L8S 4L8, Canada

Tzvi Ganel
Department of Psychology
Ben-Gurion University of the Negev
Beer-Sheva, 84105, Israel

Angela L. Gee
Mahoney Center for Brain and Behavior
Columbia University
1051 Riverside Dr., Unit 87
New York, NY 10032, USA

Golijeh Golarai
Department of Psychology
Stanford University
Stanford, CA 94305, USA

Michael E. Goldberg
Mahoney Center for Brain and Behavior
Columbia University
1051 Riverside Dr., Unit 87
New York, NY 10032, USA

Melvyn A. Goodale
CIHR Group on Action and Perception
Department of Psychology
University of Western Ontario
London, Ontario N6A 5C2, Canada

Diana Gorbet
Department of Kinesiology
University of Waterloo
200 University Ave. W
Waterloo, Ontario N2L 3G1, Canada

Kalanit Grill-Spector
Department of Psychology
Stanford University
Stanford, CA 94305, USA

Laurence R. Harris
Centre for Vision Research and
Department of Psychology
York University
4700 Keele St.
Toronto, Ontario M3J 1P3, Canada

Kari L. Hoffman
Centre for Vision Research and
Department of Psychology
York University
4700 Keele St.
Toronto, Ontario M3J 1P3, Canada

Adria E. N. Hoover
Department of Psychology
York University
4700 Keele St.
Toronto, Ontario M3J 1P3, Canada

Jens-Max Hopf
Dept. of Neurology II, Otto-von-Guericke
University,
Leibniz-Institute for Neurobiology,
Magdeburg Leipziger Strasse 44
39120 Magdeburg, Germany

Anna E. Ipata
Mahoney Center for Brain and Behavior
Columbia University
1051 Riverside Drive, Unit 87
New York, NY 10032, USA

Michael Jenkin
Centre for Vision Research and
Department of Computer Science and Engineering
York University
4700 Keele Street
Toronto, Ontario M3J 1P3, Canada

Heather Jordan
Department of Psychology
York University
4700 Keele St.
Toronto, Ontario M3J 1P3, Canada

Aarlenne Khan
Smith-Kettlewell Institute
2318 Fillmore Street
San Francisco, CA 94115, USA

B. Suresh Krishna
Mahoney Center for Brain and Behavior
Columbia University
1051 Riverside Drive, Unit 87
New York, NY 10032, USA

David J. Logan
Broad Institute
MIT
Cambridge, MA 02142, USA

Jonathan J. Marotta
Department of Psychology
University of Manitoba
190 Dysart Rd.
Winnipeg, Manitoba R3T 2N2, Canada

Bogdan Neagu
School of Kinesiology and Health Science
York University
4700 Keele St.
Toronto, Ontario M3J 1P3, Canada

Shima Ovaysikia
Department of Psychology
York University
4700 Keele St.
Toronto, Ontario M3J 1P3, Canada

William K. Page
University of Rochester Medical Center
601 Elmwood Avenue
Rochester, New York 14642-0673, USA

Martin Paré
Centre for Neuroscience Studies
Queen's University
Kingston, Ontario K7L 3N6, Canada

Laure Pisella
Espace et Action
16 avenue du doyen Lépine
69500, Bron, Rhone-Alpes, France

Yves Rossetti
Espace et Action
16 avenue du doyen Lépine
69500, Bron, Rhone-Alpes, France

Bruno Rossion
Center for Neuroscience
Université catholique de Louvain
1348 Louvain-la-Neuve, Belgium

Lauren Sergio
School of Kinesiology and Health Science
York University
4700 Keele St.
Toronto, Ontario M3J 1P3, Canada

Kelly Shen
Centre for Neuroscience Studies
Queen's University
Kingston, Ontario K7L 3N6, Canada

Khalid Tahir
Department of Psychology
York University
4700 Keele St.
Toronto, Ontario M3J 1P3, Canada

Alzahir Tharani
Department of Psychology
York University
4700 Keele St.
Toronto, Ontario M3J 1P3, Canada

Cibu Thomas
Department of Psychology
Carnegie Mellon University
Pittsburgh, PA 15213, USA

Neil W. D. Thomas
Centre for Neuroscience Studies
Queen's University
Kingston, Ontario K7L 3N6, Canada

William John Tippett
Neuroscience Research Unit
Sunnybrook Health Sciences Centre
2075 Bayview Ave.
Toronto, Ontario M4N 3M5, Canada

Michael Vesia
School of Kinesiology and Health Science
York University
4700 Keele Street
Toronto, Ontario M3J 1P3, Canada

Hugh R. Wilson
Department of Biology and
Centre for Vision Research
York University
4700 Keele Street
Toronto, Ontario M3J 1P3, Canada

Steven P. Wise
Laboratory of Systems Neuroscience
National Institute of Mental Health
49 Convent Dr., MSC 4401
Bethesda, MD 20892-4401, USA

Xiaogang Yan
Centre for Vision Research
York University
4700 Keele Street
Toronto, Ontario M3J 1P3, Canada

1 Cortical mechanisms of vision

L. R. Harris and M. Jenkin

The history of the evolution of our understanding of cortical mechanisms of vision can be traced back to the *Edwin Smith Surgical Papyrus*. Written around the year 1700 BC this papyrus contains the first known written account of the anatomy of the brain (Brandt-Rauf, P. W. and Brandt-Rauf, S. J., 1987). The papyrus documents a number of medical cases which involved trauma to the brain and spinal cord, and also enumerates gross structural components. This document related for the first time how damage to specific portions of the brain were reflected in specific functions.

By the nineteenth century the idea that function follows structural form within the brain had been well established. Observational work coupled with selective stimulation of portions of the brain via electrical stimulation demonstrated conclusively that certain functions were localized to specific regions of the brain. By the mid 1970s large-scale studies with specific patient groups (e.g. Penfield's work with patients with epilepsy, Penfield, 1975) had been conducted using this technique.

With the development of microelectrodes capable of recording intrinsic electrical activity within the brain more detailed study became possible. Vernon Mountcastle identified a highly organized columnar structure within the neocortex (see Mountcastle, 1997 for a review). Neurocomputational units were demonstrated to have a complex but repeated structure. Linkages between and among these columnar units define a distributed computational structure with individual units potentially contributing to multiple computations.

Starting in the late fifties David Hubel and Torsten Wiesel published a series of papers in the *Journal of Neurophysiology* on the behavior of cells in the anesthetized cat's visual cortex (see Hubel and Wiesel, 2005 for comprehensive review). Hubel and Wiesel described the cells they recorded as having clearly definable properties suggesting that they appeared to be looking for particular visual features. Further, although there are millions of cells in the visual cortex, Hubel and Wiesel suggested that they could all be divided into a mere three classes. Their work gave hope and

Cortical Mechanisms of Vision, ed. M. Jenkin and L. R. Harris. Published by Cambridge University Press.
©Cambridge University Press 2009.

tangibility to the notion that neurophysiology, started only some twenty years earlier with the invention of the microelectrode, could actually answer the question of how the brain works, or at least that it was possible to understand the cortical mechanisms of vision.

Some of the limitations of single cell recording were overcome through the use of less invasive technologies that monitor activities within the brain. Magnetoencephalography (MEG) measures the magnetic field associated with the electrical currents flowing in neurons. Magnetic Resonance Imaging (MRI) uses magnetic fields to align some of the protons within the brain with a magnetic field. Radio waves are used to knock these protons out of alignment. As the protons realign, radio waves are emitted and these waves are used to reconstruct the three-dimensional structure. Functional Magnetic Resonance Imaging (fMRI) uses a conventional MRI scanner but takes advantage of the fact that when parts of the brain are active they require more blood. Blood molecules contain iron which disrupts the local magnetic field and these disruptions can be detected. MEG, MRI and fMRI technologies have revolutionized the study of cortical function. Given their noninvasive nature and the relatively high degree of spatial localization they can obtain, it is possible to conduct studies with awake human observers and to watch information flow within the three-dimensional structure of the brain. This book brings together researchers at the forefront of the study of cortical mechanisms of vision. We are at an exciting moment in our understanding of how information is processed by the brain and the chapters that follow provide a view of our understanding of cortical structure and the involvement of the cortex in visual information processing.

In the present volume there are very few references to Hubel and Wiesel. The issue of understanding cortical mechanisms has become far more ambitious than aiming to understand the processing of only the earliest stages of the visual pathways. Once we leave the primary visual cortex, the anatomical connections become extremely complex, but a simplifying concept that has proved helpful is the notion that there are two broad types of visual information to be extracted from the visual image and that there are two broad pathways that specialize in processing these categories. The two broad categories of information are (i) vision that is important in controlling action (such as guiding walking and reaching out for something) and (ii) vision that is important for what we more traditionally regard as vision: that is the ability to recognize things by seeing them. The two visual pathways involve two of the association cortices: the parietal cortex on the dorsal part of the brain, and the temporal lobes in the ventral region. Mortimer Mishkin and Leslie Ungerleider described the anatomy of these dorsal and ventral pathways (Ungerleider and Mishkin, 1982) but their functional significance was brought to the fore by the patient studies of Mel Goodale and David Milner, reviewed in their two books Milner and Goodale (1995) and Goodale and Milner (2004).

The division in the structure of the visual brain is reflected in the structure of this volume which has sections on the dorsal and ventral streams. Two additional sections deal with the role of the other association cortex: the frontal lobe, and with attention and consciousness.

The dorsal stream section of the book deals with the parietal cortex and action. It starts with Chapter 2 by James Bisley and colleagues on the lateral intraparietal cortex in which the authors suggest that this area serves as a priority map for the control of actions. Damage to the dorsal stream, especially the right side, produces the complex syndrome of visuospatial agnosia. One aspect of this syndrome is a hemispatial neglect. Neglect has been worked on extensively as an access point to understanding the role of the parietal cortex in coding space. Neglect implies not interacting with space, and Chapter 3 by Florin Feloiu and colleagues describes how this intriguing ability to ignore a whole half of the world can be overcome by the simple use of displacing prisms. Chapter 4, by Aarlenne Khan and colleagues, continues the theme of parietal cortical damage as a window to understanding its normal function by considering optic ataxia. Optic ataxia is the part of visuo-spatial agnosia syndrome in which patients find themselves unable to reach out and interact with objects in space even though they report being able to see them. The control of reaching to objects seen in space (there is an area in the parietal known as the parietal reach area) is reviewed in Chapter 5 by Lauren Sergio and colleagues. And lastly the parietal's role in coding whole body movement is considered in Chapter 6 by Charles Duffy and colleagues.

The ventral stream section of the book starts with Chapter 7, a review of the development of the temporal lobes by Kalanit Grill-Spector and Golijeh Golarai. The temporal lobes are not homogeneous in their organization but appear to be divided into small areas specializing in particular functions. How this dividing up occurs with the maturation of the organism provides insight not only into the structural organization of the brain but also into the role of experience in defining and determining brain function. The technique of functional magnetic resonance imaging has contributed enormously to our understanding of the specializations within all parts of the brain. In this chapter it is used to track the development of subdivisions of the temporal lobes that process faces, places and objects. Some of the first clues to the localization of function in the brain came from studies of the effects of discrete brain injuries. The world wars pushed forward our understanding of brain organization considerably by providing small, circumscribed, bullet-sized lesions of all parts of the brain. Small lesions of an area in the front part of the temporal lobes resulted in a very specific deficit of not being able to recognize faces. This condition is called prosopagnosia. In Chapter 8, Bruno Russion uses a combination of lesions (created not by bullets but as a result of hypoxia) and fMRI to reveal some of the principles by which the healthy human brain is able to recognize faces.

Prosopagnosia can also arise not from lesions but as a congenital condition. What has gone wrong in the temporal lobe face areas in such patients is considered by Galia Avidan and colleagues in Chapter 9. The last chapter concerning the function of the temporal lobes, Chapter 10 by Raymundo Báez-Mendoza, and Kari L. Hoffman, considers the functions of the temporal lobes *not* just in humans but in other primates.

The third section of this book considers the frontal lobes. Although not traditionally regarded as a part of even the "extended" visual system, the frontal lobes are considered in this book because of their integral executive role. For example, the frontal lobes, especially the area called the frontal eye fields, are intimately involved in the control of eye movements. The prefrontal cortex (at the anterior poles of the frontal region) in contrast is involved more in not making movements. It is almost as important to not make movements (one cannot orient to everything in the visual scene!) as it is to make them. Damage to the frontal lobes produces a syndrome called Kluver-Bucy syndrome in which actions are repeated indefinitely. The first chapter in this section, Chapter 11 by Shima Ovaysikia and colleagues, reviews how the frontal lobes are involved in the important function of not doing anything.

The frontal lobes are beyond the two divisions of the visual system and as such are involved in executive functions that involve both of them. The cortical basis of deciding where to look is supported here. The simple act of looking in a particular direction is important to ventral stream functioning by selecting a particular object for perception. At the same time information concerning where one is looking (e.g. the position of the eyes in the orbits) is essential for decoding the location of objects relative to the viewer. And of course one needs to know an object's location in space in order to interact with it (a dorsal stream function). These intricate interactions are considered by Stephen Wise in Chapter 12. The direct role of the frontal lobes in controlling eye position is reviewed by Martin Paré and colleagues in Chapter 13. The role of the frontal eye fields in selecting objects is a functional implementation of attention. Martin Paré et al. consider this aspect of saccadic control which is returned to in more detail in Section 4 of the book. In Chapter 14 Maz Fallah and Heather Jordan look not just at individual saccades but at the whole process of visual search – that is how targets are selected (or not selected) as targets for visual attention. Jens-Max Hopf considers the neural mechanisms of visual search in Chapter 15.

The last section of this book deals with issues of attention and consciousness. It might be thought that consciousness is beyond the scope of a book on the cortical mechanisms of vision. However, Mel Goodale, in Chapter 16, traces the origin of the "two visual systems" (the dorsal and ventral streams) pointing out that information processed by the ventral pathway is perhaps more important for day-to-day survival but that it is information of which we are usually but dimly aware. "Consciousness" usually refers to our ability to be aware of the outside world in terms of what we see out there (ventral stream processing), so does this mean that consciousness resides in the temporal lobes? This theme is developed to give a fitting final chapter for the book by Hugh Wilson, the director of the Centre for Vision Research that hosted the Centre for Vision Research Conference on Cortical Mechanisms of Vision in June 2007 on which this book is based. In Chapter 17 he considers the cortical basis for conscious vision and puts it into both a philosophical and neurophysiological context.

References

Brandt-Rauf, P. W. and Brandt-Rauf, S. J. (1987). History of occupational medicine: relevance of Imhotep and the Edwin Smith papyrus. *Brit. J. Industrial Med.*, 44: 68–70.

Goodale, M. A. and Milner, A. D. (2004). *Sight Unseen*. Oxford, UK: Oxford University Press.

Hubel, D. and Wiesel, T. (2005). *Brain and Visual Perception: The Story of a 25-year Collaboration*. Oxford, UK: Oxford University Press.

Milner, A. D. and Goodale, M. A. (1995). *The Visual Brain in Action*. Oxford, UK: Oxford University Press.

Mountcastle, V. (1997). The columnar organization of the neocortex. *Brain*. 120: 701.

Penfield, W. (1975). *The Mystery of the Mind*. Princeton, NJ: Princeton University Press.

Ungerleider, L. G. and Mishkin, M. (1982). Two cortical visual systems. In D. G. Ingle, M. A. Goodale and R. J. W. Mansfield (eds.) *Analysis of Visual Behaviour*. Cambridge, MA: MIT Press, pp. 549–586.

Part I

Dorsal stream

2 The lateral intraparietal area: a priority map in posterior parietal cortex

J. W. Bisley, A. E. Ipata, B. S. Krishna, A. L. Gee and M. E. Goldberg

To decide what we will pay attention to, our brains must balance our goals and intentions with changes in the visual scene. One suggestion is that bottom-up visual information is combined with top-down influences to create a map of visual space in which features or locations are represented by levels of activity related to the attentional priority at that location. Using this system, our attention goes to the highest point on the map. Here we suggest that the lateral intraparietal area (LIP) of posterior parietal cortex behaves in such a fashion. Using a dual task paradigm, we will show that when eye movements are forbidden, covert attention is allocated to the peak on the priority map. Using a free-viewing visual search paradigm, we will show that when eye movements are allowed, the activity in LIP is used for overt attention to guide these eye movements. Finally, we will also show evidence of top-down and bottom-up influences on the activity in LIP and we will discuss how this interpretation of LIP neatly unites the broad array of results previously garnered from studies of this area.

2.1 Introduction

Each time we shift our gaze, our eyes are flooded with information from the rich tapestry that is the visual world. In order to manage this onslaught of information we limit detailed neural analyses to a small number of objects or regions of space. The information about these attended objects or locations can then be used for perception, learning, memory, and for planning motor commands to interact with the world. In the lab, focusing of attention improves visual processing (Yeshurun and Carrasco, 1999;

Cortical Mechanisms of Vision, ed. M. Jenkin and L. R. Harris. Published by Cambridge University Press.
© Cambridge University Press 2009.

Pestilli and Carrasco, 2005) and speeds up reaction times (Posner, 1980), and neural correlates of the effect of attention have been seen in a number of visual cortical areas (Moran and Desimone, 1985; Luck et al., 1997; Treue and Maunsell, 1999; Li et al., 2004; Williford and Maunsell, 2006), yet the mechanisms the brain uses to decide what to attend to is unclear.

2.2   Attention

Our visual attention can be allocated in one of two ways – overtly and covertly (Posner, 1980). Overt attention refers to changes in gaze, such that the item or location of interest lands on the high acuity region of the retina – the fovea. Covert attention refers to enhanced processing of visual information that is represented in the visual periphery (Carrasco et al., 2004). Intuitively, one may think that we primarily use overt attention to study the world; however covert attention is constantly being utilized to help decide where to look, and is automatically allocated to the goal of an eye movement once that eye movement has been planned, but before it is executed (Shepherd et al., 1986; Kowler et al., 1995; Deubel and Schneider, 1996).

Most of the decisions underlying the guidance of attention, both overt and covert, occur automatically. Occasionally, we may consciously decide to pay attention to an object, particularly if it is pointed out to us, but in the majority of cases it just "seems to happen". Two main groups of influences are thought to play important roles in the process of deciding where to attend: bottom-up influences and top-down influences (Treisman and Gelade, 1980; Duncan and Humphreys, 1989; Egeth and Yantis, 1997). Bottom-up influences refer to features within the visual input that are inherently salient. These tend to be features that are so different from their surrounds that they pop out from the background; thus in the natural world, in which things tend to be stationary, flashing or moving stimuli appear salient. Other features, such as color or luminance can also be strong enough to make a stimulus salient, thus a bright yellow balloon will pop out from among a bunch of dull gray ones. Top-down influences refer to cognitive signals that help guide the allocation of attention based on prior knowledge or future aims. These signals represent what we deem as important, relevant or just interesting and can be under conscious control or automatically implemented based on training or experience.

The question of how top-down and bottom-up influences are used to influence the decision about where to attend has led to the creation of a large number of models based on behavioral and physiological data (for examples see Koch and Ullman, 1985; Cave and Wolfe, 1990; Tsotsos et al., 1995; Deco and Schurmann, 2000; Hamker, 2004; Walther and Koch, 2006). A common theme throughout many of these models is the inclusion of a map of the visual world, from which attention is allocated to the object or region in space represented by the greatest activity. We will refer to such a map as a priority map (Fecteau and Munoz, 2006; Serences and Yantis, 2006). We have shied away from the use of the term salience map (Itti and Koch, 2000), since it may be incorrectly construed to imply stimulus-related properties alone (Serences and Yantis, 2006). In our view, a priority map must contain a spatial representation of the visual world, must balance both top-down and bottom-up influences, and must be used for the allocation of visual attention. Thus, to be a priority map, a cortical area should have strong responses to features that pop out. It should also have strong responses to features that are important for behavior and low responses to the same features if they are unimportant for behavior. Finally there must be a correlation between the activity and measures of attention.

A number of cortical or subcortical areas have been proposed as being salience or priority maps (Robinson and Petersen, 1992; Gottlieb et al., 1998; Li, 2002; McPeek and Keller, 2002; Mazer and Gallant, 2003; Fecteau et al., 2004; Thompson and Bichot, 2005). Rather than argue that one is the priority map and the rest are not, we will focus on a single area and show that it has all the hallmarks of a priority map. This area is the lateral intraparietal area (LIP) in macaque posterior parietal cortex.

2.3   Why look at LIP?

It is well known that posterior parietal cortex in humans is important for spatial aware-ness and attention. Classical evidence from lesions inducing spatial neglect or ex-tinction has now been supplemented by imaging studies that continue to identify the intraparietal lobule as an important component in spatial attention (Corbetta and Shul-man, 2002; Serences et al., 2005; He et al., 2007). As such, it seems that a homologous region in the monkey brain would be a good place to look for a priority map.

LIP is anatomically well situated to be involved in the allocation of attention. It receives input from visual areas (Figure 2.1, black lines), such as V3A, V4, TEO and MST, and the ventral region of LIP (LIPv) also receives input from V3, MT and the peripheral region of V2 (Blatt et al., 1990; Baizer et al., 1991; Distler et al., 1993; Lewis and Van Essen, 2000). Thus, LIP's inputs are composed of both the traditional ventral and dorsal streams of visual processing (Ungerleider and Mishkin, 1982), providing a representation of visual space predominantly in the contralateral visual field. Despite these varied inputs, neurons tend to have reasonably constrained receptive fields (Ben Hamed et al., 2001) and have not been shown to have specific tuning properties that are unrelated to training (Gottlieb et al., 1998; Kusunoki et al., 2000; Toth and Assad, 2002; Gottlieb et al., 2005 although see also Sereno and Maunsell, 1998). In addition, LIP receives a short latency initial response to sudden onsets (Bisley et al., 2004), which is ideal for the rapid allocation of attention to a flashed object. LIP also feeds back to all of these visual areas, with the exception of V2, and is thus in an excellent position to act as a priority map and bias the activity in these areas (Andersen et al., 1990; Blatt et al., 1990).

In addition to its interconnections with the visual system, LIP is also well connected to the oculomotor system (Figure 2.1, gray lines). LIP projects both to the frontal eye field (FEF) and the superior colliculus (SC) (Andersen et al., 1985, 1990; Paré and Wurtz, 1997; Ferraina et al., 2002) and receives feedback from FEF (Blatt et al., 1990). Because of its position at a node between the visual system and the oculomotor system, it is in an ideal location to influence the visual guidance of eye movements.

Neuronal activity in LIP displays more than just a visual response. Early studies of response properties of LIP neurons suggested that they had three distinct response components: a visual response; a memory response; and a saccade related response

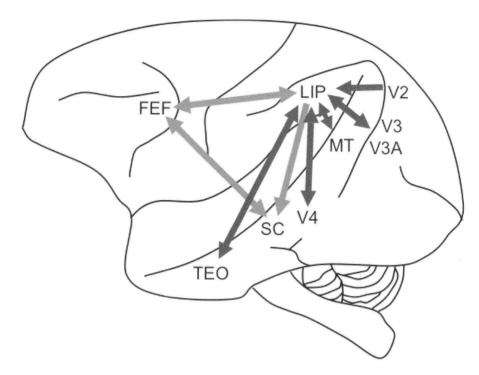

Figure 2.1. Anatomical connections of LIP. A subset of direct connections of LIP with visual areas V2, V3, V3A, MT, V4 and TEO (dark arrows) and oculomotor areas FEF and SC (light gray arrows). Arrow directions indicate flow of information.

(Barash et al., 1991). This activity is shifted from neuron to neuron as the eyes move, meaning that there is a representation of the visual world in LIP that accounts for eye movements (Duhamel et al., 1992).

Activity of LIP neurons can also be modulated by a variety of behavioral instructions. For instance, the response to a flashed spot is greater if the animal has to respond to it than if he has to ignore it (Bushnell et al., 1981), and is greater if the response is in the form of an eye movement rather than an arm movement (Snyder et al., 1997). Furthermore, the activity to a stimulus in the receptive field is also related to cognitive influences tagged to that stimulus, such as reward expectancy (Platt and Glimcher, 1999; Dorris and Glimcher, 2004; Sugrue et al., 2004), probabilistic reasoning (Yang and Shadlen, 2007), and how likely the monkey is to look at the stimulus in a decision task (Shadlen and Newsome, 2001; Roitman and Shadlen, 2002; Leon and Shadlen, 2003). Perhaps the most extreme example of these influences, and the one that first described LIP as a salience map, came from a study by Gottlieb et al. (1998). In this study, an array of stimuli was left on the monitor at all times – it became the background. When a stimulus entered the receptive field by virtue of an eye movement, there was very little response at all, for a static background is, by definition, not salient. However, when the animal was instructed that a particular stimulus was important, then the response to that stimulus became strong and robust (Gottlieb et al., 1998). In other words, LIP only responded to a stimulus when its attentional priority increased.

In the experiments described below, we aimed to test the hypothesis that LIP acts as a priority map, specifically focusing on spatial attention, in which locations in space are attended. First we tested whether LIP activity was related to covert attention. Secondly, we tested whether LIP activity was related to overt attention. While testing these two specific hypotheses, we also found strong evidence of active top-down modulation of activity in LIP.

2.4 LIP and covert attention

Early studies of monkey posterior parietal cortex suggested that the activity in area 7a, which included LIP, was modulated by attention (Robinson et al., 1978; Bushnell et al., 1981). However, a number of apparently contradictory results called this assumption into question, the most convincing of which was the finding that an identical stimulus induced a greater delay response when it was the target of a saccade compared with when it was the target of an arm movement (Snyder et al., 1997, 1998). Thus, it was asked, if activity in LIP represents attention, then why should the activity be different when presumably an equal amount of attention was present, but different effectors were to be used? While a reasonable question, this, in addition to more recent statements about the relationship between activity and the locus of attention (Quian Quiroga et al., 2006), makes an invalid assumption: namely that the experimenter knew where attention was (e.g. simultaneously at both the reach and saccade goals (Snyder et al., 1997, 1998)). Rather than make any assumptions, we felt it was of utmost importance to identify the actual locus of attention and thus have something other than a guess with which to correlate activity.

2.4.1 A dual task paradigm to study covert attention

To show convincingly that the activity in LIP is related with the allocation of covert attention, we needed to identify the monkeys' spatial locus of attention. To do this, we trained monkeys on a dual task paradigm in which the animals had to perform a memory-guided saccade as well as discriminating the orientation of a Landolt ring (Figure 2.2). The animals initiated a trial by fixating a small spot in the center of the screen. After 1–2 s, a second spot (the target) would appear in 1 of 4 possible locations for 100 ms. The target indicated the location in space to which the monkey would have to make a memory-guided saccade when the fixation point was extinguished at the end of the trial. After a variable delay, an array of 4 rings appeared for 1 video frame ($\approx$17 ms), with one at each of the possible target locations. One of these rings, the probe, was a Landolt ring, and the animals' task was to indicate whether the gap was on the right or left of the ring. The animals would indicate their choice by either making the memory-guided saccade to the remembered target location, if they thought the gap was on the left, or, if they thought the gap was on the right, by canceling the saccade plan and maintaining fixation when the fixation point was extinguished at the end of the trial. The animals had 500 ms following the appearance of the probe array before the fixation spot was extinguished, so they had plenty of time to cancel their saccade if

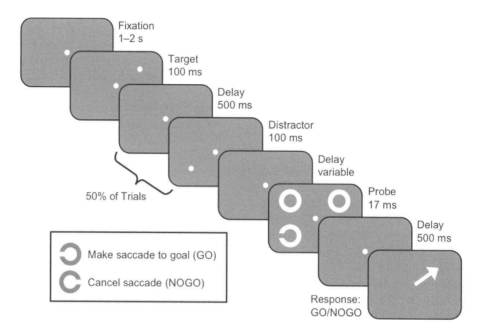

Figure 2.2. Covert attention behavioral task. The monkey initiated a trial by fixating a small spot and after a short delay a second spot (the saccade target) appeared for 100 ms at one of four possible positions. At some time after the saccade target disappeared, a Landolt ring (the probe) and three complete rings of identical luminance to the probe flashed for one video frame (≈17ms) at the four possible saccade target positions. 500 ms after the probe appeared the fixation point disappeared, and the animal had to indicate the orientation of the Landolt ring by either maintaining fixation for 1000 ms (nogo trial) or making a saccade to the goal and remaining there for 1000 ms (go trial). The Landolt ring could appear at any of the four positions. In half of the trials a task-irrelevant distractor, identical to the saccade target, was flashed 500 ms after the target either at or opposite the saccade goal.

they decided the gap was on the right (Hanes and Schall, 1995). In half of the trials, a distractor, which was identical to the target, flashed at the target location or opposite it. These trials were randomly interleaved and the monkeys were adept at maintaining fixation after the distractor was presented. Within this basic task design, we varied three parameters in addition to the target location and distractor location relative to the target. First, the location of the probe relative to the target changed randomly from trial to trial and the animal could not predict its location. In the example in Figure 2.2, the probe was presented in the location opposite the target location. Second, from trial to trial, we varied the luminance of all four rings. We used the method of constant stimuli, so the monkey could not predict the contrast of the stimuli on any given trial. By varying the luminance, we were able to record performance at different contrasts and thus create a contrast function of performance. Because attention enhances contrast sensitivity (Cameron et al., 2002), we knew that if we found a probe location that shows enhanced performance on the task, then this would be a locus of attention. The third parameter we varied was the time between stimulus onset (the target or distractor, whichever was last to appear) and the probe array onset. By measuring contrast sensitivities at different stimulus onset asynchronies (SOAs), we would be able to identify the locus of attention over time.

The locus of attention was identified by a shift in the contrast psychometric function. Data from a single session and from trials in which no distractor was flashed are shown in Figures 2.3A and B. The squares (Figure 2.3A) show performance at six contrast levels when the probe was placed at the location where the target had appeared (the saccade goal), and the circles (Figure 2.3B) show performance for the same six contrast levels when the probe was placed in any of the three locations away from the saccade goal. In this session, and across the gamut of sessions from both monkeys, performance was better at the saccade goal (Bisley and Goldberg, 2003). This is illustrated in the data by a leftward shift of the psychometric function, giving a lower (i.e. better) threshold in the case in which the probe was at the saccade goal. This result is consistent with the idea that covert attention is pinned to the goal of a saccade (Shepherd et al., 1986; Kowler et al., 1995; Deubel and Schneider, 1996), and showed that the task was suitable for identifying the locus of attention.

On trials in which the distractor was flashed away from the saccade goal, attention shifted from the saccade goal to the distractor and then back again. This pattern can be seen in the upper panel of Figure 2.3C, which plots the normalized contrast threshold against the SOA following the onset of the distractor. A normalized threshold of 1 indicates the contrast threshold at the three non-target locations from trials in which there was no distractor, and values less than 1 show lower thresholds and, thus, indicate where there is a perceptual advantage and a locus of attention. As described above, prior to the distractor flashing, attention was pinned at the saccade goal. Within 200 ms of the distractor flashing, there was a perceptual advantage at the site of the distractor (first red triangle, Figure 2.3C), and no advantage at the saccade goal (first blue open triangle, Figure 2.3C), but 700 ms following the distractor onset, attention had returned to the saccade goal (second blue open triangle), and had disappeared from the distractor site (second red triangle).

2.4.2   Neural activity in LIP correlates with the locus of attention

The neural activity from a population of LIP neurons followed the pattern of attentional allocation. The response of a population of LIP neurons from trials in which the target appeared in the receptive field (blue line) and from trials in which the distractor appeared in the receptive field (red line) is shown in the lower panel of Figure 2.3C. This plot shows 700 ms of activity starting at the onset of the distractor (this time is indicated by the thick horizontal red bar). Initially, the burst of activity to the distractor was greater than the delay response from the target, but after about 100 ms it began to decline. At approximately 340 ms, the activity from the distractor became lower than the delay activity from the target (indicated by the vertical gray bar). We noted that the activity in LIP acted like a priority map – when the activity at the saccade goal was highest, there was a perceptual advantage at the target location, and when the activity at the distractor site was highest, there was a perceptual advantage at the distractor

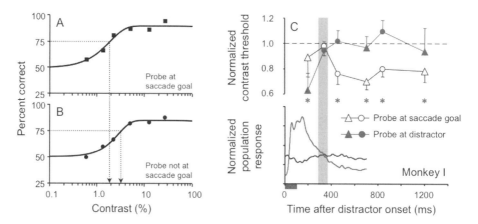

Figure 2.3. Behavioral and neural data from the covert attention task. Psychometric functions from trials in which the probe appeared at the saccade goal (A) and trials in which the probe appeared at one of the three other locations that were away from the saccade goal (B). In both cases, data from saccade target locations in all four locations were pooled. The solid lines show the best fitting Weibull functions. We defined the contrast threshold to be the 75% correct level, indicated by the dotted lines. (C) The top section shows the behavioral performance of a monkey when the probe appeared at the saccade target (open blue points) or distractor (solid red points) location in trials in which the saccade target and distractor were in opposite locations. Points that are significantly below the dashed line illustrate an attentional advantage at that site (color coded asterixes show $p < 0.05$ significance tested with Wilcoxon signed rank tests). The triangles are results collected before recording from LIP neurons and the circles are results collected after. The lines in the lower section are mean normalized spike density functions from a population of 23 neurons. The vertical gray column represents the time during which the activity in the two traces was not different. (Reprinted with permission from Bisley and Goldberg, 2006.) See accompanying CD-ROM for color version.

location. Based on this apparent winner-take-all result, we predicted that at the time when the two traces were crossing (i.e. the time in which there was no winner), the monkey's attention should be shifting from the distractor location back to the saccade goal. So based on the neural activity, we ran new psychophysical experiments (circles in Figure 2.3C) and found that at the time when there was no winner (vertical gray column), neither location showed a perceptual advantage. This was true in two monkeys, and because the time at which the traces crossed was significantly different, we were able to show a double disassociation – when attention was shifting in the first monkey, it had not shifted in the second monkey, and when attention was shifting in the second monkey, it had already shifted in the first monkey (Bisley and Goldberg, 2003).

The relationship between the neural activity in LIP and the behavioral effects of attention suggests that LIP could act as a priority map using a winner-take-all mechanism to choose the locus of attention. In both monkeys, we found that the strength of the perceptual benefit was always similar at the attended location. Whereas the difference in activity between the attended location and the non-attended location ranged from great, shortly after a stimulus flashed, to small, such as when there was only delay activity at the saccade goal and baseline activity at the distractor site (Figure 2.3C). This suggests that once the peak is chosen, attention is allocated to that location. This is consistent with the idea that for very short stimulus presentations, such as the ones we used (only one video frame, 17 ms), attention is in fact quantal, e.g. binary and indivisible (Joseph and Optican, 1996). However, it is worth noting that the day-to-day perceptual benefits were small and data had to be collected over many weeks to show significant differences. Thus, subtle differences in performance may not be resolvable in our data and there may actually be a relationship between the relative level of neural activity and the relative strength of the perceptual advantage, particularly if this relationship is not linear. Unfortunately, we do not have enough data with varying relative levels of neural activity to differentiate between these possibilities.

Given these results, we can return to the question posed in the beginning of this section that initially threw a cloud over the hypothesis that LIP activity was related to the allocation of attention: Why should activity be different when presumably an equal amount of attention was present, but different effectors were to be used? This question was driven by the result that an identical stimulus induced a greater response when it was the target of a saccade compared with when it was the target of an arm movement (Snyder et al., 1997, 1998; Quian Quiroga et al., 2006). We would now argue that had Snyder and colleagues actually measured attention, they would have found that during trials in which only an arm or eye movement target was presented, then attention would have always gone to the target, independent of which effector was to be used, because in an environment with no other stimuli, each response would be the peak of the priority map. We also would hypothesize that in the task in which both arm and eye movement targets appeared, they would have found attention distributed between both locations, because the initial neural responses were similar at both locations (Quian Quiroga et al., 2006). But had they measured attention during the delay period, they would have found that attention had left the reach goal, since the mean response at the saccade goal was higher than at the reach goal. A similar experiment has been done in humans by Deubel and Schneider (2003) who showed that attention, as measured by perceptual acuity, leaves the reach goal 300 ms after the appearance of the saccade and reach stimuli, but remains at the saccade goal for the duration of the delay period.

2.5   LIP and overt attention

A number of prior studies have implied that LIP is involved in the planning of eye movements (Gnadt and Andersen, 1988; Barash et al., 1991; Colby et al., 1996; Platt and Glimcher, 1997; Snyder et al., 1997); however these studies had always restricted eye movements and thus had never shown direct correlations between saccade target selection and LIP activity. For many years, it was argued that posterior parietal cortex, and LIP specifically, was a control center for saccadic eye movements (Mountcastle et al., 1975, Gnadt and Andersen, 1988, Barash et al., 1991). This hypothesis was

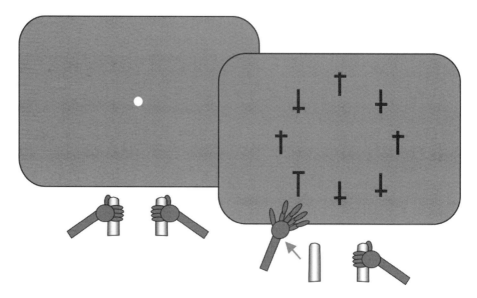

Figure 2.4. Free-viewing visual search task. The monkeys began the task by grabbing two bars attached to the primate chair. A fixation point appeared, which the monkey had to look at for 1–1.75 s, after which time it disappeared and was replaced by an array of stimuli positioned along an imaginary circle so that one member of the array was in the center of the receptive field of the neuron under study. One of the stimuli was the target, an upright or inverted T, and the monkeys had three seconds to report the orientation of the target by releasing one of the two bars. During recording, one of the distractor stimuli was green and brighter than the others. No constraints were imposed on the monkeys' eye movements; they were not required to fixate the target before giving the response and were not penalized for not fixating the target.

later refined, arguing that LIP activity represented the planning or intention to make a saccade (Bracewell et al., 1996; Mazzoni et al., 1996; Platt and Glimcher, 1997; Snyder et al., 1997; Andersen and Buneo, 2002). The problem was that a number of studies produced data that were incompatible with this hypothesis. Such inconsistencies have been seen in distractor tasks in which eye movements are not affected by the sudden onset of a distractor just before the eye movement (Robinson et al., 1995; Powell and Goldberg, 2000), in nogo tasks in which the greatest activity is seen when canceling a saccade than making it (Bisley and Goldberg, 2003, 2006) and, more recently, in a stop-signal task (Brunamonti and Paré, 2005). Yet in all cases, from studies arguing both for and against the hypothesis, the animals' eye movements were restricted, so it is possible that the lack of correlations or the apparent exceptions to the rule could be due to the fact that the monkeys were not free to move their eyes.

To test whether LIP activity is related to saccade planning, we examined the responses of LIP neurons from monkeys performing a visual search task in which they were free to move their eyes (Ipata et al., 2006a, b). In this task (Figure 2.4), monkeys initiated a trial by grasping each of two bars, after which a central spot appeared which they had to fixate for 1–1.75 s. After this time, the fixation point disappeared and an array of crosses appeared. In each array there was a target, either an upright or inverted capital T. The remaining stimuli were distractors and were composed of the same horizontal and vertical components, but differed in the relative heights at which the components crossed. The monkey's job was to indicate the orientation of the target by releasing one of the two bars within three s. If the target was an upright T, then the monkey had to release the left bar; if the target was an inverted T, then the monkey had to release the right bar. There were no other restrictions on the task, thus the monkey could look wherever he wanted, whenever he wanted after the array appeared. This means that he did not have to fixate the target to get the reward. Conversely, he did not get punished, by means of a reduced reward or timeout, if he looked at any other stimulus. Thus, the task mimics more natural viewing conditions than in previous studies, and the activity in LIP should be more akin to the activity under natural viewing conditions.

2.5.1   Monkey performance on the free-viewing visual search task

When the monkeys started working on the free-viewing visual search tasks, they were run on three different blocks of trials randomly ordered within each session. In one block of trials, a randomly chosen distractor popped out on each trial. This was identical to the behavioral task the monkeys performed while activity was recorded from LIP. In the second block of trials, no stimuli popped out. In this task, all the distractors were the same luminance and color as the target on every trial. In the final block of trials, the target popped out on every trial. Both monkeys performed all three tasks exceedingly well; monkey Z released the correct bar on over 99% of target-popout trials and on 96.2 and 96.3% of distractor-popout and non-popout trials respectively, and monkey R released the correct bar on over 99% of trials on all three tasks.

Manual reaction time on the three tasks, defined as the time from the array onset to the release of the bar, varied with set-size in similar ways seen in humans (Zelinsky and Sheinberg, 1997; Maioli et al., 2001). In the target-popout task, manual reaction time did not vary much as set-size increased from 8 to 16 (Figure 2.5). In the distractor-popout and no-popout tasks, manual reaction time increased with set-size in both monkeys. Thus, as the number of search targets increased, the monkey took longer to respond. This effect was significant in both monkeys.

Although the task only required the monkeys to indicate the orientation of the target by bar release, like humans the monkeys ended up moving their eyes and foveating the target on most trials (Maioli et al., 2001). Over 90% of all saccade endpoints lay within 2 degrees of a stimulus center. This distance is comparable to the stimulus dimensions (1.0° wide and 2.9° tall) and was considerably less than half the interstimulus distance for set-sizes of 8 and 12 stimuli, indicating that saccades were stimulus-directed and were rarely directed towards blank regions of space in between or away from stimuli.

The monkeys tended to make few saccades before identifying the target and releasing the correct bar. In blocks in which the target popped out on every trial, the monkeys made only 1 saccade on the vast majority of trials (Figures 2.6A and B). Furthermore, in the distractor-popout and no-popout blocks, the monkeys still predominantly made three or fewer saccades. These data show that the monkeys successfully found the tar-

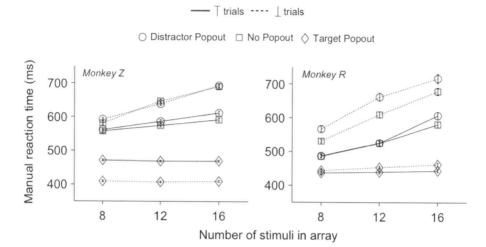

Figure 2.5. The relationship between manual reaction time and number of stimuli in the array. Manual reaction time was independent of set-size for the target-popout task (diamonds) and positively correlated with set-size for the distractor-popout (circles) and no-popout (squares) tasks in both monkeys Z and R. Error bars are standard-error of the mean (SEM). The differences between the two target-types are a result of a higher salience of the upright-T in both monkeys relative to the inverted-T.

get with their first saccade on over half of the trials in these blocks and, thus, were not performing the task in a completely serial fashion. It is worth noting that the manual reaction times were strongly correlated with the total number of saccades made within a trial (Figures 2.6C and D). Independent of whether the trials came from blocks in which the target popped out, a distractor popped out or nothing popped out, the correlation was still the same. This means the time between saccades is not dependent on the task.

2.5.2 Neural activity in LIP can guide overt attention

After a short indiscriminate response, the goal of the first saccade was represented by higher activity in LIP. During the initial visual response to the onset of the search array, LIP neurons did not differentiate between target and distractor, nor did they differentiate between whether the stimulus would be the target of the first saccade or not (Thomas and Paré, 2007). Approximately 90 ms after the array appeared (Figure 2.7A), the neuronal responses started to differentiate between whether the stimulus would be the goal of the first saccade or not, independently of what the identity of the stimulus in the receptive field was (Ipata et al., 2006a). To see if the time when LIP first identified the goal of the saccade was related to the time the saccade was made, we split the trials collected within a single session evenly into those with short saccadic latencies, those with long saccadic latencies and those with intermediate saccadic latencies (Thompson et al., 1996). By dividing the data into these groups we could ask whether the represen-

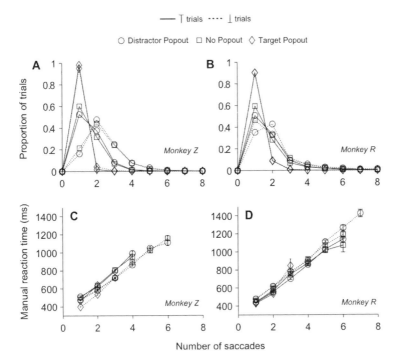

Figure 2.6. Analysis of the number of saccades per trial. (A and B) Distribution of the number of saccades for each task type for monkeys Z and R respectively. Saccades made after foveating the target but before releasing the appropriate bar were not included in this analysis. (C and D) The relationship between manual reaction time and the number of saccades for monkeys Z and R respectively. Only points with at least ten trials per condition were plotted.

tation of the saccade goal in LIP was related to the timing of the saccade, by examining whether the onset of the differential response correlated with the saccadic latency (Figure 2.7B). If the activity was completely unrelated to the actual saccade then the time when the saccade target activity splits from the remaining activity (the "split time", Figure 2.7A) as calculated from array onset, should be the same in shorter and longer saccadic latency trials (compare short latency data with gray long latency data in upper panel of Figure 2.7B). Under these conditions, the split time calculated relative to array onset is constant, so the split time will not be correlated with the saccade latency and linear regression will give a slope of 0 (gray line, lower left panel of Figure 2.7B). This would mean that all the variation in saccadic latency would be introduced independent of the LIP split time and would be apparent in the time between the split time and saccade onset. If this time is calculated for the two latency groups, then it will have a slope of 1 (gray lines, lower right panel of Figure 2.7B). However, if the identification of the saccade goal in LIP is tied to the initiation of the saccade, then the time between array onset and the split time should correlate with saccadic latency (black line, lower left panel of Figure 2.7B) and the duration from split time to saccade onset should be constant (black line, lower right panel of Figure 2.7B). Of course, it is possible that LIP neurons account for some, but not all, of the variation in saccadic latency timing, in which case there would be correlations between saccadic latency and both split times (calculated from array onset and saccade onset), but ideally the two slopes would then add to one.

We found that activity identifying the saccade goal in LIP predicted the latency of the saccade. The mean slope for the split time, calculated from array onset, plotted against saccadic latency was close to one (compare thick red line to dotted line in Figure 2.7C). In contrast, the mean slope for the split time, calculated from saccade onset, was close to 0 (Figure 2.7D). These data are similar to the black lines in Figure 2.7B, suggesting that the split time can account for the variation in saccadic latency, and thus, the initial representation of the saccade goal in LIP is related to the saccadic latency. Furthermore, the almost flat line in Figure 2.7D shows that once the saccade goal is identified in LIP, then there is an almost constant time before the saccade is made. This suggests that once a peak is identified in LIP, then a saccade is programmed to be made to that location in space. This is exactly what is predicted if LIP acts as a priority map for overt attention.

Although the mean activity in LIP appears to predict saccadic latency, there was some variation in the single neuron data (thin black lines in Figures 2.7C and D). It is clear from Figure 2.7C, that not all neurons had slopes of 1, nor did all neurons have slopes of 0 in Figure 2.7D. It is possible that this variation is due to noise inherent in our calculations of slope. But if the measurements are accurate, then the combined slopes from a single neuron should add to 1. To test this, we converted the slopes into degrees, so that they would be best visualized on a linear scale, and then plotted the slopes for the data aligned by array onset, against the slopes for the data aligned by saccade onset for each neuron. These data are plotted in Figure 2.7E. Although not all of the points cluster around $45°$ on the x-axis and $0°$ on the y-axis (see histograms), they show a remarkable correlation with a slope close to -1 that intercepts the x-axis close to $45°$. This means that when the two slopes are summed, their sum is approximately $45°$. Thus, we have shown that in the majority of cells and in the population as a whole, when activity at one location peaks above the rest, it may be used to target and then drive the first saccade under unconstrained viewing conditions (Ipata et al., 2006a; Thomas and Paré, 2007).

2.6   Active top-down suppression in LIP

The majority of studies that have examined the effect of top-down influences on activity in putative priority maps have usually shown enhancements in activity to a location that is to be attended (for examples see: Bushnell et al., 1981; Gottlieb et al., 1998; Thompson et al., 2005). However, one could interpret these results, particularly those of Gottlieb et al. (1998), as showing top-down suppression of locations that are not

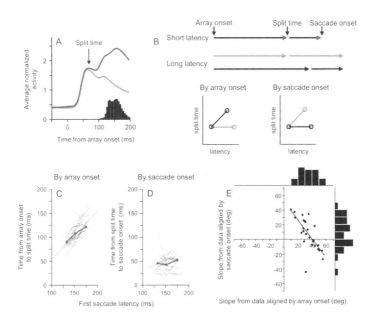

Figure 2.7. Relationship between LIP activity and first saccadic latency. (A) Average normalized activity is plotted against time. Activity from trials in which the first saccade was made away from the receptive field is shown in light blue. Activity from trials in which the first saccade was made toward the receptive field is shown in dark red. Trials in which the target was in the receptive field have been pooled with trials in which the distractor was in the receptive field. Histograms show the distribution of first saccade latencies relative to array onset. The split time was the time at which the two traces became significantly different (Ipata et al., 2006a). (B) An example short latency trial is compared with two possible long latency trials showing the two extreme possibilities in how the extra time is added to latency. In the upper (gray) example, the time from array onset until the split time is identical, so the variability in latency time does not result from the variability in split time. This would suggest LIP is not driving the saccade and is not involved in saccadic initiation. In the lower (black) example, the variability in latency time comes from the variability in split time in LIP. This would suggest that LIP is driving the saccade. The two sets of hypothesized results (gray and black) are plotted in the small panels comparing the split time calculated by array onset and split time calculated by saccade onset. (C) The time from array onset to split time is plotted against the mean first saccadic latency for each group for each cell. The dotted line shows an example slope of 1. (D) The time from the split time to saccade onset is plotted against the mean first saccadic latency for each group for each cell. For (C) and (D), the black lines connect points from the same cell and the thick red lines connect the population means. (E) The scatter plot shows the slopes (in deg) from the data aligned by saccade onset plotted against the slopes from the data aligned by array onset. The solid line shows the best fit linear regression to the data. The histograms show the distributions of the slopes under the two conditions. All data are from monkey R. (Reproduced with permission from Ipata et al., 2006a. Copyright 2006 by the Society for Neuroscience.) See CD-ROM for color version.

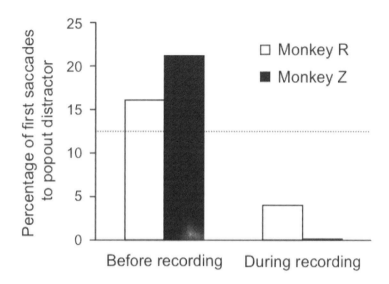

Figure 2.8. Percentage of first saccades to the popout distractor before and during recording. In sessions before recording, blocks in which the popout was the target were occasionally presented. The data on the left show the proportion of saccades to the popout distractor from these sessions, but only from blocks in which the popout was always a distractor. The data on the right were taken from recording sessions, in which the popout was never the target. Chance is shown by the dotted line at 12.5%. (Reproduced from Ipata et al., 2006b.)

of interest, particularly given the strong inhibitory connections within LIP (Zhang et al., 2007). Conversely, bottom-up influences have also been shown to give enhanced responses in LIP (Balan and Gottlieb, 2006), area 7a (Constantinidis and Steinmetz, 2001), FEF (Thompson et al., 2005) and SC (McPeek and Keller, 2002). One might imagine that the popout distractor in our visual search task should be highly salient given its bottom-up properties, however, the monkey also knew that it would never be the target, so we may expect that this could be influenced by top-down signals as well.

In the free-viewing visual search task, we found that in early training and testing monkeys did not ignore the popout distractor. When the monkeys started working on the free-viewing visual search tasks, they were run on the three different blocks of trials randomly ordered within each session (distractor popout, target popout and no popout). During this initial testing, we found that the monkeys made their first saccade towards the popout distractor significantly more often than chance performance of 12.5% (Figure 2.8, left columns; $p = 0.03$, monkey R; $p < 0.001$, monkey Z). This metric is a measure of attentional priority; the monkeys were free to move their eyes, so they should move them to the stimulus with the highest priority. If we take into account the knowledge that almost 50% of first saccades were made to the target (Figures 2.6A

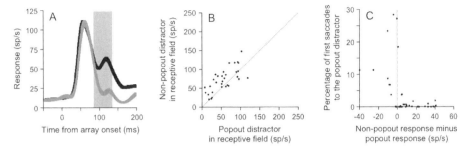

Figure 2.9. LIP responses to the popout distractor. (A) Responses of a single cell to the appearance of an array object in the receptive field are plotted against time from target onset. Black trace: response to a non-popout distractor in the receptive field when the monkey made a saccade to the target elsewhere. Light green trace: response to the popout distractor in the receptive field when the monkey made a saccade to the target elsewhere. The gray vertical column represents the approximate epoch from which the data in (B) and (C) were taken. (B) The response of each cell from a 50 ms epoch, starting 40 ms after the latency, to the non-popout distractor is plotted against the response of the same cell to the popout distractor. (C) Cell by cell correlation of response difference with saccade suppression. The percentage of trials in which the first saccade went to the popout distractor for each cell is plotted against the difference in the number of spikes between the responses (80–130 ms) to the non-popout and popout distractors for the cell recorded in that session. (Reproduced from Ipata et al., 2006b.) See CD-ROM for color version.

and B), then we can calculate the probability that the monkey would go to the popout first as a 1 in 7 chance over the remaining proportion of trials. This makes the values represented in Figure 2.8 even more striking, because, based on how often each monkey looked at the target with their first saccade, chance levels become 6.2 and 8.9% for monkeys R and Z respectively.

With training, the monkeys learned to ignore the distractor overtly. The right columns in Figure 2.8 show how often each monkey foveated the popout distractor with their first saccade once we started recording the neural activity from LIP. Once recording began, they were only exposed to trials in which the popout was a distractor (30–40,000 trials over the course of recording). For both monkeys, this metric was significantly less than theoretical chance (12.5%) and actual chance of 6.3% and 8.0% for monkeys R and Z respectively (with actual chance levels based on how often each monkey looked at the target with their first saccade in the recording sessions). The lack of attentional priority is highlighted in the data from monkey Z who went from having his overt attention grabbed by the popout on 21% of trials to almost never looking at the popout (150 out of 31,923 trials). This suggests that the popout went from having a high attentional priority in the initial testing, most likely due to its bottom-up salience, to having a very low attentional priority in the recording sessions, presumably due to top-down influences overriding the bottom-up salience. If this is the case, then the neural response to the popout should be suppressed on the priority map.

After the initial visual response, activity to the popout was suppressed when the animals successfully ignored it (Ipata et al., 2006b). Figure 2.9A shows the mean response from a single neuron to the non-popout distractors (black) and to the popout distractor (green) from trials in which the monkey made a single saccade directly to the target and released the correct bar. This means that these responses represent the activity in LIP when all the distractors were successfully ignored. For approximately the first 80 ms, the neuronal response was similar to the popout and non-popout distractors, but following this, the activity in response to the popout decayed to almost baseline levels. Both the initial equal response (Ipata et al., 2006b), and the later lower response to the popout (Figure 2.9B) were seen in most neurons in this monkey. However, it is clear from Figure 2.9B that some neurons had stronger responses to the popout than to the non-popout distractors (points below the dotted line). We hypothesized that this stronger response to the popout would be reflected in some aspect of the monkey's oculomotor behavior during the session in which the neuron's activity was recorded. To test this, we plotted our metric of attentional priority, that is, the number of times that the monkey made his first saccade towards the popout distractor, against the difference in response between the popout and non-popout distractors for each cell recorded in LIP (Figure 2.9C). In this case, our metric comes from the total behavior within a single recording session, whereas the activity comes only from those trials in which the monkey made his first saccade towards the search target and released the appropriate bar and thus all the distractors were successfully ignored. We can think of this as asking how the popout was represented on average in sessions in which the monkey either successfully ignored it (when the proportion of first saccades to the popout was very low) or could not ignore it (when the proportion of first saccades to the popout was high). The data in Figure 2.9C clearly show that in sessions in which the monkey successfully ignored the popout, the responses to the popout were lower than the responses to the non-popout distractors. However, in sessions in which the monkey looked at the popout distractor more often, the responses to the popout distractor were equal to or stronger than the responses to the non-popout distractors. Because the sessions in which the popout distractor was enhanced occurred throughout the animal's recording history, we also conclude that this represents an active top-down influence on the response of LIP to the popout distractor – on some days when the monkey was not "focused" enough and the LIP neural response to the popout was higher, his attention (and eyes) were concurrently attracted towards the popout. These data are consistent with the concept of LIP as a priority map – when the response to the popout distractor was suppressed, the monkey was able to ignore it, but when it was enhanced, it would grab his overt attention, resulting in more saccades to the popout distractor.

2.7   LIP as a priority map: a unifying role

We have shown that the representation of visual space in LIP is influenced by top-down and bottom-up influences and that the resultant map can be used to guide the allocation of covert or overt attention. But, rather than claiming a specific role for the output, such as the allocation of attention (Bisley and Goldberg, 2003) or saccade intention (Snyder et al., 1997), we suggest that LIP specifies the attentional priority of the different parts of the visual field in an agnostic manner. The map can thus be used by areas to which LIP projects in a manner specific to those recipient areas. The oculomotor system can use the priority map to choose the goal of saccadic eye movements when saccades are appropriate (Ipata et al., 2006a; Thomas and Paré, 2007), and the visual system simultaneously uses it to determine the locus of visual attention (Bisley and Goldberg, 2006).

Further evidence for LIP being involved in the allocation of attention comes from microstimulation and reversible inactivation studies. The results discussed in this chapter have shown a range of neuronal correlates with behavioral measures of attention, but these do not show causality. However, other studies have shown that microstimulation of LIP affects reaction time in attentional tasks (Cutrell and Marrocco, 2002), and that reversible inactivation biases both reaction time (Davidson and Marrocco, 2000) and behavior in visual search tasks (Wardak et al., 2004). These data are consistent with LIP acting as a priority map and being involved in the allocation of visual attention. Biases in performance, similar to those induced by attention, have also been seen after stimulating the frontal eye field (Moore and Fallah, 2001; Moore and Armstrong, 2003) and the superior colliculus (Cavanaugh and Wurtz, 2004; Müller et al., 2005). These two areas are interconnected with LIP and together are part of the parieto-frontal network that has been identified in fMRI studies of attention (Corbetta et al., 1998; Kastner and Ungerleider, 2000).

A wide range of other signals have been identified in LIP, yet they complement the idea of LIP as a priority map rather than accumulating evidence against it. Many of these signals have been related to cognitive processes, such as the reward value of the stimulus in the receptive field (Platt and Glimcher, 1999; Dorris and Glimcher, 2004; Sugrue et al., 2004), the category of the stimulus in the receptive field (Freedman and Assad, 2006), or the accrual of information in decision making (Shadlen and Newsome, 2001; Roitman and Shadlen, 2002; Leon and Shadlen, 2003; Huk and Shadlen, 2005). Others are related to more basic influences, such as stimulus motion (Williams et al., 2003), stimulus shape (Sereno and Maunsell, 1998) or effector choice (Snyder et al., 1998; Dickinson et al., 2003; Oristaglio et al., 2006). We suggest that any analysis of an object in the visual field will increase the attentional priority of the spatial location of that object, and that increased priority will be reflected in the increased activity in the representation of that location in LIP. The various cognitive exercises shown to increase activity in LIP may therefore reflect top-down inputs to the priority map, rather than participation by LIP in the decisions underlying those exercises.

Acknowledgments

The work described here was supported by grants to Michael E. Goldberg from the National Eye Institute, the Human Frontiers Science Project, the James S. MacDonnell Foundation, the W.M. Keck Foundation, and the Whitehall Foundation. JWB is supported by the Kirchgessner Foundation, the Gerald Oppenheimer Family Foundation, and has a Klingenstein Fellowship Award in the Neurosciences and an Alfred P. Sloan Foundation Research Fellowship. We thank Fabrice Arcizet for his insightful comments on the manuscript.

References

Andersen, R. A. and Buneo, C. A. (2002). Intentional maps in posterior parietal cortex. *Ann. Rev. Neurosci.*, 25: 189–220.

Andersen, R. A., Asanuma, C. and Cowan, W. M. (1985). Callosal and prefrontal associational projecting cell populations in area 7A of the macaque monkey: a study using retrogradely transported fluorescent dyes. *J. Comp. Neurol.*, 232: 443–455.

Andersen, R. A., Asanuma, C., Essick, G. and Siegel, R. M. (1990). Corticocortical connections of anatomically and physiologically defined subdivisions within the inferior parietal lobule. *J. Comp. Neurol.*, 296: 65–113.

Baizer, J. S., Ungerleider, L. G. and Desimone, R. (1991). Organization of visual inputs to the inferior temporal and posterior parietal cortex in macaques. *J. Neurosci.*, 11: 168–190.

Balan, P. F. and Gottlieb, J. (2006). Integration of exogenous input into a dynamic salience map revealed by perturbing attention. *J. Neurosci.*, 26: 9239–9249.

Barash, S., Bracewell, R. M., Fogassi, L., Gnadt, J. W. and Andersen, R. A. (1991). Saccade-related activity in the lateral intraparietal area. I. Temporal properties; comparison with area 7a. *J. Neurophysiol.*, 66: 1095–1108.

Ben Hamed, S., Duhamel, J. R., Bremmer, F. and Graf, W. (2001) Representation of the visual field in the lateral intraparietal area of macaque monkeys: a quantitative receptive field analysis. *Exp. Brain Res.*, 140: 127–144.

Bisley, J. W. and Goldberg, M. E. (2003). Neuronal activity in the lateral intraparietal area and spatial attention. *Science*, 299: 81–86.

Bisley, J. W. and Goldberg, M. E. (2006). Neural correlates of attention and distractibility in the lateral intraparietal area. *J. Neurophysiol.*, 95: 1696–1717.

Bisley, J. W., Krishna, B. S. and Goldberg, M. E. (2004). A rapid and precise on-response in posterior parietal cortex. *J. Neurosci.*, 24: 1833–1838.

Blatt, G. J., Andersen, R. A. and Stoner, G. R. (1990). Visual receptive field organization and cortico-cortical connections of the lateral intraparietal area (area LIP) in the macaque. *J. Comp. Neurol.*, 299: 421–445.

Bracewell, R. M., Mazzoni, P., Barash, S. and Andersen, R. A. (1996). Motor intention activity in the macaque's lateral intraparietal area. II. Changes of motor plan. *J. Neurophysiol.*, 76: 1457–1464.

Brunamonti, E. and Paré, M. (2005). Neural control of saccade production studied with the counter-manding paradigm: parietal cortex area LIP. *Soc. Neurosci. Abst.*, 35: 166.18.

Bushnell, M. C., Goldberg, M. E. and Robinson, D. L. (1981). Behavioral enhancement of visual responses in monkey cerebral cortex. I. Modulation in posterior parietal cortex related to selective visual attention. *J. Neurophysiol.*, 46: 755–772.

Cameron, E. L., Tai, J. C. and Carrasco, M. (2002). Covert attention affects the psychometric function of contrast sensitivity. *Vision Res.*, 42: 949–967.

Carrasco, M., Ling, S. and Read, S. (2004). Attention alters appearance. *Nature Neurosci.*, 7: 308–313.

Cavanaugh, J. and Wurtz, R. H. (2004). Subcortical modulation of attention counters change blindness. *J. Neurosci.*, 24: 11236–11243.

Cave, K. R. and Wolfe, J. M. (1990). Modeling the role of parallel processing in visual search. *Cogn. Psychol.*, 22: 225–271.

Colby, C. L., Duhamel, J. R. and Goldberg, M. E. (1996). Visual, presaccadic, and cognitive activation of single neurons in monkey lateral intraparietal area. *J. Neurophysiol.*, 76: 2841–2852.

Constantinidis, C. and Steinmetz, M. A. (2001). Neuronal responses in area 7a to multiple-stimulus displays: i. neurons encode the location of the salient stimulus. *Cerebral Cortex*, 11: 581–591.

Corbetta, M. and Shulman, G. L. (2002). Control of goal-directed and stimulus-driven attention in the brain. *Nature Rev. Neurosci.*, 3: 201–215.

Corbetta, M., Akbudak, E., Conturo, T. E., Snyder, A. Z., Ollinger, J. M., Drury, H. A., Linenweber, M. R., Petersen, S. E., Raichle, M. E., Van Essen, D. C. and Shulman, G. L. (1998). A common network of functional areas for attention and eye movements. *Neuron*, 21: 761–773.

Cutrell, E. B. and Marrocco, R. T. (2002). Electrical microstimulation of primate posterior parietal cortex initiates orienting and alerting components of covert attention. *Exp. Brain Res.*, 144: 103–113.

Davidson, M. C. and Marrocco, R. T. (2000). Local infusion of scopolamine into intraparietal cortex slows covert orienting in rhesus monkeys. *J. Neurophysiol.*, 83: 1536–1549.

Deco, G. and Schurmann, B. (2000). A hierarchical neural system with attentional top-down enhancement of the spatial resolution for object recognition. *Vision Res.*, 40: 2845–2859.

Deubel, H. and Schneider, W. X. (1996). Saccade target selection and object recognition: evidence for a common attentional mechanism. *Vision Res.*, 36: 1827–1837.

Deubel, H. and Schneider, W. X. (2003). Delayed saccades, but not delayed manual aiming movements, require visual attention shifts. *Ann. New York Acad. Sci.*, 1004: 289–296.

Dickinson, A. R., Calton, J. L. and Snyder, L. H. (2003). Nonspatial saccade-specific activation in area LIP of monkey parietal cortex. *J. Neurophysiol.*, 90: 2460–2464.

Distler, C., Boussaoud, D., Desimone, R. and Ungerleider, L. G. (1993). Cortical connections of inferior temporal area TEO in macaque monkeys. *J. Comp. Neurol.*, 334: 125–150.

Dorris, M. C. and Glimcher, P. W. (2004). Activity in posterior parietal cortex is correlated with the relative subjective desirability of action. *Neuron*, 44: 365–378.

Duhamel, J. R., Colby, C. L. and Goldberg, M. E. (1992). The updating of the representation of visual space in parietal cortex by intended eye movements. *Science*, 255: 90–92.

Duncan, J. and Humphreys, G. W. (1989). Visual search and stimulus similarity. *Psycholog. Rev.*, 96: 433–458.

Egeth, H. E. and Yantis, S. (1997). Visual attention: control, representation, and time course. *Ann. Rev. Psychol.*, 48: 269–297.

Fecteau, J. H. and Munoz, D. P. (2006). Salience, relevance, and firing: a priority map for target selection. *Trends Cogn. Sci.*, 10: 382–390.

Fecteau, J. H., Bell, A. H. and Munoz, D. P. (2004). Neural correlates of the automatic and goal-driven biases in orienting spatial attention. *J. Neurophysiol.*, 92: 1728–1737.

Ferraina, S., Paré, M. and Wurtz, R. H. (2002). Comparison of cortico-cortical and cortico-collicular signals for the generation of saccadic eye movements. *J. Neurophysiol.*, 87: 845–858.

Freedman, D. J. and Assad, J. A. (2006). Experience-dependent representation of visual categories in parietal cortex. *Nature*, 443: 85–88.

Gnadt, J. W. and Andersen, R. A. (1988). Memory related motor planning activity in posterior parietal cortex of macaque. *Exp. Brain Res.*, 70: 216–220.

Gottlieb, J., Kusunoki, M. and Goldberg, M. E. (2005). Simultaneous representation of saccade targets and visual onsets in monkey lateral intraparietal area. *Cerebral Cortex*, 15: 1198–1206.

Gottlieb, J. P., Kusunoki, M. and Goldberg, M. E. (1998). The representation of visual salience in monkey parietal cortex. *Nature*, 391: 481–484.

Hamker, F. H. (2004). A dynamic model of how feature cues guide spatial attention. *Vision Res.*, 44: 501–521.

Hanes, D. P. and Schall, J. D. (1995). Countermanding saccades in macaque. *Visual Neurosci.*, 12: 929–937.

He, B. J., Snyder, A. Z., Vincent, J. L., Epstein, A., Shulman, G. L. and Corbetta, M. (2007). Breakdown of functional connectivity in frontoparietal networks underlies behavioral deficits in spatial neglect. *Neuron*, 53: 905–918.

Huk, A. C. and Shadlen, M. N. (2005). Neural activity in macaque parietal cortex reflects temporal integration of visual motion signals during perceptual decision making. *J. Neurosci.*, 25: 10420–10436.

Ipata, A. E., Gee, A. L., Goldberg, M. E. and Bisley, J. W. (2006a). Activity in the lateral intraparietal area predicts the goal and latency of saccades in a free-viewing visual search task. *J. Neurosci.* 26: 3656–3661.

Ipata, A. E., Gee, A. L., Gottlieb, J., Bisley, J. W. and Goldberg, M. E. (2006b) LIP responses to a popout stimulus are reduced if it is overtly ignored. *Nature Neurosci.*, 9: 1071–1076.

Itti, L. and Koch, C. (2000). A saliency-based search mechanism for overt and covert shifts of visual attention. *Vision Res.*, 40: 1489–1506.

Joseph, J. S. and Optican, L. M. (1996). Involuntary attentional shifts due to orientation differences. *Percept. Psychophys.*, 58: 651–665.

Kastner, S. and Ungerleider, L. G. (2000). Mechanisms of visual attention in the human cortex. *Ann. Rev. Neurosci.*, 23: 315–341.

Koch, C. and Ullman, S. (1985). Shifts in selective visual attention: towards the underlying neural circuitry. *Human Neurobiol.*, 4: 219–227.

Kowler, E., Anderson, E., Dosher, B. and Blaser, E. (1995). The role of attention in the programming of saccades. *Vision Res.*, 35: 1897–1916.

Kusunoki, M., Gottlieb, J. and Goldberg, M. E. (2000). The lateral intraparietal area as a salience map: the representation of abrupt onset, stimulus motion, and task relevance. *Vision Res.*, 40: 1459–1468.

Leon, M. I. and Shadlen, M. N. (2003). Representation of time by neurons in the posterior parietal cortex of the macaque. *Neuron*, 38: 317–327.

Lewis, J. W. and Van Essen, D. C. (2000). Corticocortical connections of visual, sensorimotor, and multimodal processing areas in the parietal lobe of the macaque monkey. *J. Comp. Neurol.*, 428: 112–137.

Li, W., Piech, V. and Gilbert, C. D. (2004). Perceptual learning and top-down influences in primary visual cortex. *Nature Neurosci.*, 7: 651–657.

Li, Z. (2002) A saliency map in primary visual cortex. *Trends Cogn. Sci.*, 6: 9–16.

Luck, S. J., Chelazzi, L., Hillyard, S. A. and Desimone, R. (1997). Neural mechanisms of spatial selective attention in areas V1, V2, and V4 of macaque visual cortex. *J. Neurophysiol.*, 77: 24–42.

Maioli, C., Benaglio, I., Siri, S., Sosta, K. and Cappa, S. (2001). The integration of parallel and serial processing mechanisms in visual search: evidence from eye movement recording. *Eur. J. Neurosci.*, 13: 364–372.

Mazer, J. A. and Gallant, J. L. (2003). Goal-related activity in V4 during free viewing visual search. Evidence for a ventral stream visual salience map. *Neuron*, 40: 1241–1250.

Mazzoni, P., Bracewell, R. M., Barash, S. and Andersen, R. A. (1996). Motor intention activity in the macaque's lateral intraparietal area. I. Dissociation of motor plan from sensory memory. *J. Neurophysiol.*, 76: 1439–1456.

McPeek, R. M. and Keller, E. L. (2002). Superior colliculus activity related to concurrent processing of saccade goals in a visual search task. *J. Neurophysiol.*, 87: 1805–1815.

Moore, T. and Armstrong, K. M. (2003). Selective gating of visual signals by microstimulation of frontal cortex. *Nature*, 421: 370–373.

Moore, T. and Fallah, M. (2001). Control of eye movements and spatial attention. *Proc. Nat. Acad. Sci. USA*, 98: 1273–1276.

Moran, J. and Desimone, R. (1985). Selective attention gates visual processing in the extrastriate cortex. *Science*, 229: 782–784.

Mountcastle, V. B., Lynch, J. C., Georgopoulos, A., Sakata, H. and Acuna, C. (1975). Posterior parietal association cortex of the monkey: command functions for operations within extrapersonal space. *J. Neurophysiol.*, 38: 871–908.

Müller, J. R., Philiastides, M. G. and Newsome, W. T. (2005). Microstimulation of the superior colliculus focuses attention without moving the eyes. *Proc. Nat. Acad. Sci. USA*, 102: 524–529.

Oristaglio, J., Schneider, D. M., Balan, P. F. and Gottlieb, J. (2006). Integration of visuospatial and effector information during symbolically cued limb movements in monkey lateral intraparietal area. *J. Neurosci.*, 26: 8310–8319.

Paré, M. and Wurtz, R. H. (1997). Monkey posterior parietal cortex neurons antidromically activated from superior colliculus. *J. Neurophysiol.*, 78: 3493–3497.

Pestilli, F. and Carrasco, M. (2005). Attention enhances contrast sensitivity at cued and impairs it at uncued locations. *Vision Res.*, 45: 1867–1875.

Platt, M. L. and Glimcher, P. W. (1997). Responses of intraparietal neurons to saccadic targets and visual distractors. *J. Neurophysiol.* 78: 1574–1589.

Platt, M. L. and Glimcher, P. W. (1999). Neural correlates of decision variables in parietal cortex. *Nature*, 400: 233–238.

Posner, M. I. (1980). Orienting of attention. *Quart. J. Exp. Psych.*, 32: 3–25.

Powell, K. D. and Goldberg, M. E. (2000.) Response of neurons in the lateral intraparietal area to a distractor flashed during the delay period of a memory-guided saccade. *J. Neurophysiol.*, 84: 301–310.

Quian Quiroga, R., Snyder, L. H., Batista, A. P., Cui, H. and Andersen, R. A. (2006). Movement intention is better predicted than attention in the posterior parietal cortex. *J. Neurosci.*, 26: 3615–3620.

Robinson, D. L. and Petersen, S. E. (1992). The pulvinar and visual salience. *Trends Neurosci.*, 15: 127–132.

Robinson, D. L., Bowman, E. M. and Kertzman, C. (1995). Covert orienting of attention in macaques. II. Contributions of parietal cortex. *J. Neurophysiol.*, 74: 698–712.

Robinson, D. L., Goldberg, M. E. and Stanton, G. B. (1978). Parietal association cortex in the primate: sensory mechanisms and behavioral modulations. *J. Neurophysiol.*, 41: 910–932.

Roitman, J. D. and Shadlen, M. N. (2002). Response of neurons in the lateral intraparietal area during a combined visual discrimination reaction time task. *J. Neurosci.*, 22: 9475–9489.

Serences, J. T. and Yantis, S. (2006). Selective visual attention and perceptual coherence. *Trends Cogn. Sci.*, 10: 38–45.

Serences, J. T., Shomstein, S., Leber, A. B., Golay, X., Egeth, H. E. and Yantis, S. (2005). Coordination of voluntary and stimulus-driven attentional control in human cortex. *Psychological Sci.*, 16: 114–122.

Sereno, A. B. and Maunsell, J. H. (1998). Shape selectivity in primate lateral intraparietal cortex. *Nature*, 395: 500–503.

Shadlen, M. N. and Newsome, W. T. (2001). Neural basis of a perceptual decision in the parietal cortex (area LIP) of the rhesus monkey. *J. Neurophysiol.*, 86: 1916–1936.

Shepherd, M., Findlay, J. M. and Hockey, R. J. (1986). The relationship between eye movements and spatial attention. *Quart. J. Exp. Psychol.*, 38: 475–491.

Snyder, L. H., Batista, A. P. and Andersen, R. A. (1997). Coding of intention in the posterior parietal cortex. *Nature*, 386: 167–170.

Snyder, L. H., Batista, A. P. and Andersen, R. A. (1998). Change in motor plan, without a change in the spatial locus of attention, modulates activity in posterior parietal cortex. *J. Neurophysiol.*, 79: 2814–2819.

Sugrue, L. P., Corrado, G. S. and Newsome, W. T. (2004). Matching behavior and the representation of value in the parietal cortex. *Science*, 304: 1782–1787.

Thomas, N. W. and Paré, M. (2007). Temporal processing of saccade targets in parietal cortex area LIP during visual search. *J. Neurophysiol.*, 97: 942–947.

Thompson, K. G. and Bichot, N. P. (2005). A visual salience map in the primate frontal eye field. *Prog. Brain Res.*, 147: 251–262.

Thompson, K. G., Biscoe, K. L. and Sato, T. R. (2005). Neuronal basis of covert spatial attention in the frontal eye field. *J. Neurosci.*, 25: 9479–9487.

Thompson, K. G., Hanes, D. P., Bichot, N. P. and Schall, J. D. (1996). Perceptual and motor processing stages identified in the activity of macaque frontal eye field neurons during visual search. *J. Neurophysiol.*, 76: 4040–4055.

Toth, L. J. and Assad, J. A. (2002). Dynamic coding of behaviourally relevant stimuli in parietal cortex. *Nature*, 415: 165–168.

Treisman, A. M. and Gelade, G. (1980). A feature-integration theory of attention. *Cognitive Psychol.* 12: 97–136.

Treue, S. and Maunsell, J. H. (1999). Effects of attention on the processing of motion in macaque middle temporal and medial superior temporal visual cortical areas. *J. Neurosci.*, 19: 7591–7602.

Tsotsos, J. K., Culhane, S. M., Wai, W. Y. K., Lai, Y. H., Davis, N. and Nuflo, F. (1995). Modeling visual-attention via selective tuning. *Artificial Intell.*, 78: 507–545.

Ungerleider, L. G. and Mishkin, M. (1982). Two cortical visual systems. In D. J. Ingle, M. A. Goodale and R. J. W. Mansfield (eds.) *Analysis of Visual Behavior*. Cambridge, MA: MIT Press, pp. 549–586.

Walther, D. and Koch, C. (2006). Modeling attention to salient proto-objects. *Neural Networks*, 19. 1395–1407.

Wardak, C., Olivier, E. and Duhamel, J. R. (2004). A deficit in covert attention after parietal cortex inactivation in the monkey. *Neuron*, 42: 501–508.

Williams, Z. M., Elfar, J. C., Eskandar, E. N., Toth, L. J. and Assad, J. A. (2003). Parietal activity and the perceived direction of ambiguous apparent motion. *Nature Neurosci.*, 6: 616–623.

Williford, T. and Maunsell, J. H. (2006). Effects of spatial attention on contrast response functions in macaque area V4. *J. Neurophysiol.*, 96: 40–54.

Yang, T. and Shadlen, M. N. (2007). Probabilistic reasoning by neurons. *Nature*, 447: 1075–1080.

Yeshurun, Y. and Carrasco, M. (1999). Spatial attention improves performance in spatial resolution tasks. *Vision Res.*, 39: 293–306.

Zelinsky, G. J. and Sheinberg, D. L. (1997). Eye movements during parallel-serial visual search. *J. Exp. Psychol.: Human Percept. Perf.*, 23: 244–262.

Zhang, M., Wang, X. and Goldberg, M. E. (2007). GABAergic inhibitory mechanisms shape the response properties of parietal neurons in the monkey. Paper presented at the Society for Neuroscience Annual Meeting.

3 Left-to-right reversal of hemispatial neglect symptoms following adaptation to reversing prisms

F. D. Feloiu, J. J. Marotta, M. Vesia, S. E. Black and J. D. Crawford

Damage to the right posterior parietal cortex may result in left visual-field deficits including hemispatial neglect and/or asymmetry in pointing accuracy (as in optic ataxia). It is unclear whether these disorders are due to deficits in retina-fixed or world/action-fixed coordinates. We trained parietal patients and age-matched controls to point at remembered visual targets while looking through left-right optical reversing prisms. If neglect remained fixed in retinal coordinates, reversing vision should reverse the baseline pointing patterns. However, if neglect was fixed in action coordinates, the prism task should not affect the baseline patterns. Remarkably, eight of the nine brain-damaged patients learned this task, compared with only six of the ten age-matched controls. Three right-parietal patients showed target neglect in pointing to the left, and this neglect reversed from the left to the right during prism training. These results suggest that parietal neglect (specific to our patients) remains fixed in visual coordinates rather than in motor coordinates.

3.1 Introduction

In everyday life, we use vision to guide movements of the hand when we perform various tasks, such as reaching to and grasping a cup of coffee, driving a car, using a tool or working on a computer. In other words, we perform eye–hand coordination

Cortical Mechanisms of Vision, ed. M. Jenkin and L. R. Harris. Published by Cambridge University Press.
© Cambridge University Press 2000.

when carrying out these tasks. Although we do many of these things with ease, such seemingly simple behavior requires a complex transformation of visual information input into the appropriate coordinated motor responses of both the eyes and hands. The question of how and where this transformation is implemented in the brain is, to a large extent, unknown.

The posterior parietal cortex (PPC) is thought to be part of the "dorsal stream" of vision and is involved in processing spatial information and directing visually guided actions (Goodale and Milner, 1992; Milner and Goodale, 1993; Jeannerod et al., 1995; Andersen et al., 1997; Colby and Goldberg, 1999; Crawford et al., 2004). Human neuroimaging techniques have been successfully used to identify regions within PPC that are activated during various tasks such as saccades and arm movements. In a functional magnetic resonance imaging (fMRI) study, Sereno et al. (2001) reported a bilateral region in the PPC that showed a contralateral topographic pattern of activations for memory-guided eye movements. In a subsequent event-related fMRI study, Connolly et al. (2003) identified a human analog of monkey's "parietal reach region," an area in the medial aspect of the PPC that responded preferentially when humans planned to point to, rather than to make a saccade to a remembered location. Medendorp and colleagues (Medendorp et al., 2003) found that the same PPC region showed contralateral topographic activations for both saccades and pointing and, furthermore, that this information in PPC was encoded and updated in a gaze-centered frame of reference.

However, these gaze-centered signals within PPC could represent either the visual stimulus (vision) or the movement command toward that stimulus (motor). Fernandez-Ruiz and colleagues (Fernandez-Ruiz et al., 2007) used a reversing prism pointing technique to test whether the gaze-centered signal in human PPC encodes the visual goal of the movement (that is, upstream from the vision-to-motor transformation) (Gottlieb and Goldberg, 1999) or the direction of the movement (downstream from this transformation) (Kalaska, 1996; Eskandar and Assad, 1999; Zhang and Barash, 2000). The authors trained healthy individuals to point in a MRI setup while looking through optical left-right reversing prisms. Without the prisms, the PPC activations were contralateral to both the visual goal and movement direction (since both were in the same visual field), in agreement with previous fMRI studies (Sereno et al., 2001; Medendorp et al., 2003). However, with the left-right reversing prisms, the activations remained contralateral to the visual goal, but were ipsilateral to the direction of movement. These results suggested that human PPC encodes visual target direction rather than movement direction. It is not known how this relates to visuospatial symptoms of parietal damage.

Disruptions within parietal lobe may lead to various parietal syndromes such as optic ataxia (misreaching), hemispatial neglect (failure to process or report information presented in the contralesional space), constructional apraxia (difficulty in drawing or constructing objects), gaze apraxia (inability to move the eyes voluntarily to objects of interest) and akinetopsia (inability to perceive movement).

Based on neuropsychological data, two main functional regions can be distinguished within the PPC. Lesions to the right inferior parietal lobule and the temporal parietal junction may induce left unilateral neglect (Vallar and Perani, 1986; Heilman et al., 2000; Marotta et al., 2003; Parton et al., 2004), a neurological deficit involving perception, attention and/or performing actions within the left side of the subject's workspace. On the other hand, lesions to the superior parietal lobule and to the region including and surrounding the intraparietal sulcus may induce a deficit in visually guided movements (e.g., reaching, grasping, pointing) known as "optic ataxia" (Perenin and Vighetto, 1988).

Hemispatial neglect is a neurological disorder characterized by a failure to attend to, report, or represent information appearing in the visual field contralateral to the location of a brain lesion, in spite of sensory processing and visual acuity being intact for that field (Heilman et al., 2000). Neglect induces many functional debilitating effects in everyday life. For example, neglect patients may eat food only from the right side of their plate, ignore people who approach from the left, miss words from the left of the page when reading, or omit details on the left when copying pictures. It was suggested that perceptual and visuomotor deficits seen in neglect patients may be due to the patient's inability to form good structural representations of the entire object for use in visual perception and visuomotor control (Marotta et al., 2003).

Neglect is often associated with contralesional hemiplegia or hemiparesis (Bisiach and Vallar, 1988; Robertson and Marshall, 1993), which has been shown to be responsible for poor functional recovery and reduced ability to benefit from treatment of impaired motor functions (Pantano et al., 1996; Katz et al., 1999).

Some parietal neglect patients may have no apparent deficit for an isolated stimulus on the affected side. Their deficit only emerges when stimuli are presented on both sides simultaneously, in which case the previously detectable contralesional stimulus is now "extinguished" from awareness by the competing ipsilesional stimulus. This phenomenon is thought to reflect an attentional rather than sensory disorder (Baylis et al., 1993; Ward et al., 1994).

Studies have shown that hemispatial neglect is not exclusively due to lesions centered on the PPC. Neglect has been also shown to occur after lesions to the parahyppocampal region of the medial temporal lobe (Mort et al., 2003), temporal-parietal-occipital junction (Leibovitch et al., 1999), superior temporal gyrus (Karnath et al., 2001, 2004), frontal lobe (Husain and Kennard, 1996) or putamen and caudate nucleus within basal ganglia (Karnath et al., 2004).

Many studies have approached the issue of separating "perceptual" components of neglect (patients could not perceive targets on the contralesional space, but were able to direct movements toward that space) from "motor" components of neglect (patients perceived targets on the contralesional space but were unable to direct movements to that space) by the use of opposition tasks, in which the perceptual and motor demands of the tasks were set in spatial opposition via, for example, a 90° angle mirror (Tegner and Levander, 1991; Bisiach et al., 1995) or an epidiascope (Nico, 1996). Although these studies show some evidence that neglect is fixed in retinal coordinates, these opposition methods are extremely incompatible tasks even for neurologically intact subjects, and the participants may give up after just a few initial attempts, therefore biasing the results.

The present study sought to address this question: do spatial errors in left hemispatial neglect as a result of the PPC damage arise in visual- or action-based coordinates? One way to test this question is to train left neglect patients with right posterior parietal damage due to stroke to point at left and right visual targets (dots) while looking through left-right optical reversing prisms (Kohler, 1962; Sugita, 1996; Marotta et al., 2005; Fernandez-Ruiz et al., 2007). We have recently shown that young healthy adults can rapidly learn to reverse their visual-motor transformation for pointing to remembered targets (Marotta et al., 2005; Fernandez-Ruiz et al., 2007).

The use of such prisms reverses the normal spatial relationship between the retinal stimulus and the direction of movement (Kohler, 1962; Sugita, 1996), placing the retinal stimulus in one visual hemifield and the direction of movement towards the other visual hemifield. This condition is called visual-motor dissociation task. Since the left-right reversing prisms reverse the horizontal position of an object across a vertical midline, a target whose actual position is on the left is seen on the right with prisms.

The correct pointing movement with reversing prisms to a particular left target seen on the right will be to the left, and in a closed loop condition subjects will see their hands going to the right (where the target was seen). At the beginning of the adaptation training, subjects will do the opposite. They will point to the apparent (seen) right position of the target and, having visual feedback, will see their pointing hands going to the left (away from the viewed target position) (Marotta et al., 2005; Fernandez-Ruiz et al., 2007). After the training period, the majority of the subjects were found to have learned to adapt their pointing so that they could successfully point to actual target location while looking through left-right reversing prisms. This visuomotor adaptation consisted of pointing in a direction that was opposite to the direction where the target was seen.

The reversing prism technique used in the present study differs from the opposition tasks by allowing a direct visual feedback of both the remembered target location and the pointing hand, promoting a more natural reaching behavior and adding only one new visuomotor transformation to be learned (left-right reversal), thus eliminating other possible confounding visuomotor transformations.

In the current study, if left neglect (quantified here as failure to respond/point to left targets) due to right PPC damage remains fixed in visual coordinates, the neglected targets should reverse from left (without prisms) to right (with prisms) in real space. On the other hand, if neglect remains fixed in motor coordinates, the prisms will not reverse the motor behavior. Prism-reversal training might reveal new adapted visuomotor pathways, or even help to alleviate the symptoms due to damage to these pathways, as observed in neglect patients after rightward displacing prism adaptation (Rossetti et al., 1998; Farnè et al., 2002; Newport and Jackson, 2006).

In summary, using a reversing prism pointing paradigm, we investigated whether unilateral right parietal patients (with or without left neglect) could be trained to point with reversing prisms (parietal cortex would normally be required to control pointing in contralesional space) and, if so, what effect the reversing prism training had on the pointing pattern of neglect patients.

3.2   Materials and methods

Subjects   Informed consent was obtained from all subjects prior to the beginning of the experiment. All procedures were approved by the York University Human Participants Review Sub-Committee and the Sunnybrook Health Sciences Centre Human

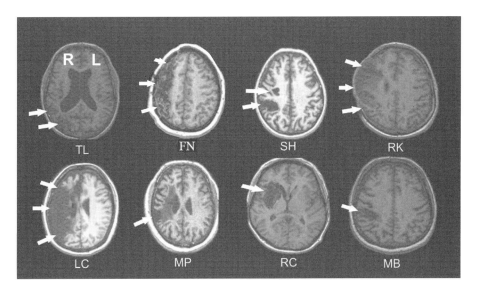

Figure 3.1. MRI imaging scans for eight of the nine patients tested. All scans confirmed that only the right hemisphere was affected by stroke, with no involvement of the left hemisphere (R, right hemisphere; L, left hemisphere; white arrows, location of the lesion(s)).

Participation Ethical Review Board. We tested nine right hemisphere stroke-affected patients (all righthanded, mean age = 55.7 ± 13.7 years, see Table 3.1). The lesion locations were obtained from patients' clinical charts, neurological assessments, and MRI imaging scans where available (scans for eight patients are shown in Figure 3.1).

Patients had no right (pointing) hand sensorimotor deficits and had normal or corrected-to-normal visual acuity. Visual fields were assessed by clinical confrontation testing. The presence of hemispatial neglect was assessed using the Sunnybrook Neglect Assessment Procedure (SNAP), consisting of four subtests: a shape cancellation task, spontaneous drawing and copying of a clock and daisy, line bisection, and a line cancellation task (Black et al., 1990; Leibovitch et al., 1998). Depending on the total score, performance is classified either as within normal limits, or as mild or severe neglect. All stroke patients were tested in the chronic stage with a mean of seven years post-stroke.

Three of the nine patients tested were diagnosed with mild hemispatial neglect prior to the testing using the SNAP. They were classified as the "neglect group" and are described in some detail in subsequent sections.

Patient TL is a right-handed 71-year-old male who had right hemisphere ischemic strokes in July 1999 and April 2000. He was admitted to the hospital for marked confusion and peripheral vision problems. On admission, TL showed severe left hemispatial neglect and left hemifield deficits. CT scans taken in February 2005 showed stroke lesions involving the right parietal, right frontal and occipital areas (Figure 3.1), with no involvement of the left cerebral hemisphere. At the time of experimental testing (Oc-

Patient	Age	Gender	Location of Stroke	Time post-stroke testing at (months)	Performed Task Without Disclosure?	Performed Task After Disclosure?	Sensorimotor Deficits	Visual Field Deficits	Other Observations
T.L.	71	M	Right frontal, parietal and occipital areas.	62	Yes	-	Normal motor and sensory findings.	Left inferior quadrantanopia by clinical confrontation testing.	Mild left hemispatial neglect and optic ataxia in the baseline testing.
M.L.	67	F	Right frontal, temporal and parietal areas.	134	Yes	-	Moderate left hemiparesis and normal sensory findings.	Normal visual fields to clinical confrontation testing.	Showed mild left hemispatial neglect in the baseline testing.
F.N.	27	F	Right temporal and parietal areas.	75	Yes	-	Moderate left hemiparesis and normal sensory findings.	Normal visual fields to clinical confrontation testing.	Showed mild left hemispatial neglect in the baseline testing.
S.H.	59	M	Right frontal, temporal, parietal and supplementary motor areas.	84	No	No	Normal motor and sensory findings.	Normal visual fields confirmed by formal testing.	Very confused when pointing with prism.
R.K.	53	M	Right frontal, temporal and parietal areas.	6	Yes	-	Mild left hemiparesis and normal sensory findings.	Normal visual fields to clinical confrontation testing.	-
M.P.	63	M	Right frontal, temporal and parietal areas and right basal ganglia.	178	No	Yes	Left arm paralysis, moderate leg paresis and normal sensory findings.	Normal visual fields to clinical confrontation testing.	-
L.C.	56	F	Right frontal, temporal and parietal areas.	135	Yes	-	Moderate left hemiparesis and left tactile extinction.	Normal visual fields to clinical confrontation testing.	-
R.C.	42	M	Right frontal, temporal and parietal areas and right basal ganglia.	28	Yes	-	Left arm paralysis, moderate leg paresis and normal sensory findings.	Normal visual fields to clinical confrontation testing.	-
M.B.	64	M	Right frontal and parietal areas and thalamus.	59	Yes	-	Normal motor function and mild sensory deficits.	Normal visual fields confirmed by formal testing.	-

Table 3.1. Characteristics of the patients tested.

tober 2004), he had fully recovered (no sensorimotor deficits) except for mild residual left neglect and left inferior quadrantanopia.

Patient ML is a right-handed 67-year-old female that had a right carotid dissection in September 1993 with right middle cerebral artery infarction involving right frontal, parietal and temporal cortices and sparing deep structures. On admission, she showed significant left hemispatial neglect and anosognosia (impaired awareness of illness). The left cerebral hemisphere was not affected by stroke. She was ambulatory with a residual left hemiparesis, but at the time of the present study, showed only mild left neglect.

Patient FN, a right-handed 27-year-old female, suffered a severe right middle cerebral artery territory stroke (temporal, parietal and frontal) with hemorrhagic transformation and malignant edema in December 1998, for which she underwent a partial right temporal lobectomy and skull removal for decompression. At the time of the present testing she was ambulatory with residual hemiparesis and showed mild left hemispatial neglect.

The other six stroke-affected patients (RK, LC, MP, RC, SH and MB) had cortical damage that included the right parietal lobe and other nonparietal areas, such as right frontal, temporal, occipital, basal ganglia and thalamus, but in every case only the right cerebral hemisphere was affected (unilateral stroke) (see Table 3.1 and Figure 3.1). They were not diagnosed with neglect prior to testing, and were classified as "brain-damaged controls."

We also tested ten neurologically intact age-matched controls (all right handed, mean age = 58.2 ± 9.7 years) (Table 3.2), in order to identify whether this healthy population could perform the reversing prism task. All subjects were naïve as to the aims of the experiment.

3.3   Apparatus and procedure

We have recently showed that pointing with reversing prisms in young healthy subjects produces a rapid task-specific visuomotor adaptation (Marotta et al., 2005). Similar methods were used here. In brief, subjects' heads were stabilized and vision was obstructed by opaque goggles, except through a rectangular tube placed in front of the right eye (Figure 3.2A). Visual stimuli were presented through the tube, in dim light, on a computer screen located 40 cm in front of the subject. Subjects were instructed to maintain visual fixation throughout the experiment on a central cross that remained on the screen at all times.

A target (5 mm dot) was presented for 500 ms at 3.2 cm (4.7° visual angle) to the left or right of the cross (Figure 3.2B) (this was considered one trial). Subjects were instructed to point-to-touch the screen where they saw the target (therefore at the actual position of the target in space) as soon as the target was off and do this as fast and as accurately as possible. If they did it correctly, they would see their pointing index finger landing where they saw the target. Six seconds were allowed for the subject to touch the remembered target location with the index finger of their right hand, and return to resting position.

Control	Age	Gender	Performed task without disclosure?	Performed task after disclosure?	Other observations
F.F.	55	M	No	No	Very confused when pointing with prism.
G.K.	46	M	Yes	-	-
T.M.	54	F	No	No	Very confused when pointing with prism.
T.F.	50	F	Yes	-	-
H.W.	57	F	No	No	Pointed to the wrong direction with prism.
I.N.	52	M	Yes	-	-
G.N.	54	F	No	Yes	-
E.L.	68	F	Yes	-	-
D.G.	71	M	No	No	Pointed to the wrong direction with prism.
S.M.	75	F	Yes	-	-

Table 3.2. Characteristics of the neurologically intact controls tested

Fifteen experimental blocks were run in total, each block consisting of 20 trials, 10 to the left and 10 to the right presented in random order. Two blocks were run in the baseline condition (no reversing prism). A dove reversing prism was then inserted into the viewing tube, and subjects were then required to point for an additional eleven blocks (subjects received the same initial pointing instructions). If subjects were not able to perform the reversing prism task after two of these blocks, we disclosed the nature of the task to them and then continued recording (see Tables 3.1 and 3.2 for details). Two more blocks were run at the end without prisms (recovery condition).

Pointing performance was recorded using an Optotrak recording system (Northern Digital, Inc., Waterloo, Canada; sampling rate = 200 Hz) and analyzed offline. We used three IRED markers placed on the distal phalanx of the pointing index finger of the right hand, arranged so that we could record the position of the finger even if subjects performed pronation/supination movements during pointing.

The initial position of the hand was not visible at all, with the hand being visible starting about half way into the pointing movement. We did not select a particular starting position for the pointing hand (which was at each patient's discretion, but as close to their bodies as possible) because we did not want patients to focus on placing their hand on a particular location on the table instead of focusing on performing the task properly (given the challenge of the task).

Because it was not possible to monitor eye movements with our goggle set-up, the subjects were instructed and tested "offline" before the beginning of experimental trials in order to ensure that they understood how to perform the task (the subjects were not, however, aware that their eyes were not monitored during the experiment). The experimenter and the subject were seated facing each other, with no other piece of equip-

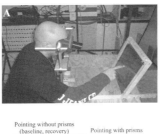

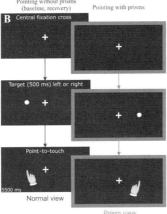

Figure 3.2. Apparatus (A) and conditions of the experiment (B). (A) The goggles-chin rest setup was affixed on a custom-built, modular aluminum pipe apparatus that was firmly attached vertically to a table. The subjects were seated in an adjustable chair in front of a tabletop with their heads at the level of the goggles-chin rest setup. They looked through the tube and pointed-to-touch a computer screen that was situated within comfortable pointing distance from their body. (B) Baseline and recovery conditions (left). Prism condition (prisms are worn) (right): the left target is viewed on the right, and, when pointing to the left, subjects will see the image of their hand reversed and moving in the opposite direction to where they pointed (right), and vice versa.

ment/set up in between. The "offline" testing began by instructing the subjects to fixate a point located in between experimenter's eyes. The experimenter then positioned his left and right index fingers at about 20 cm to either side of the subject's fixation point. The fingers were moved briefly up and down, one at a time and in random order, without moving the hands, while the experimenter kept looking at the subject's gaze, and the subjects were instructed to point-to-touch the experimenter's moving index finger while maintaining the fixation. The experimenter observed the subject's gaze direction during these pointing tasks, and the "offline" testing was considered successful if the subject made five consecutive pointings without shifting their gaze. All of our subjects met this condition.

3.4   Data analyses

Pointing errors in the x (left-right) and y (up-down) directions were computed for each trial, relative to the coordinates of the two target positions. We counted the number of trials that subjects failed to point to the presented target ("neglected" trials) in each of the three conditions of the experiment.

3.5   Results

Target neglect related to our task was considered present when patients consistently failed to point (move their pointing hand) to targets presented in their contralesional visual field in the baseline condition (Heilman et al., 2000).

3.5.1   Neurologically intact controls

Half (five) of our age-matched, neurologically intact control subjects (Table 3.2) were able to rapidly learn the prism reversal task. The other half of intact controls failed to perform the prism-reversal task after two blocks of visually guided trials. The latter subjects were then informed of the nature of the prism reversal task, but still, only one additional subject was then able to perform the task. During experiments with the four remaining "nonlearning" intact controls, we often observed that they began pointing in the wrong direction and, after the pointing hand became visible, they continued to make movements further and further in the same (wrong) direction.

3.5.2   Stroke-affected subjects

Seven of the nine stroke patients learned the prism reversal task quickly. Of the re-maining two patients, one learned the task after we disclosed its nature, so only one patient (SH) was not able to learn the task (he kept pointing to the perceived location of the targets, and not to their reversed spatial location).

The "brain-damaged control group" (six subjects) did not fail to point to any tar-get presented in their contralesional visual field in the baseline testing. Regardless of whether they learned or not how to perform the prism task, they did not fail to point to any target presented on the screen during prism training as well.

All (three) subjects in the "neglect group" failed to respond (point) to some of the trials presented in their left (contralesional) visual hemifield during baseline testing (we defined this deficit within the parameters of our task as left target neglect, see Figure 3.3). For example, TL neglected 5% of the trials presented on the left, ML neglected 10% of trials and FN neglected 25% of them. All three subjects pointed to all targets presented in their right (ipsilesional) visual field.

The question posed was what would happen to the left inattention (specific to our task) when these three patients pointed while looking through the left-right reversing prisms, where the left targets would then be seen on the right, and the right targets would be seen on the left (subjects still had to point toward their actual location). If target neglect remained fixed in visual coordinates, reversing vision should reverse

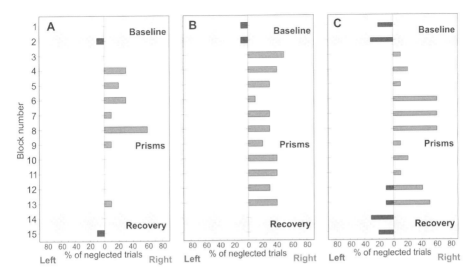

Figure 3.3. Target neglect patients' performances. These three patients (A, patient TL; B, patient ML; C, patient FN) neglected left targets in the baseline condition (darker bars), right targets in the prism condition (lighter bars) and left targets in the recovery condition (darker bars). Bars represent percentage of neglected trials in each block; horizontal axis, percentage of neglected trials; vertical axis, conditions of the experiment.

neglect to rightward-positioned targets. On the other hand, if target neglect stayed fixed in motor coordinates, then reversing the vision should not affect the subject's overt behavior.

During reversing prism training, target neglect reversed from left to right in the "neglect group": all three patients failed to respond to some targets that they viewed on the left, although they were presented on the right (ipsilateral to the lesion) (Figure 3.3). TL neglected 15.45%, ML 32.72% and FN 31.81% of the right-positioned targets. TL and ML did not neglect any of the left targets with prisms, and FN neglected only two (out of 110). There was an increase in the percentage of overall neglected trials for each patient during prism training compared with trials neglected in the baseline condition; the increase was from 5% to 15.45% for TL, from 10% to 32.72% for ML and from 25% to 31.81% for FN.

In the recovery condition, the left/right neglect pattern reversed again in the "neglect group": TL and FN failed to point to some targets presented only on the left (5% and 25% of the trials, respectively). ML did not neglect any targets in the recovery condition.

3.6   Discussion

Our three right parietal patients diagnosed pre-testing with mild left neglect showed signs of some type of left neglect in the baseline condition, defined in relation to our task as target neglect (i.e. they consistently failed to point toward some of the leftward targets). This type of left neglect reversed to the right with prisms and then it reversed back to the left when the prisms were taken off. These results support the hypothesis that target neglect (related to our task) obeys visual coordinates rather than motor coordinates.

A remarkable observation is the high capacity of our "recovered" unilateral parietal patients – in particular our brain-damaged controls with extensive lesions including much of the right cerebral hemisphere – to accurately perform this particular memory-guided pointing task. How could patients with so much brain damage be similar to age-matched controls at performing/learning the prism task? The answer may be in the nature of the mechanisms required to point with reversing prisms. To do this task, the subjects must learn to reverse the feedforward motor command, based on the visual information and memory of performance in previous trials (Marotta et al., 2005). They must also ignore direct visual feedback from the hand during pointing, because it (being reversed) provides inappropriate information to guide the hand. We did not consistently observe problems with this in our previous study, which employed young adult subjects (Marotta et al., 2005), but it is thought that older adults (like those used here) may differ in their use of visual feedback (Collins et al., 1995; Baugh and Marotta, 2007). If some of our neurologically intact subjects were unable to disengage the use of (inappropriate) visual feedback during the prism task, this would account for the anti-corrective movements that we observed in subjects who failed to learn the task. On the other hand, parietal cortex is thought to be an important target for these visual feedback signals (Pisella et al., 2000; Prablanc et al., 2003). Thus, it is possible that in parietal-damaged patients the visual control may be compromised, which in this special case – pointing with reversing prisms – could be an advantage.

Anti-pointing paradigms may also seem to produce a left-right reversal in visuomotor coordinates. However, reversing prism tasks and anti-pointing tasks are different. In anti-pointing tasks, subjects are instructed to point in a direction opposite to the perceived location of the target (Hallett, 1978; Connolly et al., 2000; DeSouza et al., 2003). The motor command produces a congruent corollary discharge, because subjects see the pointing hands (vision) going to the same direction where the motor commands were (motor). Moreover, anti-pointing does not alter subjects' perception of the target (Fischer and Weber, 1992). In contrast, in reversing prism pointing task, the subjects are not given any specialized instructions, except to point where the target was. The motor command with prisms produces an incongruent corollary discharge, because the subjects see the pointing hands (vision) going to the opposite direction where the motor commands were (motor) (dissociation between vision and proprioception). Reversing prism pointing task provides direct visual feedback of pointing errors and affects perception.

The apparent increase in the number of neglected trials in the prism condition compared to trials neglected in the baseline condition may be due to a phenomenon similar to extinction, or it could be due to the increased difficulty of the prism task and subsequent shift of attentional resources. In contrast to neglect, extinction is defined as the inability to process or attend to the more contralesionally located stimulus when two stimuli are simultaneously presented (Rapcsak et al., 1987). Mattingley et al. (1997) showed that extinction can occur with two simultaneous stimuli from different sensory modalities (one visual and the other one tactile). In our study, in the prism condition, for pointing to right targets, the visual goal was on the left (contralesional) hemifield, and the required motor command was towards right (ipsilesional) space. The two "stimuli" (left-viewed target and right motor command) were not presented simultaneously per se. But, because of the nature of the prism task, some phenomenon similar to extinction may have occurred: the two stimuli may have competed with each other, resulting in the "extinction" of the stimulus located in the left (contralesional) visual hemifield (visual goal). Without a visual goal, there was no subsequent pointing movement (to the right).

Although we could not monitor subjects' eye movements during experiments (which would have been ideal), it is less likely that eye movements would change the results significantly due to the nature of the neglect itself. Subjects with left neglect will ignore stimuli presented on their left visual field even when they are allowed full head and eye movements. Therefore, we consider that lack of fixation would not influence the results.

Visual field deficit may be a confounding factor in this experiment, as patient TL was diagnosed with left inferior quadrantanopia prior to testing. Patients with this condition will not see/perceive all targets presented on a fixed area within their left visual hemifield, area that has the same spatial location relative to patient's gaze. In our experiment, had it been an overlap between TL's left quadrantanopic field and the location of left targets, TL should not have been able to perceive all left targets. However, all baseline leftward targets were presented on the same left location with respect to his gaze and he did not perceive only some (not all) of them. Therefore, it seems that the omitted baseline targets on the left in patient TL were due to some form of neglect rather than due to left visual field loss.

In short, our results from the prism task suggest quite clearly that this form of neglect remained fixed in visual coordinates. Of course, this is a very special type of neglect: we cannot directly conclude that all types of neglect that have been tested experimentally and clinically (Behrmann and Tipper, 1999) would show the same reversal. Further studies are warranted regarding this issue.

Acknowledgments

The authors would like to thank subjects for their kind participation in the experiments, as well as the Heart and Stroke Foundation Centre for Stroke Recovery for infrastructure support, Valerie Closson for help with recruiting subjects, Farrell Leibovitch and Fuqiang Gao for help with preparing the brain images, Gerald Keith, Farshad Farshadmanesh and Alina Constantin for their help with experiments and data analyses, Aarlenne Khan for help and comments on the manuscript, and Saihong Sun for help with technical programming. This work was supported by grants from the Canadian Institute of Health Research (CIHR) and Ontario Graduate Scholarship in Science and Technology (OGSST). JDC holds a Canada Research Chair.

References

Andersen, R. A., Snyder, L. H., Bradley, D. C. and Xing, J. (1997). Multimodal representation of space in the posterior parietal cortex and its use in planning movements. *Ann. Rev. Neurosci.*, 20: 303–330.

Baugh, L. A. and Marotta, J. J. (2007). Differential effects of aging on a visuomotor paradigm. In Society for Neuroscience Program 397.16. Washington, DC: Society for Neuroscience.

Baylis, G. C., Driver, J. and Rafal, R. D. (1993). Visual extinction and stimulus repetition. *J. Cogn. Neurosci.*, 5: 453–466.

Behrmann, M. and Tipper, S. P. (1999). Attention accesses multiple reference frames: evidence from visual neglect. *J. Exp. Psychol.. Hum, Percept. Perf.*, 25: 83–101.

Bisiach, E. and Vallar, G. (1988). Hemineglect in humans. In F. Boller and J. Grafman (Eds.) *Handbook of Neuropsychology, Vol. 1*, Amsterdam: Elsevier, pp. 195–222.

Bisiach, E., Tegner, R., Làdavas, E., Rusconi, M. L., Mijovic, D. and Hjaltason, H. (1995). Dissociation of ophthalmokinetic and melokinetic attention in unilateral neglect. *Cereb. Cortex*, 5: 439–447.

Black, S. E., Vu, B., Martin, D. K. and Szalai, J. P. (1990). Evaluation of a bedside battery for hemispatial neglect in acute stroke. *J. Clin. Exp. Neuropsyc.*, 12: 109.

Colby, C. L. and Goldberg, M. E. (1999). Space and attention in parietal cortex. *Ann. Rev. Neurosci.* 22: 319–349.

Collins, J. J., De Luca, C. J., Burrows, A. and Lipsitz, L. A. (1995). Age-related changes in open-loop and closed-loop postural control mechanisms. *Exp. Brain Res.*, 104: 480–492.

Connolly, J. D, Andersen, R. A. and Goodale, M. A. (2003). FMRI evidence for a 'parietal reach region' in the human brain. *Exp. Brain Res.*, 153: 140–145.

Connolly, J. D., Goodale, M. A., DeSouza, J. F., Menon, R. S. and Vilis, T. (2000). A comparison of frontoparietal fMRI activation during anti-saccades and anti-pointing. *J. Neurophysiol.*, 84: 1645–1655.

Crawford, J. D., Medendorp, W. P. and Marotta, J. J. (2004). Spatial transformations for eye-hand coordination. *J. Neurophysiol.*, 92: 10–19.

DeSouza, J. F., Menon, R. S. and Everling, S. (2003). Preparatory set associated with pro-saccades and anti-saccades in humans investigated with event-related FMRI. *J. Neurophysiol.*, 89: 1016–1023.

Eskandar, E. N. and Assad, J. A. (1999). Dissociation of visual, motor and predictive signals in parietal cortex during visual guidance. *Nature Neurosci.*, 2: 88–93.

Farnè, A., Rossetti, Y., Toniolo, S. and Làdavas, E. (2002). Ameliorating neglect with prism adaptation: visuo-manual and visuo-verbal measures. *Neuropsychologia*, 40: 718–729.

Fernandez-Ruiz, J., Goltz, H. C., DeSouza, J. F., Vilis, T. and Crawford, J. D. (2007). Human parietal "reach region" primarily encodes intrinsic visual direction, not extrinsic movement direction, in a visual-motor dissociation task. *Cereb. Cortex*, 17: 2283–2292.

Fischer, B. and Weber, H. (1992). Characteristics of "anti" saccades in man. *Exp. Brain Res.*, 89: 415–424.

Goodale, M. A. and Milner, A. D. (1992). Separate visual pathways for perception and action. *Trends Neurosci.*, 15: 20–25.

Gottlieb, J. and Goldberg, M. E. (1999). Activity of neurons in the lateral intraparietal area of the monkey during an antisaccade task. *Nature Neurosci.*, 2: 906–912.

Hallett, P. E. (1978). Primary and secondary saccades to goals defined by instructions. *Vision Res.*, 18: 1279–1296.

Heilman, K. M., Valenstein, E. and Watson, R. T. (2000). Neglect and related disorders. *Seminars in Neurology*, 20: 463–470.

Husain, M. and Kennard, C. (1996). Visual neglect associated with frontal lobe infarction. *J. Neurol.*, 243: 652–657.

Jeannerod, M., Arbib, M. A., Rizzolatti, G. and Sakata, H. (1995). Grasping objects: The cortical mechanisms of visuomotor transformation. *Trends Neurosci.*, 18: 314–320.

Kalaska, J. F. (1996). Parietal cortex area 5 and visuomotor behavior. *Can. J. Physiol. Pharmacol.*, 74: 483–498.

Karnath, H. O., Ferber, S. and Himmelbach, M. (2001). Spatial awareness is a function of the temporal not the posterior parietal lobe. *Nature*, 411: 950–953.

Karnath, H. O., Fruhmann Berger, M., Kuker, W. and Rorden, C. (2004). The anatomy of spatial neglect based on voxelwise statistical analysis: a study of 140 patients. *Cereb. Cortex*, 14: 1164–1172.

Katz, N., Hartman-Maeir, A., Ring, H. and Soroker, N. (1999). Functional disability and rehabilitation outcome in right hemisphere damaged patients with and without unilateral spatial neglect. *Arch. Phys. Med. Rehab.*, 80: 379–384.

Kohler, I. (1962). Experiments with goggles. *Sci. Am.*, 206: 62–72.

Leibovitch, F. S., Black, S. E., Caldwell, C. B., Ebert, P. L., Ehrlich, L. E., Szalai, J. P. (1998) Brain-behavior correlations in hemispatial neglect using CT and SPECT: the Sunnybrook stroke study. *Neurologia*, 50: 901–908.

Leibovitch, F. S., Black, S. E., Caldwell, C. B., McIntosh, A. R., Ehrlich, L. E. and Szalai, J. P. (1999). Brain SPECT imaging and left hemispatial neglect covaried using partial least squares: the Sunnybrook stroke study. *Hum. Brain Mapp.*, 7: 244–253.

Marotta, J. J., Keith, G. P. and Crawford, J. D. (2005). Task-specific sensorimotor adaptation to reversing prisms. *J. Neurophysiol.*, 93: 1104–1110.

Marotta, J. J., McKeeff, T. J. and Behrmann, M. (2003). Hemispatial neglect: its effects on visual perception and visually guided grasping. *Neuropsychologia*, 41: 1262–1271.

Mattingley, J. B., Driver, J., Beschin, N. and Robertson, I. H. (1997). Attentional competition between modalities: extinction between touch and vision after right hemisphere damage. *Neuropsychologia*, 35: 867–880.

Medendorp, W. P., Goltz, H. C., Vilis, T. and Crawford, J. D. (2003). Gaze-centered updating of visual space in human parietal cortex. *J. Neurosci.*, 23: 6209–6214.

Milner, A. D. and Goodale, M. A. (1993). Visual pathways to perception and action. *Prog. Brain Res.*, 95: 317–337.

Mort, D. J., Malhotra, P., Mannan, S. K., Rorden, C., Pambakian, A., Kennard, C. and Husain, M. (2003). The anatomy of visual neglect. *Brain*, 126: 1986–1997.

Newport, R. and Jackson, S. R. (2006). Posterior parietal cortex and the dissociable components of prism adaptation. *Neuropsychologia*, 44: 2757–2765.

Nico, D. (1996). Detecting directional hypokinesia: the epidiascope technique. *Neuropsychologia*, 34: 471–474.

Pantano, P., Formisano, R., Ricci, M., Di Piero, V., Sabatini, U., Di Pofi, B., Rossi, R., Bozzao, L. and Lenzi, G. L. (1996) Motor recovery after stroke: morphological and functional brain alterations. *Brain*, 119: 1849–1857.

Parton, A., Malhotra, P. and Husain, M. (2004). Hemispatial neglect. *J. Neurol., Neurosurg. Psyc.*, 75: 13–21.

Perenin, M. T. and Vighetto, A. (1988). Optic ataxia: a specific disruption in visuomotor mechanisms. I. Different aspects of the deficit in reaching for objects. *Brain*, 111: 643–674.

Pisella, L., Gréa, H., Tilikete, C., Vighetto, A., Desmurget, M., Rode, G., Boisson, D. and Rossetti, Y. (2000). An 'automatic pilot' for the hand in human posterior parietal cortex: toward reinterpreting optic ataxia. *Nature Neurosci.*, 3: 729–736.

Prablanc, C., Desmurget, M. and Gréa, H. (2003). Neural control of on-line guidance of hand reaching movements. *Progress Brain Res.*, 142: 155–170.

Rapcsak, S. Z., Watson, R. T. and Heilman, K. M. (1987). Hemispace-visual field interactions in visual extinction. *J. Neurol., Neurosur. Psyc.*, 50: 1117–1124.

Robertson, I. H. and Marshall, J. C. (1993). *Unilateral Neglect: Clinical and Experimental Studies*. Hove, UK: Lawrence Erlbaum.

Rossetti, Y., Rode, G., Pisella, L., Farnè, A., Li, L., Boisson, D. and Perenin, M.-T. (1998). Prism adaptation to a rightward optical deviation rehabilitates left hemispatial neglect. *Nature*, 395: 166–169.

Sereno, M. I., Pitzalis, S. and Martinez, A. (2001). Mapping of contralateral space in retinotopic coordinates by a parietal cortical area in humans. *Science*, 294: 1350–1354.

Sugita, Y. (1996). Global plasticity in adult visual cortex following reversal of visual input. *Nature*, 380: 523–526.

Tegner, R. and Levander, M. (1991). Through a looking glass. A new technique to demonstrate directional hypokinesia in unilateral neglect. *Brain*, 114: 1943–1951.

Vallar, G. and Perani, D. (1986). The anatomy of unilateral neglect after right-hemisphere stroke lesions. A clinical/CT-scan correlation study in man. *Neuropsychologia*, 24: 609–622.

Ward, R., Goodrich, S. and Driver, J. (1994). Grouping reduces visual extinction: neuropsychological evidence for weight-linkage in visual selection. *Vis. Cognit.*, 1: 101–129.

Zhang, M. and Barash, S. (2000). Neuronal switching of sensorimotor transformations for antisaccades. *Nature*, 408: 971–975.

4 Sensorimotor aspects of reach deficits in optic ataxia

A. Z. Khan, L. Pisella, A. Blangero, Y. Rossetti and J. D. Crawford

The classical description of the behavioral deficit in optic ataxia patients is limited to errors in reaching and pointing to visual targets, thus involving a deficit in visuomotor transformation processes. However, recent studies have shown that optic ataxia patients also have deficits in a number of additional mechanisms involved in a more general sensorimotor transformation process such as maintaining spatial constancy, integrating visual and proprioceptive information about hand position and performing online adjustments of movements. Here we review the details of how these mechanisms are disrupted in optic ataxia and outline some clinical and functional implications.

4.1 Introduction

The deficit known as optic ataxia was first identified by Rezsõ Bálint as part of the syndrome named after him (Bálint, 1909; Hécean and Ajuriaguerra, 1954; Rizzo and Vecera, 2002; Pisella et al., 2007). Bálint first described the syndrome as a result of "visual binding deficits" and comprising three separate deficits, optic ataxia, gaze apraxia and simultanagnosia. Optic ataxia is classically defined as the inability to guide the hand toward an object using visual information (Perenin and Vighetto, 1988). Gaze apraxia describes a deficit in directing gaze appropriately and simultanagnosia describes an attentional deficit involving integrating multiple objects in a visual scene (Pisella et al., 2007).

Bálint's syndrome, with all three deficits, results mostly from extensive bilateral lesions to the posterior parietal cortex. With less extensive or unilateral lesions, optic ataxia can occur without the accompanying deficits in Bálint's syndrome (Garcin et al., 1967; Rondot and Recondo, 1974; Rondot et al., 1977; Levine et al., 1978; Perenin

Cortical Mechanisms of Vision, ed. M. Jenkin and L. R. Harris. Published by Cambridge University Press.
© Cambridge University Press 2009.

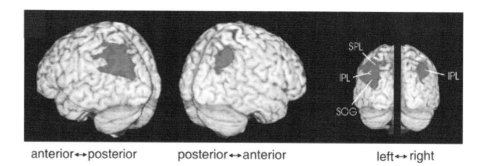

anterior↔posterior   posterior↔anterior   left↔right

Figure 4.1. Damaged areas in optic ataxia. The figure shows three (left side of the brain, right side of the brain and the view from behind from left to right) views of the regions of damage related to optic ataxia superimposed on an average brain. The areas shown are lesions of unilateral left and right brain-damaged optic ataxia patients. These are subtracted plots, in which lesions of a second group of patients with parietal damage, but without optic ataxia have been removed, thus showing only lesions related specifically to optic ataxia. The darker purple areas (larger areas) show areas in which there is a 40% overlap in the lesioned areas across the patient groups, whereas the brighter pink (smaller areas) are regions in which there is a 60% overlap. SPL, superior parietal lobule; IPL, inferior parietal lobule; SOG, superior occipital gyrus. (Reprinted with permission from Karnath and Perenin, 2005.) See CD-ROM for color version.

and Vighetto, 1988; Pisella et al., 2000). These lesions have been widely acknowledged to be mostly limited to the superior part of the posterior parietal cortex (Perenin and Vighetto, 1988) although there is some evidence that areas involving the inferior parietal lobule and the superior occipital cortex are also involved (Karnath and Perenin, 2005). Figure 4.1 shows overlay plots of the damage from 16 unilateral optic ataxia patients, 10 of which had left hemisphere damage, subtracted from damage from a control group with left or right hemisphere damage but who did not show optic ataxia. The figure shows damage related to optic ataxia in the superior parietal lobule (SPL), the inferior parietal lobule (IPL) and the superior occipital gyrus (SOG).

One of the first quantitative analyses of the reach deficits of unilateral optic ataxia was written by Perenin and Vighetto (1988). In this influential paper, they describe reaching and grasping deficits in optic ataxia as a specific visuomotor deficit, resulting from combining visual and motor information, excluding primary motor, visual or attentional effects (for a definition of "visuomotor" – see Box 4.1. They suggest that the deficit results from damage to the superior parietal cortex and areas surrounding the intraparietal sulcus. Additionally, they report both field and hand effects of unilateral damage to these areas; reaching deficits arise from reaching to visual targets in the contralesional visual field using both hands as well as reaching to visual targets in both visual fields using the contralesional visual field. We will elaborate on this in Section 4.2.

Recently, there has been growing controversy as to whether the label "optic ataxia" is appropriate (e.g. Rossetti et al., 2003). Specifically, with more extensive and creative

Box 4.1 The visuomotor transformation

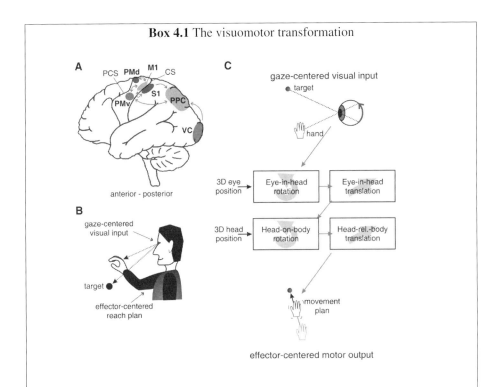

Figure 4.2 Visuomotor transformation. (A) Brain regions involved in the visuomotor transformation. VC, visual cortex; PPC, posterior parietal cortex; S1, primary sensory cortex; M1, primary motor cortex; PMd, dorsal premotor cortex; PMv, ventral premotor cortex. The precentral sulcus (PCS) as well as the central sulcus (CS) are also shown. Arrows depict the direction of information flow. (B) Visuomotor transformation. Visual information about the hand and the target (dotted arrows) enters the eye in a gaze-centered reference frame. This is transformed into an effector-centered reach plan, e.g. the arm. (C) Schematic of the computations involved in the visuomotor transformation. Visual information about the hand and the target is transformed into the movement plan by taking into account rotations such as the rotation of the eye in the head, and the rotation of the head on the body. The relative translations of the eye in the head and the head relative to the body are also taken into account. These rotations and translations are extracted from the 3-D eye and head positions. (Reproduced with permission from Blohm and Crawford, 2007.)

Box 4.1 continued The visuomotor transformation

The term visuomotor defines the interface between visual input and motor output. The visuomotor transformation is a process by which visual information entering our eyes is converted into the appropriate motor action to interact with the environment. Although we refer specifically to visual input, the need for such a transformation is not limited to vision alone. Rather, other forms of sensory information can also be used, e.g. auditory or haptic. While we only describe the visuomotor transformation this may be generalized to other sensory modalities given the correct sensory information is provided.

Visuomotor is neither visual nor motor. It does not refer to the purely visual information present in areas such as the visual cortex (VC) (Figure 4.2A). Nor does it refer to motor commands such as those found in the primary motor cortex (M1) – reflecting muscle commands, etc (Figure 4.2A). Rather, it is the process by which the information about the visual location of a target is transformed into the appropriate action, e.g. a reach movement. The visuomotor transformation involves a number of different areas in the brain, namely the posterior parietal cortex (PPC), and the premotor areas (PMd and PMv) (Figure 4.2A). These areas gradually transform the visual information encoded on the retina to a motor plan for the arm. Information entering the retina is encoded in gaze-centered reference frames, i.e. relative to the line of sight (a description of reference frames can be found in Box 4.1). This information then needs to be converted into a reference frame appropriate for the effector, e.g. a shoulder-centered reference frame (Figure 4.2B). This reference frame transformation requires integrating information about the positions of the body parts relative to one another e.g. the position of the eyes in the head, and about how body parts move relative to each other, e.g. the rotations and translations of the eyes and head. Since the visual input is encoded relative to the line of sight, the brain must take the eye-in-head position as well as the head orientation relative to the body into account in order to know where the visual target is in space or relative to the effector. This is shown in Figure 4.2C above, which provides a schematic of how this transformation could take place and what information is used for it. For more details, see Crawford et al. (2004) as well as Blohm and Crawford (2007).

experiments, patients diagnosed with optic ataxia show myriad deficits that include but are not limited to visually guided actions such as reaching, grasping and pointing. They all however seem to be related to transforming sensory information about the environment into appropriate actions. Indeed, this is one of the most fundamental functions of the human brain – to allow us to interact with our environment. Analyzing the impaired system is crucial in investigating the role of the parietal cortex in sensorimotor transformations in the healthy brain. Therefore it is not surprising that optic ataxia is a pathology that has gained huge interest over the past years. In addition, optic ataxia provides crucial insight into the functions of the dorsal stream in the context of the model of the double stream of visual information processing (Goodale and Milner, 1992; Jeannerod and Rossetti; 1993, Milner and Goodale, 1995; Pisella et al., 2006).

Here we argue that lesions of the parietal cortex result in deficits that are far more wide ranging than simply a "deficit of visual orientation" (Holmes, 1918), which in turn reflects the important function of the parietal cortex in visuomotor transformations. In the following pages, we will show that optic ataxia can be viewed as a deficit in a number of different processes in visuomotor as well as sensorimotor transformations such as (i) maintaining spatial constancy, (ii) the visuomotor transformation itself, (iii) spatial integration, and (iv) feedback and online movement control. We end by discussing the clinical implications of these findings.

4.2   Classical deficits described in optic ataxia

Patients with optic ataxia tend to make directional errors when reaching for objects in peripheral vision (Perenin and Vighetto, 1988; Karnath et al., 1997; Revol et al., 2003), they incorrectly adjust their grip to the size of the object (Jakobson et al., 1991; Roy et al., 2004) and they have problems orienting their hand appropriately to grasp the object (Perenin and Vighetto, 1988). These various deficits are shown in Figure 4.4. Optic ataxia cannot be explained exclusively in terms of a basic visual or motor perturbation since optic ataxia patients are capable of performing tasks such as identifying or remembering objects or reaching towards their own body parts with their eyes closed (Perenin and Vighetto, 1988). Therefore, optic ataxia can be defined as a disorder involving a visuomotor transformation deficit for peripersonal visually guided movements (Perenin and Vighetto, 1988; Milner and Goodale, 1993; Rossetti and Pisella, 2002; Rossetti et al., 2003).

The main argument for a deficit involving the visuomotor transformation process comes from *unilateral* optic ataxia patients, specifically in the interaction between deficits related to reaching in the different visual fields (known as a field effect) and those related to reaching with either hand (known as a hand effect) (Vighetto and Perenin, 1981; Perenin and Vighetto, 1988). This interaction is such that reaching with the contralesional hand (the hand opposite to the damaged hemisphere) in the contralesional visual field (the visual field opposite to the damaged hemisphere) produces extensive directional errors. This is shown in the bottom right panel in Figure 4.4A. On the other hand, reaching with the ipsilateral hand in the ipsilateral field reveals errors that are comparable to neurologically intact controls (top left panel in Figure 4.4A). Finally, the patients show intermediate errors between these two extremes when reaching to targets in the ipsilesional field with the contralesional hand or the contralesional field with the ipsilesional hand (top right and bottom left panels respectively) (Perenin and Vighetto, 1988; Blangero et al., 2007). This modulation of reach errors reveals an interaction between a hand effect of the contralesional hand and a field effect of the contralesional visual field. Given this interaction, it has been difficult to disentangle the relative roles of visual and motor factors involved in this disorder (Vighetto and Perenin, 1981; Perenin and Vighetto, 1988; Battaglia-Mayer and Caminiti, 2002).

The visuomotor transformation is complex and requires many extraretinal signals about the position of body parts, e.g. eye-in-head position (Crawford et al., 2004; Blohm and Crawford, 2007). There is considerable neurophysiological evidence that the parietal cortex is a key area involved in this sensorimotor transformation, thus it is not surprising that one of the main disorders in optic ataxia is reaching errors (Perenin and Vighetto, 1988; Rossetti, 1998; Milner et al., 1999, 2001, 2003; Pisella et al., 2000; Gréa et al., 2002; Revol et al., 2003; Khan et al., 2005a, b). It is likely that these errors result in part from deficits in integrating extraretinal signals appropriately for the sensorimotor transformation (Blohm and Crawford, 2007).

The disorder of optic ataxia fits well with the current framework of a dissociation between the visual pathways for action and perception (Jeannerod and Rossetti 1993; Milner and Goodale, 1995; Goodale, 1996). For example, although these patients are often unable to correctly reach or grasp an object (dorsal stream) (Figure 4.4B), they can nevertheless describe the properties of the object quite well (ventral stream) (Figure 4.4E). This ability is in stark contrast to patients with visual agnosia, who have damage to their temporal cortex (ventral stream), and who are unable to describe a visually viewed object but can reach or grasp it correctly (Goodale et al., 1994). However, the idea that a double dissociation can be established between these two conditions has been recently reevaluated (Pisella et al., 2006).

Studies investigating the visual field deficit in unilateral patients tend to be limited to peripherally viewed targets (Garcin et al., 1967; Jeannerod, 1986a; Perenin and Vighetto, 1988; Ratcliff, 1990; Pisella et al., 2000; Revol et al., 2003; Blangero et al., 2007), where reaching errors increase with retinal eccentricity (Holmes, 1918; Ratcliff, 1990; Milner et al., 1999, 2003; Rossetti et al, 2003, 2005). For example, Figure 4.4C shows the reaching endpoints made by a unilateral optic ataxia patient with damage to the right parietal cortex (shown by the "X"). The patient was asked to fixate on the red central cross and reach to a target presented at one of the blue crosses. The patient's reaching endpoints as well as 95% confidence interval ellipses are shown for reaching to targets presented in the left and right visual fields. As can be seen, the patient reached with very small errors to the targets in his ipsilesional visual field (not different from controls) but reached with much larger errors to targets presented in his contralesional visual field. Most optic ataxia patients show relatively unimpaired reaching errors in central vision (Buxbaum and Coslett, 1998; Rossetti et al., 2003) but a few patients do show reach errors even in the central visual field (Perenin and Vighetto, 1988; Buxbaum and Coslett, 1998). Based on the dissociation between centrally and peripherally viewed reaching errors, optic ataxia has been divided into two groups: foveal optic ataxia, where patients show deficits when reaching to targets in both the peripheral and central visual fields, and nonfoveal optic ataxia, where patients' reaching errors are limited to the peripheral visual field (Buxbaum and Coslett, 1998).

Box 4.2 Reference frames

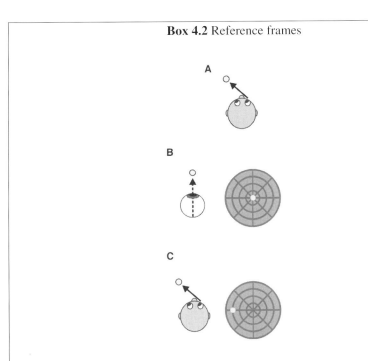

Figure 4.3 Reference frames. (A) Viewed target location (above view). The subject views a target (yellow dot) that is located to the left of the head. The eyes are foveated on the target. (B) Gaze-centered internal representation. The left panel depicts the location of the target relative to the fovea. Because the subject is looking at the target, the target is straight ahead of the eye. This is schematically represented as being in the center of a gaze-centered internal representation. (C) Head-centered internal representation. In a head-centered representation, the target is represented relative to the straight-ahead position of the head. In this case, it is internally represented as to the left. (Reproduced with permission from Khan, 2006).

We refer to a specific perspective on our surroundings as a reference frame. Mathematically, a reference frame is composed of a reference position and reference orientations (axes) with respect to which we measure the location, direction, speed, etc. of objects. Reference frames are important in all spatial aspects of sensorimotor transformations, because information (whether sensory or motor-related) always has to be expressed relative to a certain reference, i.e. in a certain reference frame. The particular choice of a reference frame has important consequences on the mathematical operations the brain needs to undertake in order to interpret sensory information correctly or generate the adequate motor output.

Box 4.2 continued Reference frames

Here, to make the point, we outline two possibilities of sensory reference frames, a gaze-centered representation or a head-centered representation. In Figure 4.4, the subject views a target presented to the left of the head. In a gaze-centered representation, all that matters is where the target is relative to the fovea (Figure 4.4). So in this case, even though the target is to the left, the target is encoded as straight-ahead relative to the fovea (left panel). A schematic of the internal representation is shown in the right panel where the target is represented at the center, which represents the foveal location. (Note: Of course, in order to make an actual movement toward the target, such as a reach, the position of the eyes in the head as well as other extraretinal information must be taken into account to establish the location of the target relative to the effector, e.g. the hand. This is addressed in Box 4.1.) On the other hand, the brain could represent objects relative to the straight ahead position of the head – meaning a head-centered representation (Figure 4.4). For example, a target is presented to the left. For the brain to represent the location of the target, it can calculate the position of the target relative to the fovea and then add the position of the eyes in the head to this information, which would result in a representation of the target relative to the head as shown in the schematic in the right panel. Because the location of the target is represented relative to the head, any eye movements will not matter and the target position is maintained accurately.

These two deficits are sometimes separately labeled as "Optische Ataxie" and "ataxie optique" respectively on the basis of German (Bálint, 1909) and French (Garcin et al., 1967; Rondot et al., 1977) papers describing them (see Pisella et al., 2008). It has been suggested that these two types of optic ataxia result from separate functional cortical streams for foveally versus peripherally viewed targets for reaching (Prado et al., 2005; Clavagnier et al., 2007).

During prehension of a visual object, an anticipatory shaping and scaling of the grip as well as an orienting of the wrist and hand is classically observed in normal subjects (Jeannerod, 1986b; Jeannerod et al., 1998). These distal components of reach and grasp movements are also adapted to the properties of the object to grasp in patient D.F. with visual agnosia (ventral stream damage), even though she is unable to recognize the identity of the object (review in Milner and Goodale, 1995). In contrast, it is widely acknowledged that the distal components of the reach-and-grasp movements are impaired in optic ataxia patients. The distal errors have been described, mainly in peripheral vision, in tasks where the patients are required to grasp a ball (Figure 4.4B – Jeannerod, 1986a) or to "post" their hand through a slot of different orientations (Figure 4.4D – Perenin and Vighetto, 1988). In addition to misreaching (errors in location, i.e. directional errors), the patients typically misorient their wrist when "posting" their hand (Figure 4.4D) and use a large scaling of grip which does not match the size of the visual object. They usually pick up the object with the palm using tactile feedback (Figure 4.4B). Further evidence for deficits in prehension comes from studies performing kinematic analyses of grasping movements (Jakobson et al., 1991; Goodale et al., 1994); subjects were asked to pick up a meaningless ovoid shape between the index finger and thumb. In contrast with the grasping movements of control subjects and the patient with visual agnosia, the grasp line (line between the index finger and thumb's points of contact with the shape) for optic ataxia patients did not pass through the center of mass of the shape, resulting in clumsiness handling the shape. Unfortunately visual perception of orientation, shape and size has not been explored as extensively in these patients as for patients with visual agnosia (see Perenin and Vighetto 1988 for analyses of perceptual discriminations of location and orientation) therefore it is unclear whether these deficits may result in part from a perceptual deficit. Interestingly however, the distal components are much improved when grasping meaningful objects (Jeannerod et al., 1994). This finding suggests that the distal components of the grasp may be planned using (preserved) knowledge of object properties stored in the ventral visual stream, an area involved in object recognition (Faillenot et al., 1997).

To summarize, optic ataxia is currently defined as errors in performing visually guided actions to targets presented in the peripheral visual space (in the case of unilateral optic ataxia – the contralesional visual space). Recent findings investigating the deficits in these patients suggest that this view should be expanded. The following sections will provide a more detailed description of these new findings.

4.3 Maintaining spatial constancy

Reaching to an object involves a number of steps, the first of which is to internally represent the target location. This is necessary in order to form the movement plan

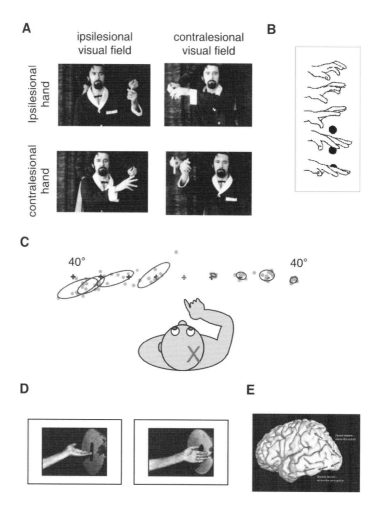

Figure 4.4. Various deficits classically related to optic ataxia. (A) Typical pattern of reaching deficits in unilateral optic ataxia. Reach errors are shown in four cases as combinations of the reaching with the ipsilesional or contralesional hand to the ip-silesional or contralesional visual field. The patient was asked to fixate at a location straight ahead and to reach and grasp a pen presented in his peripheral vision by the experimenter. (Copied and modified with permission from Vighetto, 1980.) (B) Ex-ample of the grasping deficit in optic ataxia. When control subjects attempt to grasp the ball shown in the figure, they adjust the configuration of their hand to match the size of the ball. In contrast, optic ataxia patients do not make adjustments for the object size. In addition, they also misreach the location of the object. (Copied with permission from Jeannerod, 1986a.). (C) Reach errors in unilateral optic ataxia. The patient performed a peripheral reaching task with his right (ipsilesional) hand. He was asked to fixate on a central red cross and reach to blue crosses located at $10°$ intervals up to $40°$ on either side. The X marks the lesioned hemisphere. The gray dots represent individual reaching endpoints and the circles are 95% confidence

ellipses. (Reproduced with permission from Revol et al., 2003.) (D) Hand orientation deficit. The left and right panels show two examples of the hand orientation deficit in unilateral optic ataxia. The task of the patient was to pass the hand through the gap in the circle. In the left panel, the patient's hand is incorrectly oriented relative to the gap but is at the correct location. In the right panel, the patient's hand is both incorrectly positioned and oriented relative to the gap. (Copied with permission from Perenin and Vighetto, 1988.) (E) Schematic of the brain with the dorsal and ventral streams outlined. The dorsal stream (passing through the posterior parietal cortex) is involved in processing vision for action, e.g. reaching to a visual object, whereas the ventral stream (passing through the infero-temporal cortex) is involved in processing vision for perception, e.g. recognizing a pen as being a pen. (Copied with permission from M. Goodale, http://psychology.uwo.ca/faculty/goodale/research/.)

for the reach. There are two important components involved in internally representing an object. First, the location of the object must be represented relative to something, e.g. on my desk, my coffee cup is ahead of the mouse (I am able to describe the location of the cup relative to the mouse). Similarly, within the brain, the location of an object is often represented relative to a specific part of the body, e.g. the fovea or the effector. This concept is known as a reference frame and is described in detail in Box 4.1. There is much evidence based on neural recordings and functional imaging that target-location information is mainly represented in gaze-centered coordinates in the extrastriate visual and parietal cortical areas (Galletti and Battaglini, 1989; Lal and Friedlander, 1990; Weyand and Malpeli, 1993; Snyder et al., 1997; Andersen et al., 1998; Batista et al., 1999; Colby and Goldberg, 1999; Cohen and Andersen, 2000; Buneo et al., 2002; Nakamura and Colby, 2002; Medendorp et al., 2003). A gaze-centered representation of reach targets means that the target's location is coded in the same manner as the target's position on the retina – that is, relative to the fovea (Box 4.1).

The second component involved in internally representing an object, is that for this internally represented location to accurately reflect the object's actual location, any movements of the body must be taken into account, e.g. eye or head movements. This is known as spatial constancy (Box 4.3). Spatial constancy is maintained through the updating of the internal location of the target. How and where could this updating take place?

Duhamel et al. (1992) were amongst the first to demonstrate how neurons in the parietal cortex could update target locations. An individual neuron in the lateral in-traparietal area (LIP) within the parietal cortex will show a change in activation if an object appears in a certain location in space (while gaze is maintained). The location in space which causes this modulation of activity is known as the neuron's receptive field. Duhamel et al. (1992) first found properties of a neuron's receptive field as seen in the left panel in Figure 4.6A. At the top of the panel are the task stimuli (i and ii)) and the neuron's activity is shown at the bottom (iii, iv and v). The neuron responds strongly when a target is presented within its receptive field (i, the asterisk). The monkey then was given a signal to move the eyes to a new fixation spot (ii, leftward arrow). Before the movement is made, the neuron shows increased activity for the new target

Box 4.3 Spatial constancy

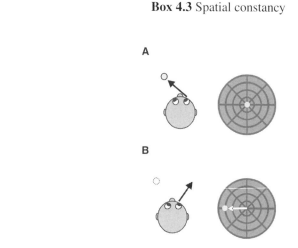

Figure 4.5 Spatial constancy. (A) Gaze-centered representation of a foveated target depicted in the same manner as Figure 4.4. (B) Updated representation of the target. After the disappearance of the target, if the subject subsequently moves the eyes, the representation of the target's location must be updated relative to the new foveal location. (Reproduced with permission from Khan, 2006).

The aim of any internal representation of a target position is to provide accurate information that can be used in the motor task – in our case a successful reach. The brain encodes incoming visual input in gaze-centered coordinates. Any gaze-centered representation, however, changes with every gaze shift. If this eye movement is not accounted for, then the internal memory of the target location becomes inaccurate. For example, if a target is foveated when the eyes are directed towards the left in the head, the location in a gaze-centered representation is encoded as being on the fovea (Figure 4.5A). If subsequently, an eye movement is made toward the right (Figure 4.5B), this movement has to be accounted for by updating the internal memory of the target location (the white arrow shows how the target representation is updated). It is believed that updating is key to what is called spatial constancy, i.e. that we experience our visual environment as being stable despite intervening eye movements.

(iv) presented at the position where the receptive field will eventually be (gray dotted circle). Note that in (ii) there is no stimulus presented in the receptive field at the current fixation position. Finally, after the eye movement, the neuron continues coding the object at the updated receptive field (v). In summary, neurons in the parietal cortex show transient shifts in their receptive fields before/during eye movements, thus showing evidence for updating of target position due to the intended movement. Further evidence for updating in the parietal cortex has also been shown through neurophysiological and functional imaging studies (Medendorp et al., 2003; Merriam et al., 2003; for a review, see Colby and Goldberg, 1999). Updating has also been shown in earlier extrastriate visual areas, such as A3A, V3 and V2 (Nakamura and Colby, 2002; see review, Merriam and Colby, 2005). Thus, there seem to be multiple areas involved in the updating of gaze-centered reach space to maintain spatial constancy including the parietal cortex.

Two studies tested the ability of unilateral and bilateral optic ataxia patients to update a memorized location of a target across eye movements for reaching (Khan et al., 2005a, b). The first study tested unilateral optic ataxia patients, who had damage to their right parietal cortex, and showed that they were able to update the location of targets across the two visual hemi-fields (Khan et al., 2005a). To do so, they had two unilateral optic ataxia patients reach to targets in space, but interposed an eye movement between viewing the target and reaching to it. Figure 4.6B shows the data from one of these patients. This updating task was compared to reaching in a control fixation task where the patient did not make an eye movement but rather reached to a remembered peripherally viewed target while maintaining fixation during the entire trial (upper panel). During the control fixation task, the patient reached to targets comparable to controls (crosses within the bars) when the reach target was in the ipsilesional visual field (left of the vertical dotted line) but reached with much larger errors when the target was in the contralesional visual field. During the updating task (lower panel), the patient showed the same pattern of reaching errors, that is, they were able to update the position of the reach target to take account of the interposing eye movement, and reached to the target in the same way as if they had viewed it peripherally. These findings suggest that unilateral optic ataxia patients are able to update the internal representation of that target, and therefore do not show a deficit in maintaining spatial constancy. Rather, they have a problem transforming this dynamically updated information into a reach plan when it aligns with the damaged field of vision in gaze-centered coordinates.

In sharp contrast however, bilateral optic ataxia patients do show a deficit in updating target location (Khan et al., 2005b). This second study asked two bilateral optic ataxia patients to perform a similar task as the one presented in Figure 4.6B and found that both subjects were unable to fully update the gaze-centered target location. Based on the findings on both groups of optic ataxia patients put together, we conclude that maintaining spatial constancy is damaged in bilateral optic ataxia but not in unilateral optic ataxia. One obvious reason for this difference is the amount of damage to the parietal/occipital cortex between the two groups. The bilateral optic ataxia patients not only had more overall damage to the parietal cortex but also, unlike the unilateral patients, they also had damage in some areas in the extrastriate cortex. As mentioned above, updating has been shown to occur in both parietal and extrastriate areas. Based on this, we can make two possible conclusions. The first is that the parietal cortex is involved in spatial constancy and somehow the undamaged hemisphere in the unilateral optic ataxia patients compensates for the damaged hemisphere, perhaps in conjunction with other preserved areas of the brain (including the extrastriate visual cortex) that are also involved in updating. The second is that the parietal cortex may not be involved in spatial constancy at all. Rather, the observed signals in PPC (Colby and Goldberg, 1999; Medendorp et al., 2003; Merriam et al., 2003) might merely be the reflection of this area receiving and using already updated information from an earlier area actually performing the updating (Nakamura and Colby, 2002; Merriam and Colby, 2005). In this case, the role of the PPC would be limited to using correctly updated signals along with effector-related information for the visuomotor transformation.

4.4   Sensorimotor integration

Given that the parietal cortex has been shown to be involved in sensorimotor integration (Rushworth et al., 1997a, b; Buneo et al., 2002; Cohen and Andersen, 2002; Medendorp et al., 2005), it is very likely that optic ataxia does also result in deficits within nonvisual realms such as proprioception. This was recently shown to be the case in two studies on optic ataxia (Blangero et al., 2007; Khan et al., 2007). The first study revealed that optic ataxia patients show impairments in reaching to both visual and proprioceptive targets, whereas the second study showed that these patients have trouble integrating the position of the hand for reaching.

The first study (Blangero et al., 2007) presented evidence that unilateral optic ataxia patients show the same pattern of reach errors toward proprioceptive targets as they do for visual targets. As mentioned in Section 4.2, unilateral optic ataxia patients show visually guided reaching errors that are a combination of hand and field effects (Figure 4.4A). Blangero et al. (2007) repeated the experiment, this time using the nonreaching hand as the reaching target, thus providing a proprioceptive target. The results are shown in Figure 4.7A for one of the two patients. The figure reveals a number of interesting findings. The left panel shows reaching errors when reaching to the ataxic hand with the nonataxic hand. As shown by the green bars, reaching errors are greater when reaching to the ataxic hand in the contralesional visual field compared with the ipsilesional visual field. This pattern follows closely that seen with visual targets (blue bars). This is also true in the right panel, where the patient reached with the ataxic hand to the nonataxic hand. Therefore there is a field effect also when pointing to a nonvisual target in the dark. A similar though minor effect of gaze eccentricity on proprioceptive pointing was also found in healthy subjects (Blangero et al., 2005). The second finding shown by the left panel is that when reaching with the nonataxic hand, reaching errors are greater when pointing to the ataxic hand than when pointing to a visual target, revealing an impairment in determining the spatial position of the ataxic hand from proprioceptive information. This high level proprioceptive deficit in integrating the hand's spatial position is observed in the absence of primary somatosensory deficits and is thus not related to a deficit in proprioception per se but rather results from an impaired use of somatosensory information. These results show that reaching to proprioceptive targets involves the same sensorimotor deficit as reaching to visual targets, indicating that optic ataxia is not limited to deficits in visually guided actions, but rather more generally to sensory-guided actions. The findings from this study suggest that optic ataxia patients have impairments in determining target positions for reaching, regardless of the sensory modality in which target position is encoded.

A reach plan requires not only knowledge about the movement goal, but rather also knowledge of the movement start position. To make an accurate reaching movement, the current position of the hand has to be compared with the target position so that the correct arm movement can be planned (Soechting and Flanders, 1992; Buneo and Andersen, 2006; Blohm and Crawford, 2007). Figure 4.7B shows why it is necessary

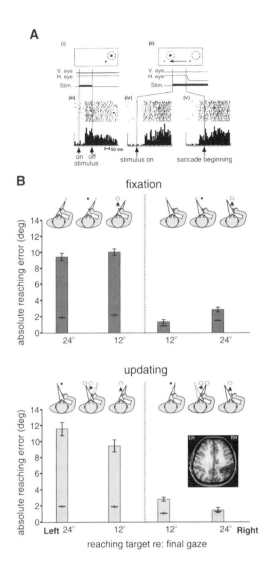

Figure 4.6. Spatial constancy (A) Neural evidence of spatial constancy. Neuronal activity in the lateral intraparietal sulcus (LIP) of the posterior parietal cortex was recorded while the monkey performed a saccadic task. In the left panel (i), neuronal activity was recorded while a stimulus (asterisk) is presented within the neuron's receptive field (black dotted circle). The monkey is fixating on the black dot. The neuronal raster plots below the task schematic (iii) shows that the neuron responds to the presentation of the stimulus inside the receptive field (neural activity increases after the stimulus is turned on). In the right panel (ii), the monkey was instructed to make a saccade from the original fixation spot (black spot) to a new one towards the right (gray dot). The visual stimulus (the asterisk) is now presented not in the current receptive (black dotted

circle) but at the location where the receptive field will be (gray dotted circle) when the monkey completes the saccade. The neural activity shows a response to this "future" stimulus even though currently there is nothing in the receptive field of the neuron (inside the black dotted circle) (iv). This activity occurs before the saccade begins (v). (Copied with permission from Duhamel et al., 1992). (B) Optic ataxia reaching errors reveal spatial constancy. Absolute reaching horizontal endpoint errors relative to the reach target (presented straight ahead) in a fixation task (upper panel) and an updating task (lower panel). The upper portion of each panel depicts the task for each visual field separately (separated by the dotted vertical line) as a function of time (left to right). As can be seen in the upper panel, the patient reached with much greater errors when the reaching target was in his left visual field (the two blue bars on the left) compared with when the reaching target was in his right visual field. The crosses in each graph depict average control data $\pm$ SEM. The lower panel depicts the updating task, where the subject first viewed the target in one visual field, then subsequently made an eye movement before reaching to the target in the opposite visual field. The reaching errors (yellow bars) are plotted as a function of the position of the reaching target relative to the final gaze position. That means that the left part of the graph with the larger errors depicts the case where the patient viewed the reaching target in his intact visual field before making an eye movement that would "update" the location of the target into his damaged visual field. In contrast, the right side of the graph depicts the case when the patient viewed the target in his damaged visual field but reached to its updated position in his intact visual field. As can be seen, reach errors follow the pattern as when the patient actually viewed the target in the same visual field (fixation task), thus showing that he was able to update the target and reached to the updated remembered target position. Error bars are SEM. (Reproduced with permission from Khan et al., 2005b.) See accompanying CD-ROM for color version.

to know hand position to make a correct reach movement. The first panel depicts the location of the visual target relative to the head. The second and third panels show how the reaching movement (black arrow) is entirely different depending on the initial hand position. Neurophysiological studies have shown evidence of an internal representation of hand position in multiple brain areas, such as the ventral and dorsal pre-motor cortices and the motor cortex and importantly, including the parietal cortex (Galletti et al., 1993; Kalaska et al., 1997; Battaglia-Mayer et al., 2001, 2003; Kakei et al., 2001, 2003; Scott et al., 2001; Buneo et al., 2002).

Khan et al. (2007) tested whether unilateral optic ataxia patients showed an influence of the initial hand position on their reaching movements. As shown in Figure 4.7C, patients reached to the same reaching target (black dot), while fixating the different fixation targets – open dot (left panel, fixation to the left; center panel, fixation at center; right panel, fixation to the right). Within each panel, the only variable that changed was the initial hand position. If the initial hand position was not involved in reach planning, then because the reaching target and fixation positions do not change (within each panel), reach errors should be the same. The figure shows the reaching errors for one unilateral optic ataxia patient. As can be seen however, reaching errors varied greatly for each fixation position, depending on the initial hand position. Reaching errors also varied for control subjects (dashed lines within each bar) for different initial hand positions, but not to the same degree as the patient. The findings from both the patient and controls suggest that information about the initial hand position is used to plan the reach movement. Further, the different pattern and magnitude of reach errors between the patient and the controls suggest that integration of the hand position is affected by the damage to the parietal cortex.

In summary, reach errors in optic ataxia can be explained by deficits involving both a sensorimotor transformation (not limited to visual targets) and integrating hand and target position to form the movement vector within the parietal cortex.

4.5 Feedback and online movement control

Recent imaging and patient studies have also proposed that the parietal cortex is involved in the online control of reaching movements (Rossetti, 1998; Milner et al., 1999, 2001; Pisella et al., 2000; Desmurget et al., 2001; Gréa et al., 2002; Glover, 2003; Revol et al., 2003). Studies on optic ataxia patients provide support for this proposal showing a temporal component in their reaching deficits – specifically, their immediate reaches to targets are impaired to a much larger degree than their delayed reaches.

Two separate lines of evidence show a deficit in optic ataxia for online reaching. First, these patients are unable to make automatic adjustments to perturbations during reaching and second, these patients tend to reach more like neurologically intact people if given a delay before having to make the reaching movement. These are described separately below.

Two studies have shown the inability of bilateral optic ataxia patients to successfully modify their ongoing reach in the presence of a perturbed target (Pisella et al., 2000; Gréa et al., 2002). The study by Gréa et al. (2002) showed that this patient was unable to correct her movement trajectory if the target was moved at movement onset. Figure 4.8 A depicts the movement trajectories for patient IG and a typical control toward three different targets, two stationary (a central target – yellow traces (C), a target located to the right – green traces (R)) and a perturbed target (a target that moved from the central to the right position at movement onset – red traces (CR)). In contrast to the control subject (top panel), the patient (bottom panel) was unable to adjust her trajectory, but rather completed the first movement to the original location of the target before undertaking a second movement to the new location of the target. A similar finding was observed in Pisella et al. (2000); the researchers showed that unlike controls, who automatically corrected ongoing movements to target perturbations, the same bilateral optic ataxia patient (IG) did not correct in the same manner. Rather she corrected movements at a much slower rate. A control task showed that her slow corrections were not due to a slowing of visuomotor processing; the task required subjects to stop their ongoing movement at a change in the color of the target and the patient performed just as controls did. These two findings suggest that fast movements toward objects requiring online guidance are disrupted in bilateral optic ataxia.

The second line of evidence shows that reaching and grasping movements improve when optic ataxia patients are given a delay before having to perform the required

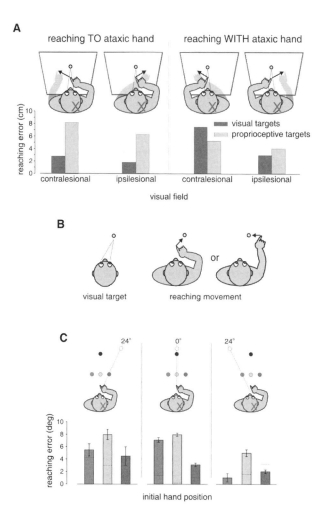

Figure 4.7. Sensorimotor integration. (A) Reaching to proprioceptive targets in optic ataxia. The top of the left and right panels depict the task for each set of bars below each image. The red cross depicts the region of damage for the patient – in his case, the left hand is the ataxic hand and the left visual field is the ataxic visual field (contralesional visual field). Reaching errors in centimeters are plotted as a function of the visual field in which the patient reached. The patient maintained fixation at the same position (straight ahead at eye level) during all tasks. The blue bars depict the case where the subject reached to a visual target presented at the same location as the hand position (the hand behind the screen as shown by the gray shape). The green bars represent reach errors when reaching to the perceived hand position (either ataxic or nonataxic). (Reproduced with permission from Blangero et al., 2007). (B) Reaching movements depend on initial hand position. The left panel depicts the location of the target relative to the head. The same visual target in the right two panels is reached with two different reaching movements (away and to the left or to the right) depending on where the hand is. (C) Reaching errors vary as a function of initial hand position in optic

ataxia. The top of each of the three panels depicts the task. The patient fixated on either the left, center or right fixation position (open circles) while reaching toward the central reaching target (black circle). His reaching movement began from one of three initial hand positions (red, green or purple). The colored bars correspond to the three initial hand positions and depict horizontal reaching error in degrees relative to the reaching target. The dotted horizontal lines crossing each bar depict the mean control errors. Standard error bars are SEM (Reproduced with permission from Khan et al., 2007.)

movement (Milner et al., 1999, 2001; Revol et al., 2003; Khan et al., 2005b; Rossetti et al., 2005). Figure 4.8 shows absolute pointing errors to targets presented in peripheral vision for two bilateral optic ataxia patients (Rossetti et al., 2005). The patients pointed to the targets in two conditions – an immediate pointing condition, where they pointed to the target as soon as it was presented (green bars), and a delayed pointing condition, where they pointed to the remembered location of the target after a 7 second delay (yellow bars). As can be seen, both subjects, reaching errors paradoxically decreased after the delay. This is in contrast to the control subject, whose errors slightly increased (Figure 4.8D). This is perhaps more intuitive in Figure 4.8E which plots typical trajectories of reaching movements of patient IG (Milner et al., 2003). As is easily apparent, reach trajectories are aimed much better towards the targets in the delayed task (lower panel) compared with the immediate task (upper panel).

This online deficit is also apparent during prehension. Milner et al. (2001) asked patient IG to grasp objects of different sizes (range of 20 to 50 mm widths). While approaching the target, control subjects normally adjust the distance between their index finger and thumb (known as the maximum grip aperture) proportional to the size of the object to be grasped. As can be seen in Figure 4.8F, this was not the case for patient IG during immediate grasping (left panel). However, if the grasping movement was delayed for 5 seconds (right panel), her maximum grip aperture showed better adjustment to the object size. More interesting perhaps was that during the delay period, if the occluded target object was replaced by an object of a different size, she showed a maximum grip aperture that was correlated with the original target object, rather than the currently viewed object. Hence, these optic ataxia patients tend to use the memorized object for grasping even if the current object is different (Milner et al., 2003).

It is suggested that the reason reaching or grasping is improved over a delay in these optic ataxia patients is because this slower visuomotor transformation may not involve the dorsal stream but rather the intact ventral stream – see Figure 4.4E (Milner and Dijkerman, 2001; Rossetti and Pisella, 2002). The ventral stream, used by optic ataxia patients for reaching, may involve the storage of target location in working memory within the ventral stream and subsequently used within this stream to plan the movement (Rossetti, 1998, 2000; Milner et al., 1999, 2001, 2003; Milner and Dijkerman, 2001).

These findings provide convincing support for a disruption in the fast, online transformation of visual information about an object's location into appropriate reaching/grasping movements in optic ataxia.

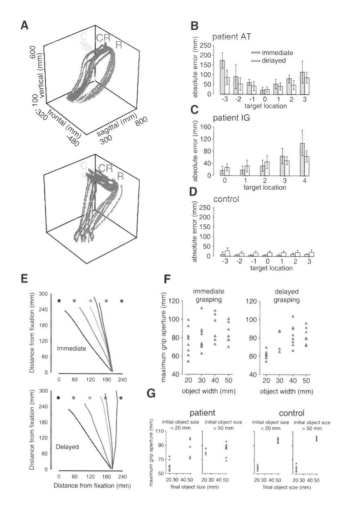

Figure 4.8. Feedback and online movement control. (A) Reaching trajectories in a perturbed target task in bilateral optic ataxia. The top panel depicts the reaching trajectories for the control subject in space (in mm) from the same starting position to one of three targets (C, central target – yellow traces; R, right target – green traces; CR, central target perturbed to right position at movement onset – red traces). As can be seen, the control subject modified the reaching trajectory during the movement to account for the target perturbation (red traces). In contrast, the bilateral optic ataxia patient (lower panel) did not modify her reaching trajectory during the movement. Rather she made an initial movement toward the original position of the target (red traces follow the yellow traces) followed by a second movement from the original to the new position of the target. (Copied with permission from Gréa et al., 2002.) (B) Delayed reaching for patient AT. Absolute reaching errors (mm) are plotted as a function of target location relative to fixation (0) for patient AT, who has extensive bilateral parietal and extrastriate damage (Jeannerod et al., 1994). Target locations $-3, -2, -1, 0, 1, 2, 3$ correspond to targets located at $30°, 20°, 10°$ left,

0° straight-ahead, 10°, 20°, 30° right of straight ahead at a distance of 55 cm from the body. The patient was asked to fixate at the central straight ahead target during the reaching movement. Reaching errors are shown for both immediate trials (green bars), where the patient reached for the target while the target remained visible, and delayed trials (yellow bars), where the patient was asked to reach for the target after it was extinguished for 5 s (target was illuminated for 2 s). (C) Delayed reaching for patient IG. Patient IG has bilateral lesions in the posterior parietal cortex as well as some lateral-occipital damage (Pisella et al., 2000). Targets 0, 1, 2, 3, and 4 correspond to targets located at 0° straight ahead, 8°, 15°, 23° and 30° right of fixation. The patient was asked to fixate at target 0 during the entire trial. The timings of the immediate and delayed trials were similar to those for patient AT. Standard errors are shown. (D) Control reaching errors. Data are plotted in the same manner as B. (Reproduced with permission from Rossetti et al., 2005.) (E) Immediate vs. delayed reaching trajectories for patient IG. Each colored trace is the reach trajectory corresponding to the colored target position during the immediate (upper) and delayed (lower) trials. The patient was asked to fixate during all trials on the leftmost black target. (Reproduced with permission from Milner et al., 2003.) (F) Immediate vs. delayed grasping in optic ataxia. Patient IG's maximum grip aperture (mm) is plotted as a function of the object width (mm) during immediate (left panel) and delayed (right panel). The patient was asked to reach out and grasp an object as soon as it was visible (immediate condition) or after a delay, where it was first presented for 2 s then was out of view for 5 s. Each triangle shape represents one trial. (G) Grasping after object switch. The task was similar to the task in (F) except that the object was switched half the time during the delay period. For example, in the leftmost panel, the initial object was 20 mm wide and during half the trials, the final object was 50 mm wide. Maximum grip apertures are shown for the patient (left two panels) and for comparison, a control subject (right two panels). (Reproduced with permission from Milner et al., 2001.) See CD-ROM for a color version.

4.6 Clinical implications

The investigations on optic ataxia thus far indicate that damage to the parietal-occipital cortex results in deficits involving the sensorimotor transformation. Reaching and grasping movements to viewed or sensed targets are made up of large localization, orientation and scaling errors. However, it is important to note that these errors are seen in an artificial laboratory environment. For example, these patients are often required to make movements to targets seen mostly in peripheral vision or are required to make very fast movements or movements to targets that are perturbed during the movement. These controlled and artificial environments allow us to investigate in detail the nature of deficits in optic ataxia. In everyday life however, these patients use multiple strategies to successfully interact with their environment. For example, like most people, they often carefully foveate an object they are reaching for, which is the best strategy to use. In addition they tend to slow their movements; as mentioned above, this decreases their reaching and grasping errors. They also make fewer errors when grasping well known objects, which is mostly the case in everyday life. Haptic information about the object being grasped is often used to appropriately adjust their scaling and grip size allowing them to successfully pick up most objects. Thus, these strategies allow them to ameliorate their deficits. Such strategies can be used as simple yet effective rehabilitative techniques that patients can take advantage of in order to improve their daily lives. But to date, no specific rehabilitation protocol is used to help optic ataxia patients to recover from their visuomotor deficits.

Optic ataxia is interesting from a pathophysiological point of view. Although optic ataxia has been largely oversimplified over the last ten years as a straightforward deficit showing a double dissociation with the deficit of visual agnosia, it is becoming clear that it is much more complex. Bilateral patients clearly show a number of deficits beyond relatively pure sensorimotor functions, including attentional and perceptual deficits; however, this is often less apparent for unilateral optic ataxia patients. It would be interesting to understand why such deficits have remained ignored for so long in the unilateral patients. On the one hand, it is possible that the contralesional hemisphere can take over some functions, but then it is surprising that it would take over all functions except sensorimotor transformations. Alternatively, one might consider that these deficits are only weaker in unilateral patients. This implies that patients with optic ataxia should be screened more carefully in search for associated attentional and perceptual deficits, since trainable strategies involving consciously shifting attention to the peripheral visual field are often successful. A better evaluation of these patients' deficits is especially crucial because patients with unilateral optic ataxia do not often complain about their sensorimotor deficits (especially when they are restricted to peripheral vision). Thus, although patients may be unaware of the cause of these sensorimotor and associated attentional and perceptual deficits, they may nevertheless pose problems in their everyday life. A more thorough evaluation of the individual patients' deficits would not only allow a better understanding of the diversity of the impairments but more importantly would give doctors a chance to propose rehabilitation techniques that are more adapted to the individual patient and thus more successful than currently used ones.

4.7   Conclusions

After many years of investigation, the syndromes of optic ataxia have turned out to be much more extensive that previously thought. Despite ongoing oversimplifications of the deficit, one cannot deny that optic ataxia is much more than just a deficit in reaching to viewed objects. Bilateral optic ataxia patients have trouble updating the internal representation of visual space. Other sensory modalities like proprioception are involved and one might even expect to find deficits related to localizing auditory stimuli in space, a task where the posterior parietal cortex has also been shown to play a role. Furthermore, optic ataxia patients also display difficulties in adjusting their movements in a fast, online manner. Finally, these more action-related deficits are often associated with perceptual deficits which remain to be investigated in more detail. Overall, the analysis of this particular deficit due to posterior parietal brain damage provides neuroscientists and clinicians with deep insight into the role and function of this brain area in the visuomotor transformation, multisensory integration, motor control and perception.

Acknowledgments

We would like to thank CF, OK, IG and AT for their kind participation in the experiments described above. We would also like to thank Dr. G. Blohm for helpful comments on the manuscript. AZK is funded by CIHR (Canada). AB, LP and YR are funded by INSERM, Université Claude Bernard Lyon and Hospices Civils de Lyon (France) and JDC is a Canada Research Chair.

References

Andersen, R. A., Snyder, L. H., Batista, A. P., Buneo, C. A. and Cohen, Y. E. (1998). Posterior parietal areas specialized for eye movements (LIP) and reach (PRR) using a common coordinate frame. *Novartis Foundation Symposium*, 218: 109–122.

Bálint, R. (1909). Seelenlähmung des "Schauens," optische Ataxie, räumliche Störung der Aufmerksamkeit. *Monatschrift für Psychiatrie und Neurologie*, 25: 51–181.

Batista, A. P., Buneo, C. A., Snyder, L. H. and Andersen, R. A. (1999). Reach plans in eye-centered coordinates. *Science*, 285: 257–260.

Battaglia-Mayer, A. and Caminiti, R. (2002). Optic ataxia as a result of the breakdown of the global tuning fields of parietal neurones. *Brain*, 125(Pt 2): 225–237.

Battaglia-Mayer, A., Caminiti, R., Lacquaniti, F. and Zago, M. (2003) Multiple levels of representation of reaching in the parieto-frontal network. *Cereb. Cortex*, 13: 1009–1022.

Battaglia-Mayer, A., Ferraina, S., Genovesio, A., Marconi, B., Squatrito, S., Molinari, M., Lacquaniti, F. and Caminiti, R. (2001). Eye-hand coordination during reaching. II. An analysis of the relationships between visuomanual signals in parietal cortex and parieto-frontal association projections. *Cereb. Cortex*, 11: 528–544.

Blangero, A., Ota, H., Delportem, L., Revol, P., Vindras, P., Rode, G., Boisson, D., Vighetto, A., Rossetti, Y. and Pisella, L. (2007). Optic ataxia is not only 'optic': impaired spatial integration of proprioceptive information. *NeuroImage*, 36 Suppl 2: T61–68.

Blangero, A., Rossetti, Y., Honoré, J. and Pisella, L. (2005). Influence of gaze direction on pointing to unseen proprioceptive targets. *Adv. Cognitive Psychol.*, 1: 9–16.

Blohm, G. and Crawford, J. D. (2007). Computations for geometrically accurate visually guided reaching in 3-D space. *J. Vision*, 7:4, 1–22.

Buneo, C. A. and Andersen, R. A. (2006). The posterior parietal cortex: sensorimotor interface for the planning and online control of visually guided movements. *Neuropsychologia*, 44: 2594–2606.

Buneo, C. A., Jarvis, M. R., Batista, A. P. and Andersen, R. A. (2002). Direct visuomotor transformations for reaching. *Nature*, 416: 632–636.

Buxbaum, L. J. and Coslett, H. B. (1998). Spatio-motor representations in reaching: evidence for subtypes of optic ataxia. *Cognitive Neuropsychol.*, 15: 279–312.

Clavagnier, S., Prado, J., Kennedy, H. and Perenin, M. T. (2007). How humans reach: distinct cortical systems for central and peripheral vision. *Neuroscientist*, 13: 22–27.

Colby, C. L. and Goldberg, M. E. (1999). Space and attention in parietal cortex. *Ann. Rev. Neurosci.*, 22: 319–349.

Cohen, Y. E. and Andersen, R. A. (2000). Reaches to sounds encoded in an eye-centered reference frame. *Neuron*, 27:647–652.

Crawford, J. D., Medendorp, W. P. and Marotta, J. J. (2004). Spatial transformations for eye-hand coordination. *J. Neurophysiol.*, 92: 10–19.

Desmurget, M., Gréa, H., Grethe, J. S., Prablanc, C., Alexander, G. E. and Grafton, S. T. (2001). Functional anatomy of non-visual feedback loops during reaching: a positron emission topography study. *J. Neurosci.*, 21: 2919–2928.

Duhamel, J. R., Colby, C. L. and Goldberg, M. E. (1992). The updating of the representation of visual space in parietal cortex by intended eye movements. *Science*, 255: 90–92.

Faillenot, I., Toni, I., Decety, J., Gregoire, M. C. and Jeannerod, M. (1997). Visual pathways for object-oriented action and object recognition: functional anatomy with PET. *Cereb. Cortex*, 7: 77–85.

Galletti, C. and Battaglini, P. P. (1989). Gaze-dependent visual neurons in area V3A of monkey prestriate cortex. *J. Neurosci.*, 9: 1112–1125.

Galletti, C., Battaglini, P. P. and Fattori, P. (1993). Parietal neurons encoding spatial locations in craniotopic coordinates. *Exp. Brain Res.*, 96: 221–229.

Garcin, R., Rondot, P. and Recondo, J. (1967). Ataxie optique localisée aux deux hémichamps visuels homonymes gauche (étude clinique avec présentation d'un film). *Revue Neurologique*, 46: 707–714.

Glover, S. (2003). Optic ataxia as a deficit specific to the on-line control of actions. *Neurosci. Biobehav. Rev.*, 27: 447–456.

Goodale, M. A. (1996). Visuomotor modules in the vertebrate brain. *Can. J. Physiol. Pharmacol.*, 74: 390–400.

Goodale, M. A. and Milner, A. D. (1992). Separate visual pathways for perception and action. *Trends Neurosci.*, 15: 20–25.

Goodale, M. A., Meenan, J. P., Bülthoff, H. H., Nicolle, D. A., Murphy, K. J. and Racicot, C. I. (1994). Separate neural pathways for the visual analysis of object shape in perception and prehension. *Curr. Biol.*, 4: 604–610.

Gréa, H., Pisella, L., Rossetti, Y., Desmurget, M., Tilikete, C., Grafton, S., Prablanc, C. and Vighetto, A. (2002). A lesion of the posterior parietal cortex disrupts on-line adjustments during aiming movements. *Neuropsychologia*, 40: 2471–2480.

Hécean, H. and de Ajuriaguerra, J. (1954). Bálint's syndrome (psychic paralysis of visual fixation) and its minor forms. *Brain*, 77: 373–400.

Holmes, G. (1918). Disturbances of visual orientation. *Brit. J. Ophthalmol.*, 2: 449–468, 506–516.

Jakobson, L. S., Archibald, Y. M., Carey, D. P. and Goodale, M. A. (1991). A kinematic analysis of reaching and grasping movements in a patient recovering from optic ataxia. *Neuropsychologia.* 29: 803–809.

Jeannerod, M. (1986a). Mechanisms of visuomotor coordination: a study in normal and brain-damaged subjects. *Neuropsychologia*, 24: 41–78.

Jeannerod, M. (1986b). The formation of finger grip during prehension. A cortically mediated visuomotor pattern. *Behav. Brain Res.*, 19: 99–116.

Jeannerod, M. and Rossetti, Y. (1993). Visuomotor coordination as a dissociable visual function: experimental and clinical evidence. *Baillière's Clinical Neurol.*, 2: 439–460.

Jeannerod, M., Decety, J. and Michel, F. (1994). Impairment of grasping movements following a bilateral posterior parietal lesion. *Neuropsychologia*, 32: 369–380.

Jeannerod, M., Paulignan, Y. and Weiss, P. (1998). Grasping an object: one movement, several components. *Novartis Foundation Symposium*, 218: 5–16.

Kakei, S., Hoffman, D. S. and Strick, P. L. (2001). Direction of action is represented in the ventral premotor cortex. *Nature Neurosci.*, 4: 1020–1055.

Kakei, S., Hoffman, D. S. and Strick, P. L. (2003). Sensorimotor transformations in cortical motor areas. *Neurosci. Res.*, 46: 1–10.

Kalaska, J. F., Scott, S. H., Cisek, P. and Sergio, L. E. (1997). Cortical control of reaching movements. *Curr. Opin. Neurobiol.*, 7: 849–859.

Karnath, H. and Perenin, M. T. (2005). Cortical control of visually guided reaching: evidence from patients with optic ataxia. *Cereb. Cortex*, 15: 1561–1569.

Karnath, H., Dick, H. and Konczak, J. (1997). Kinematics of goal-directed arm movements in neglect: control of hand in space. *Neuropsychologia*, 35: 435–444.

Khan, A. Z. (2006). *Spatial representations for visually-guided movements in intact subjects and neurological patients.* PhD Dissertation, York University, Toronto, Canada.

Khan, A. Z., Crawford, J. D., Biohm, G., Uzquizar, C., Rossetti, Y. and Pisella, L. (2007). Effects of initial hand position on reach errors in optic ataxic and normal subjects. *J. Vis.*, 7: 8, 1–16.

Khan, A. Z., Pisella, L., Rossetti, Y., Vighetto, A. and Crawford, J. D. (2005a). Impairment of gaze-centered updating of reach targets in bilateral parietal-occipital damaged patients. *Cereb. Cortex*, 15: 1547–1560.

Khan, A. Z., Pisella, L., Vighetto, A., Cotton, F., Luaute, J., Boisson, D., Salemme, R., Crawford, J. D. and Rossetti, Y. (2005b). Optic ataxia errors depend on remapped, not viewed, target location. *Nature Neurosci.*, 8: 418–420.

Lal, R. and Friedlander, M. J. (1990). Effect of passive eye position changes on retino-geniculate transmission in the cat. *J. Neurophysiol.*, 63: 502–522.

Levine, D. N., Kaufman, K. J. and Mohr, J. P. (1978). Inaccurate reaching associated with a superior parietal lobe tumor. *Neurology*, 28: 556 561

Medendorp, W. P., Goltz, H. C., Crawford, J. D. and Vilis, T. (2005). Integration of target and effector information in human posterior parietal cortex for the planning of action. *J. Neurophysiol.*, 93: 954–962.

Medendorp, W. P., Goltz, H. C., Vilis, T. and Crawford, J. D. (2003). Gaze-centered updating of visual space in human parietal cortex. *J. Neurosci.*, 23: 6209–6214.

Merriam, E. P., Genovese, C. R. and Colby, C. L. (2003). Spatial updating in human parietal cortex. *Neuron*, 39: 361–373.

Merriam, E. P. and Colby, C. L. (2005). Active vision in parietal and extrastriate cortex. *Neuroscientist*, 11: 484–493.

Milner, A. D. and Dijkerman, H. C. (2001). Direct and indirect routes to visual action. In B. de Gelder, E. H. F. de Haan, and C. A. Heywood (eds.) *Out of Mind. Varieties of Unconscious Processing: New Findings and New Comparisons.* Oxford: Oxford University Press, pp. 241–264.

Milner, A. D. and Goodale, M. A. (1993). Visual pathways to perception and action. In T. P. Hicks, S. Molotchnikoff, and T. Ono (eds.) *Progress in Brain Research, Vol. 95 The Visually Responsive Neuron: From Basic Neurophysiology to Behavior,* Amsterdam: Elsevier, pp. 317-337.

Milner, A. D. and Goodale, M. A. (1995). *The Visual Brain in Action.* Oxford: Oxford University Press.

Milner, A. D., Dijkerman, H. C., McIntosh, R. D., Rossetti, Y. and Pisella, L. (2003). Delayed reaching and grasping in patients with optic ataxia. *Prog. Brain Res.*, 142: 225–242.

Milner, A. D., Dijkerman, H. C., Pisella, L., McIntosh, R. D., Tilikete, C., Vighetto, A. and Rossetti, Y. (2001). Grasping the past. Delay can improve visuomotor performance. *Curr. Biol.*, 11: 1896–1901.

Milner, A. D., Paulignan, Y., Dijkerman, H. C., Michel, F. and Jeannerod, M. (1999). A paradoxical improvement of misreaching in optic ataxia: new evidence for two separate neural systems for visual localization. *Proc. Biol. Sci. / Roy. Soc.*, 266: 2225–2229.

Nakamura, K. and Colby, C. L. (2002). Updating of the visual representation in monkey striate and extrastriate cortex during saccades. *Proc. Nat. Acad. Sci.*, 99: 4026–4031.

Perenin, M. T. and Vighetto, A. (1988). Optic ataxia: a specific disruption in visuomotor mechanisms. I. Different aspects of the deficit in reaching for objects. *Brain*, 111: 643–674.

Pisella, L., Binkofski, F., Lasek, K., Toni, I. and Rossetti, Y. (2006). No double-dissociation between optic ataxia and visual agnosia: multiple sub-streams for multiple visuo-manual integrations. *Neuropsychologia*, 44: 2734–2748.

Pisella, L., Gréa, H., Tilikete, C., Vighetto, A., Desmurget, M., Rode, G., Boisson, D. and Rossetti, Y. (2000). An 'automatic pilot' for the hand in human posterior parietal cortex: toward reinterpreting optic ataxia. *Nature Neurosci.*, 3: 729–736.

Pisella, L., Ota, H., Vighetto, A. and Rossetti, Y. (2008). Optic ataxia and Bálint syndrome: neurological and neurophysiological prospects. In G. Goldenberg and B. Miller (eds.) *Handbook of Clinical Neurology: Neuropsychology and Behavioral Neurology, 88*. Amsterdam: Elsevier.

Prado, J., Clavagnier, S., Otzenberger, H., Scheiber, C., Kennedy, H. and Perenin, M. T. (2005). Two cortical systems for reaching in central and peripheral vision. *Neuron*, 48: 849–858.

Ratcliff, G. (1990). Brain and space: some deductions from the clinical evidence. In J. Paillard (ed.) *Brain and Space*. Oxford: Oxford University Press.

Revol, P., Rossetti, Y., Vighetto, A., Rode, G., Boisson, D. and Pisella, L. (2003). Pointing errors in immediate and delayed conditions in unilateral optic ataxia. *Spatial Vision*, 16: 347–364.

Rizzo, M. and Vecera, S. P. (2002). Psychoanatomical substrates of Bálint's syndrome. *J. Neurol., Neurosurg. Psychiat.*, 72: 162–178.

Rondot, P. and Recondo, J. (1974). Ataxie optique : trouble de la coordination visuo-motrice. *Brain Res., Amsterdam*, 71: 367–375.

Rondot, P., Recondo, J. and Ribadeau-Dumas, J. L. (1977). Visuomotor ataxia. *Brain*, 100: 355–376.

Rossetti, Y. (2000). Implicit perception in actions: short-lived representations of space. In P. G. Gorrsenbacher (ed.) *Finding Consciousness in the Brain*, Amsterdam: Benjamins, pp. 131-179.

Rossetti, Y. (1998). Implicit short-lived motor representations of space in brain damaged and healthy subjects. *Conscious. Cogn.*, 7: 520–558.

Rossetti, Y. and Pisella, L. (2002). Several 'vision for action' systems: a guide to dissociating and integrating dorsal and ventral functions. In W. Prinz and B. Hommel (eds.) *Attention and Performance XIX: Common Mechanisms in Perception and Action*. Oxford: Oxford University Press, pp. 62–119.

Rossetti, Y., Pisella, L. and Vighetto, A. (2003). Optic ataxia revisited: visually guided action versus immediate visuomotor control. *Exp. Brain Res.*, 153: 171–179.

Rossetti, Y., Revol, P., McIntosh, R., Pisella, L., Rode, G., Danckert, J., Tilikete, C., Dijkerman, H. C., Boisson, D., Vighetto, A., Michel, F. and Milner, A. D. (2005). Visually guided reaching: bilateral posterior parietal lesions cause a switch from fast visuomotor to slow cognitive control. *Neuropsychologia*, 43: 162–177.

Roy, A. C., Stefanini, S., Pavesi, G. and Gentilucci, M. (2004). Early movement impairments in a patient recovering from optic ataxia. *Neuropsychologia*, 42: 847–854.

Rushworth, M. F., Nixon, P. D. and Passingham, R. E. (1997a). Parietal cortex and movement. I. Movement selection and reaching. *Exp. Brain Res.*, 117: 292–310.

Rushworth, M. F., Nixon, P. D. and Passingham, R. E. (1997b). Parietal cortex and movement. II. Spatial representation. *Exp. Brain Res.*, 117: 311 323.

Scott, S. H., Gribble, P. L., Graham, K. M. and Cabel, D. W. (2001). Dissociation between hand motion and population vectors from neural activity in motor cortex. *Nature*, 413: 161–165.

Snyder, L. H., Batista, A. P. and Andersen, R. A. (1997). Coding of intention in the posterior parietal cortex. *Nature*, 386: 167–170.

Soechting, J. F. and Flanders, M. (1992). Moving in three-dimensional space: frames of reference, vectors, and coordinate systems. *Ann. Rev. Neurosci.*, 15: 167–191.

Vighetto, A. (1980). Etude neuropsychologique et psychophysique de l'ataxie optique. PhD dissertation, Université Claude Bernard Lyon I.

Vighetto, A. and Perenin, M. T. (1981). Optic ataxia: analysis of eye and hand responses in pointing at visual targets (author's transl). *Revue Neurologique (Paris)*, 137: 357–372.

Weyand, T. G. and Malpeli, J. G. (1993). Responses of neurons in primary visual cortex are modulated by eye position. *J. Neurophysiol.*, 69: 2258–2260.

5   When what you see isn't where you get: cortical mechanisms of vision for complex action

L. E. Sergio, D. J. Gorbet, W. J. Tippett, X. Yan and B. Neagu

Picture the following: You have once again been overly enthusiastic with your efforts during a recreational soccer match. The tearing sound before you go down suggests that more than some ice and a week off will be required. Your physician, looking grave, explains that indeed, your anterior cruciate ligament will require rebuilding. Fortunately for you, she adds brightly, the arthroscopic surgery will leave little scarring and has a fairly short recovery time. On the big day, the medical team obligingly gives you an advance peek at the surgical set-up: a stainless steel table, a complicated apparatus with wavy metallic tubes and handles, and a monitor positioned upright on a cart stationed along the wall of the room, opposite to the equipment. You don't dwell on it again until after the anaesthetic has started, when you are counting backwards, and a little thought pops up before the darkness engulfs you: *"Shouldn't that monitor be lying flat, right over the spot where those knives and drills are swirling about inside my knee joint??!"*

5.1   The neural control of reaching under increasingly arbitrary conditions: an introduction

Hundreds of times per day we find ourselves reaching for and interacting with objects in our environment. Most of these visually guided reaching movements begin with a

Cortical Mechanisms of Vision, ed. M. Jenkin and L. R. Harris. Published by Cambridge University Press.

redirection of the eyes to the target of interest, followed by the initiation of an arm movement made in the direction of the gaze. In other words, we often directly interact with an object in the environment using visual information provided by the object itself. An example of such a direct interaction could include noticing a tea cup on a table and then using this visual information (among other signals) to perform a movement that results in your hand grasping the cup's handle. Visual-to-motor transformations such as these can be considered "standard" or "direct" because the visual stimulus guiding the action is itself the target of the action. However, the evolution of the capacity for tool-use in primates has resulted in situations where the correspondence between vision and action is not direct. Rather, the mapping between stimulus and response must be learned and calibrated. This situation has been referred to as "nonstandard" sensorimotor mapping (Wise et al., 1996). In nonstandard visual-to-motor transformations, the visual information used to perform a motor task does not come from the object one's arm is interacting with. Thus, such nonstandard tasks can require the spatial dissociation of aspects of visuomotor control including gaze, attention and the overt motor output.

In everyday life, we perform these types of transformations routinely. A common example is the use of a computer mouse to move a pointer on a monitor. Such a skill requires a remapping of motor output from a frontal to a horizontal plane. In this example, in order to displace the pointer upward vertically on the screen one has to move the hand forward in a horizontal plane. Another example is the difference between picking up an apple and driving a car; the first is standard, the second is nonstandard. In comparing standard with nonstandard movements, the relationships between sensory input, motor output, and motor consequences are all fundamentally different. In the former, action is directed toward the sensory stimulus and the target of the action corresponds to the spatial location of the stimulus. In the latter, the goal is to control the motion of an object by following arbitrary transformation rules. The incorporation of arbitrary sensory information when planning a movement is not innate, developing only in the second year of life (Piaget, 1965). Following damage to the cerebral cortex in the form of stroke or disease, the ability to perform these complex visuomotor transformations may be compromised. While such arbitrary sensorimotor associations underlie much of human tool-use, and indeed are made without thought in much of our everyday lives, the basic cortical mechanisms underlying this type of visual-to-motor transformation are far from fully understood.

In this chapter we will review the basic terms associated with what we will refer to as "dissociated" nonstandard reaching movements. That is, reaching movements in which the guiding visual information is dissociated at some level from the required motor output. We will also provide a brief review of some of the behavioral and neurophysiological work that has been done in this area to date. The remainder of the chapter will summarize and contextualize our laboratory's recent research into the neural control of visually guided dissociated movement, and how this control is affected by sex, age, and disease.

5.2 Visuomotor compatibility and visually guided movements

In the literature, nonstandard visuomotor mappings are divided into two different categories: "arbitrary" and "transformational" (Wise et al., 1996). As the name suggests, arbitrary visuomotor transformations occur when the relationship between a visual stimulus and the motor response it guides is completely arbitrary. For example, drivers know that a red light indicates that they should apply force to the brake pedal, while a green light indicates that the accelerator pedal should be pressed instead. These learned associations between the colors of a light and the choice of moving to the accelerator or brake pedal are arbitrary (e.g. there is no reason that the colors used could not be reversed or even changed altogether). In contrast, while transformational visuomotor mappings also involve dissociated visual cues and motor responses, they use a specific spatial algorithm to relate the position of visual cues to the direction of an action. Again using our computer mouse example given above, a mouse is typically used on a horizontal tabletop to control a cursor displayed on a vertical monitor. In order to control the cursor in this scenario, one must learn the spatial rule that moving the cursor vertically "upward" on the screen requires the hand to move the mouse "forward" horizontally on the desk.

Two further terms are relevant to this realm of motor behavior. In many of the studies that will be reviewed here, nonstandard transformational mappings (as opposed to arbitrary mappings) can take two forms: a change in the physical location of the visual stimulus relative to plane of the limb movement, and a cue that signals a required movement in some direction (often opposite) to the cued target location. These different levels of visuomotor compatibility represent two fundamentally different levels of sensorimotor mapping. Adapting to spatial orientation differences (e.g. those where the hand moves in a different location relative to the visual target) is referred to as *sensorimotor recalibration*. Such a recalibration requires a coordinated remapping between different sensory modalities such as vision and proprioception (Bedford, 1993; Lackner and Dizio, 1994; Clower and Boussaoud, 2000), and will produce after-effects if the source of the recalibration is removed. This represents a different type of information compared with the more cognitive "mental rotation" conditions. Adapting to a situation which requires a mental rotation in order to realign the required hand movement relative to the spatial location of the target is referred to as *visuomotor adaptation*. Visuomotor adaptation can include having to integrate various rules for correctly acquiring a new skill, and does not produce after-effects. Multiple mappings of this sort can be learned at once, something that is more difficult for perceptual recalibration tasks such as prism adaptation. For the purposes of this chapter, we will rely on these categorizations. However, it behooves us to point out that these terms are not universally agreed upon. One may also come across the terms *spatial realignment* or *perceptual recalibration* – versions of sensorimotor recalibration – and *strategic control* – a version of visuomotor adaptation (Redding and Wallace, 1996; Redding et al., 2005). Untangling the subtleties of these concepts, and the determinants of what calls forth behavior appropriate to one category versus another, remains an active and important area of research.

An example of the distinction between the three levels of visuomotor compatibility discussed here would be a North American driving a car in Britain, where the cars are driven on the opposite side of the road. On one level, the driver must learn where the left front bumper is relative to the driver's position on the right side of the car so as not to hit the curb. This sensorimotor/perceptual recalibration involves incorporating a new allocentric spatial awareness which encompasses the vehicle. On another level the driver must incorporate the explicit rule that when turning a corner, she must keep the right side of the car along the double yellow lines (visuomotor adaptation/strategic control). On a third level, she must reformulate the arbitrary relationship between a red light and a motor act, this time reaching with the left hand to put the gear shift into neutral at a stoplight, rather than the right hand. Throughout this chapter we will advance the notion that these different levels of dissociation are subserved by distinct yet interdependent neural substrates.

Other examples of motor behaviors that use nonstandard, dissociated mapping include operating vehicles such as cars and airplanes, playing video games, and the performance of laparoscopic or arthroscopic surgery (in which a mechanical interface such as a joystick is used to remotely control a surgical tool-wielding robot arm). Clearly, given our hypothetical situation discussed at the opening of this chapter, it is important to know how nonstandard mapping, and different levels of dissociation between vision and action, will affect the motor behavior of the operator. Will having small, sharp surgical instruments moving in one location while the brain controlling the instruments is receiving its sensory signals from a different location cause a few millimeters deviation in the desired tool movement, compared with when the gaze and the hands are directed toward the same place? If these few millimeters make up your anterior cruciate ligament, this becomes a very important question!

5.3 A (very) brief history of research on nonstandard visuomotor mapping: behavioral and neurophysiological studies

Previous psychophysical studies have revealed that movement kinematics can change as the sensorimotor mappings vary. In an elegant and influential study, Messier and Kalaska (1997) had subjects reach to locations on a horizontal workspace. In some trials, subjects touched targets directly using their index fingers. In other trials, subjects displaced a cursor reflecting finger location to targets displayed on a vertical screen. Patterns of spatial errors (direction and extent) of final endpoint position were found to differ between the two conditions in spite of the fact that movements made in each condition were biomechanically identical. Others have observed changes in reaction time (Dassonville et al., 1999; Ghilardi et al., 2000a), handpath curvature (Goodbody and Wolpert, 1999) and learning processes (Clower and Boussaoud, 2000) when subjects were required to perform nonstandard sensorimotor tasks (compared with standard transformations). These changes may reflect differences in processing used by the brain to account for variations in the correspondence between sensory input and motor responses. Patient studies (Ghilardi et al., 1999, 2000a), and oculomotor studies

(Munoz et al., 1998, 2003; Connolly et al., 2000; Everling and Munoz, 2000) also suggest that regions of the brain are differently involved in sensorimotor transformations depending on the task alignment. A comprehensive review of anti-saccade movement control (in which the eyes move in a direction opposite to a cued target location) and anti-pointing movement control (in which the eyes remain fixated at a certain location while the hand moves in a direction opposite to a cued target location) is beyond the scope of the present chapter. These behaviors are relevant to the current topic, since eye and hand movements are typically tightly coupled (Neggers and Bekkering, 2000), and indeed comprise an important line of research in our lab (Gorbet and Sergio, 2006; Ma et al., 2006). We refer the reader to excellent papers by Connolly et al. (2000), Johnson et al. (2002), and Munoz and Everling (2004) for a discussion of neural control when eye and/or hand movements are uncoupled from each other and from their guiding visual information.

Current research suggests that the parallel networks formed via reciprocal connections between premotor and parietal areas have important roles in transforming sensory information about limb and target position into movement (see Figure 5.1). These networks are heavily involved in coordinating both the reaching movement that transports the arm to an object of interest, and the grasping movements for interacting with that object once the hand has arrived at its destination. It is thus reasonable to assume that these same areas are heavily involved in the planning and execution of reaching movements under conditions of dissociated visuomotor relationships. Indeed, examinations of the neural correlates of nonstandard visual-to-motor transformations over the last couple of decades have begun to reveal a network of specific brain regions involved in nonstandard mapping. In particular, areas of the brain thought to be vital for the learning and/or performance of these tasks include the prefrontal cortex (PF), the dorsal premotor cortex (PMd), and nuclei of the basal ganglia (BG) (Hadj-Bouziane et al., 2003) .

PMd has a role in using sensory information from different modalities, integrated and sent forward from the parietal cortex, in order to plan reaching movements. A great deal of evidence demonstrates that part of this role involves choosing appropriate motor responses within the context of nonstandard visuomotor responses. Of the brain regions implicated in processes associated with nonstandard mapping, the PMd region is decidedly the most thoroughly studied. Among the first experimental evidence of PM's role in nonstandard transformations was an ablation study by Petrides (1982). This study demonstrated that after bilateral removal of the PMd region, monkeys could not learn an arbitrary visuomotor task in which the presentation of a green bottle cap instructed the animals to grasp a manipulandum handle, while the presentation of a toy truck instructed the animals to press a button. The lesioned animals were unable to perform the task at levels greater than chance after 34 days of training, suggesting that PMd is necessary for acquisition of new arbitrary visuomotor associations.

Since this initial ablation study by Petrides, neurophysiological examinations of cell activity in PMd have demonstrated that a substantial proportion of these cells show modulations of activity as monkeys learn new arbitrary visuomotor associations (Passingham, 1988; Mitz et al., 1991; Wise et al., 1996; Petrides, 1997; Shen and Alexander, 1997; Lee and van Donkelaar, 2006). Furthermore, the amplitude of this modulation often correlates strongly with task proficiency (Mitz et al., 1991). An interesting exception to the general rule of PMd's involvement in nonstandard visuomotor skills was demonstrated by Passingham and his colleagues in 1986. They observed that monkeys who had had their PMd region ablated were able to perform these nonstandard tasks if the color cue instructing the response was presented on the manipulandum itself (the actual object to be manipulated). Thus, PMd involvement in nonstandard mapping performance could be a consequence of dissociating the spatial locations of gaze or attention from the location of a reaching movement. Indeed, other examinations have revealed that the activity of PMd cells is highly affected by the angle of gaze (Boussaoud et al., 1998; Boussaoud and Bremmer, 1999; Boussaoud and Wise, 1993).

The mechanism by which PMd exerts its influence on nonstandard movement control may be temporal in nature. In tasks that spatially dissociate the location of visual cues and the targets of reaching responses, the activity of individual cells has been observed to initially coincide with the direction of the cue but to then shift so that it better corresponds to the direction of the target prior to movement initiation (Crammond and Kalaska, 1994; Johnson et al., 1999; Shen and Alexander, 1997). This observation suggests that the PMd's role in nonstandard mapping could involve taking the contextual information provided by a visual cue and then transforming it into signals more closely related to the motor output required to achieve a correct response.

The connections between PMd and the basal ganglia may have an important role in nonstandard visuomotor tasks as well. For example, ablation of the globus pallidus (internal segment) in one hemisphere and the dorsal premotor cortex in the other hemisphere effectively disconnects PMd-basal ganglia loops bilaterally. Monkeys that were lesioned in this manner were no longer able to recall associations between arbitrary visual cues and movement direction of a joystick handle in spite of being proficient at this task prior to surgery (Nixon et al., 2004). These animals were also severely impaired when attempting to relearn the lost conditional associations. Furthermore, bilateral lesions of the thalamic regions through which signals from the BG are sent to the premotor cortex also induce deficits in the performance of prelearned arbitrary visuomotor associations and impair relearning of these tasks. In contrast, lesions of thalamic regions that project BG output to the primary and medial supplementary motor cortices do not (Canavan et al., 1989).

Simultaneous recording of activity in PMd and the putamen (part of the striatum region of the basal ganglia) has demonstrated that as monkeys learn arbitrary associations between visual cues and motor responses, neurons in these two regions change their rates of firing at approximately the same time (Brasted and Wise, 2004). This evolution of firing rates also paralleled the monkeys' increasing proficiency in performing the task over the learning period. Examinations of the specific contribution of BG activity to the formation of links between visual cues and motor responses in nonstandard tasks suggest that these nuclei may be involved in forging the link between individual stimuli and the correct motor responses these stimuli signify. For example, the observation that increased putamen activity following a movement to an arbitrary cue, and a maintenance of that augmented activity during the reward period (Buch et al., 2006), suggests that activity in the BG could provide the PMd with information about the "correctness" of a particular cue-response pairing. Such correctness would presumably be deduced by the brain depending on the consequence (reward or no reward) of the chosen action.

Areas of the prefrontal cortex have also been implicated as necessary regions for nonstandard mapping tasks. In particular, the ventral and orbital components of the prefrontal cortex (PFv+o, not the more dorsal regions) seem to have the most direct involvement in these processes. This distinction is demonstrated by lesion studies, which demonstrate that while lesions of the PFv+o interfere with the learning of new arbitrary visuomotor mappings (Murray et al., 2000), lesions of the prefrontal regions dorsal to this area (e.g. the dorsolateral prefrontal cortex) only result in a slight increase in the amount of time required to learn these kinds of mappings (Petrides, 1982). PFv+o appears to be less involved in the retrieval of well-learned arbitrary mappings (Murray et al., 2000).

The specific role of the ventral prefrontal region in the acquisition of nonstandard mapping skills remains relatively unknown. However, recent studies by Wise and his colleagues have begun to provide some clues regarding what these functions might include. We will not review these studies here, but rather refer the reader to Chapter 12 in this volume by Steven Wise for a more thorough discussion.

The studies described in the preceding sections provide evidence that the dorsal premotor cortex, the basal ganglia, and the ventral prefrontal cortex are essential members of a functional network that is crucial for the performance of nonstandard visuomotor tasks. The majority of the studies described above were conducted in nonhuman primates (with the exception of the Petrides 1982 study, which examined the effect of frontal lobe lesions on arbitrary mapping in humans). However, imaging studies have begun to confirm that these regions also have roles in nonstandard mapping in human subjects. Learning to associate arbitrary cues to specific hand movements (either finger tapping, wrist flexion or grasping) has revealed learning-related changes in activity in the prefrontal cortex (Toni and Passingham, 1999; Toni et al., 2001; Eliassen et al., 2003; Hanakawa et al., 2006), premotor cortex (Grafton et al., 1998; Eliassen et al., 2003; Hanakawa et al., 2006), and basal ganglia (Toni and Passingham, 1999) in human subjects.

Figure 5.1 provides a schematic summary of the behavior and related brain areas associated with dissociated visually guided reaching. In this schematic (which is not at all meant to be a comprehensive summary of reaching control), we propose different-but-interconnected pathways processing information related to the different types of visuomotor compatibility. One pathway integrates different types of sensory information with spatial awareness, and performs the transformations necessary for implicit sensorimotor recalibration. We suggest that such a pathway would involve parietal and premotor cortical areas. A second pathway would integrate sensory information with more explicit, cognitively related information in order to guide action. We suggest that such a pathway would involve parietal and prefrontal cortical areas. Both pathways would ultimately converge upon the primary motor cortex and spinal cord, which then incorporates the various dynamic factors and biomechanical details needed for final movement production (Sergio and Kalaska, 2003). While subcortical structures are not specifically drawn into the schematic, cerebellar-cortical and basal ganglia-cortical loops would of course be involved heavily in dissociated reaching production. These subcortical-cortical pathways have a well-known topographic parallel arrangement. We

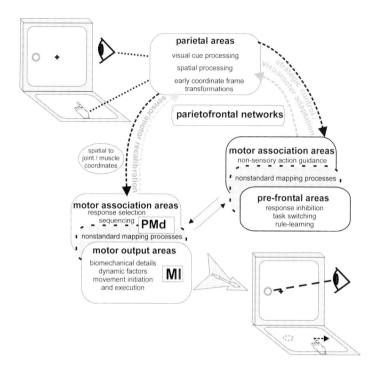

Figure 5.1. Schematic diagram of proposed brain networks underlying dissociated reaching movements. Different types of visuomotor compatibility are processed independently, to some extent. The list of functions related to dissociated reach for the different cortical areas is not meant to be comprehensive.

presume that these loops would also be separate for the different types of visuomotor processing discussed here, mirroring the segregated cortical pathways that we have proposed.

All of the cortical areas discussed above may be involved in the more complex visuomotor transformations needed for eye-hand coordination when the guiding sensory information is not in direct alignment with the required motor action. However, to date cortical mechanisms of visuomotor control under increasingly dissociated, or nonstandard conditions have not been systematically studied. In the remainder of this chapter, we will review a number of studies undertaken in our lab to fill this void.

5.4   Cortical mechanisms of visually guided reaching under increasingly dissociated conditions: the basic network

We first used a human neuroimaging approach to characterize both the basic network associated with visually guided reaching movements, and how this network changed with increasing levels of dissociation between vision and action (Gorbet et al., 2004). Our hypothesis was that activity in task-related regions throughout the brain would increase as the sensorimotor tasks became increasingly dissociated. As we discuss ahead, however, this did not prove to be the case. Event-related BOLD fMRI was collected in a 4.0 Tesla scanner and used to identify those neural regions involved in the integration of cognitive information into a motor act. Examinations of human brain activity associated with various types of skilled movement are rare, partially because imaging techniques (such as fMRI), are often sensitive to movement. We minimized the contribution of movement artifacts to our data by using an event-related paradigm, and by restricting our analysis to the long preparatory period before the actual movement onset. Thus, subject motor output or somatosensory feedback did not contribute significantly to the observed activity. In this initial study, we tested nine females (pilot work revealed sex-related differences, see ahead). We will take a moment to review the task conditions thoroughly, since they are similar to those used for all of the other studies discussed in the remainder of this chapter.

Subjects performed four progressively dissociated sensorimotor transformations. These tasks were all as kinematically similar as possible and included a direct reaching task, a rotated reaching task, a joystick task, and a rotated joystick task. Specifically, during imaging data collection, subjects lay supine in the scanner with their heads tilted forward approximately $30°$ so that they could directly see and touch a plastic screen suspended in front of them. In the "hand movement" (HM) condition, subjects used their right index fingers to first touch directly a center target and then a cued peripheral target projected onto the screen. Note that this is the only "standard" condition in the task. The "rotated hand movement" (RHM) condition was as above except that subjects touched first the center target and then a peripheral location $180°$ opposite to the cued target. In the "joystick movement" (JM) condition, subjects used their right index fingers to move a joystick handle that controlled the movement of a cursor on the screen. Subjects moved the cursor first to the center target and then to a cued peripheral target. Finally, in the "rotated joystick movement" (RJM) condition, subjects used the joystick to move a cursor onto the center target and then onto a cued peripheral target. However, after reaching the center target, the cursor movement was programmed to reflect movement opposite to the direction of joystick handle movement (e.g. rightward movement of the joystick handle produced a leftward cursor movement; see supplemental Note 1 and Figure 1 associated with this chapter on the accompanying CD-ROM for more detail on the experimental paradigm). Thus, the visual stimuli in all conditions were identical but the required motor outputs were increasingly dissociated from this visual input. All of the experimental conditions were presented in random order within the course of three imaging runs per subject (the name of the condition to be performed was projected onto the screen before the onset of trials for each condition). Hand movements made in all conditions were similar; all used motion at the wrist and contact with either the screen or the joystick was made with the right index finger. Subjects were instructed to perform identical eye movements from the center target to the cued peripheral target in all conditions. The stimulation protocol used during imaging data collection was event-related. In this way we were able to exclude from our analysis portions of the fMRI time series in which overt movements were made in order to help prevent motion artifacts. Therefore, our analyses focused on the preparation of movement during an instructed delay period that occurred in each trial prior to the "go signal" instructing subjects to generate the required motor output.

We made three basic observations. First, we observed that there were some areas of activity common to all or most of the experimental conditions. This basic network included many of the "usual suspects," or predictable areas for a reaching task: the contralateral primary, premotor, and medial motor regions, and the postcentral gyrus. The left medial frontal gyrus was apparent in the HM, RHM, and JM conditions relative to controls, while the HM, JM, and RJM conditions had activity in the ipsilateral superior frontal gyrus and superior parietal lobule (Figure 5.2A, and Table 1 associated with this chapter on the accompanying CD-ROM). Second, we observed that additional active regions over this basic pattern of activity appeared as the required sensorimotor transformations became increasingly dissociated. For the most dissociated task (rotated joystick feedback), there were significant clusters of additional activity in the left precuneus, the right superior frontal and middle temporal gyri and bilaterally in the angular gyri relative to the standard task (direct target touching). The spatially dissociated joystick tasks were associated with a large increase (relative to the direct hand tasks) in both overall and bilateral activity, prominent across the inferior parietal lobule (IPL) region in both hemispheres. Activity in this area has been associated with tool use in humans (Inoue et al., 2001). Third, we observed something that on the outset is very odd: the amount of activity in the basic brain network when preparing the standard task was greater than the activity in the nonstandard task. We had predicted that we would see greater activity throughout the cortex as subjects' movements became more dissociated from the visual information. In actuality, direct contrasts between experimental conditions revealed many regions of increased activity in less dissociated visuomotor tasks, relative to tasks in which sensory and motor components were more greatly dissociated (Figure 5.2B).

The active areas that were common to most or all of these tasks can be thought of as a basic, default parietofrontal network required for complex eye-hand coordination. That there were small amounts of activity in additional areas while preparing for more dissociated tasks is not surprising, given subjects' use of a tool and their additional attention requirements. What was surprising was the reduced activity in many components of this parietofrontal network as the tasks became more dissociated. However, upon reflection, if one thinks of this phenomenon as reflecting an inhibition of a network established to control direct interaction with objects, it is perhaps less surprising. There is ample behavioral evidence of the strong tendency to pair eye and hand movement (Prablanc et al., 1979; Vercher et al., 1994; Carey et al., 1997; Henriques et al., 1998; Neggers and Bekkering, 2001; Scherberger et al., 2003). Thus, when comparing the same network active for the standard task, in the nonstandard task those particular areas may be inhibited to halt the natural tendency to move the hand to the same spatial location as the visual stimulus. In our hypothetical knee-surgery patient, such a direct-to-viewed target movement would have disastrous results! The brain may thus overcome its programming for direct interaction by a combination of an inhibition in a default eye-hand coordination network, and an increase in brain activity in other attention- and tool-related areas.

5.5 The effects of sex on skilled movement performance. We mean being male or female

At this point we were happy to have characterized a basic network for dissociated reaching and were intrigued by what we thought might be inhibition of this basic network for direct, natural eye-hand coordination. Still, there was that small detail about having only looked at female brains. Could there really be basic differences in the way male and female brains process identical movements? The following event only bolstered our determination to explore this idea further. It was June of 2004, and a few members of the lab were collecting data for another line of research that we pursue examining the effects of experience on unimanual and bimanual eye-hand coordination. Specifically, we were testing the top 100 National Hockey League draft picks for the NHL's central scouting. It was a mutually beneficial arrangement: the scouts got their eye-hand coordination score, we got our data, these 17-year-olds got a shot at the NHL, everybody's happy. During a break in the testing, Monica – the EEG technician assisting with the medical exams – came over to our set-up and asked if she could try the bimanual coordination task (a variation on the washer-peg assembly task, see McCullough et al., 2006). On her first try she blew away pretty much every superstar, pampered, elite NHL draft pick in the building. It took a few minutes for the lead author of this chapter to return her jaw to its default position. To our astonishment, this observation held: in a controlled follow-up study, females, regardless of whether they were professional hockey players or not, fared considerably better on a bimanual coordination task, while males (particularly the NHL hopefuls) fared better on the unimanual task (McCullough et al., 2006). Monica's performance was so striking that we wondered: for some eye-hand coordination tasks, could biology trump skill? Was there something inherently different in the neural control of movement between males and females that might explain this behavioral result? Before delving into our imaging study on the topic, we will first review some previous work in this area.

5.5.1 Sex-based differences in eye-hand coordination

Performance asymmetries between males and females in eye-hand coordination tasks have been documented, and may arise from sex-based differences in hemispheric asymmetry and interhemispheric connectivity (Davatzikos and Resnick, 1998; Roalf et al., 2006; Gorbet and Sergio, 2007). Historically, it has been demonstrated that women outperform men in fine motor skill tasks, while men outperform women in motor tasks assessing reaction time (Kimura and Harshman, 1984; Fozard et al., 1994). Men tend to adopt strategies emphasizing speed, while women tend to adopt strategies emphasizing accuracy (Kimura, 1993). Greater interhemispheric connectivity in females allows greater transmission across hemispheres and increased capacity for one hemisphere to inhibit the other. This suggests an enhanced ability to decouple the arms in bimanual movements, translating into better performance on novel bimanual motor tasks

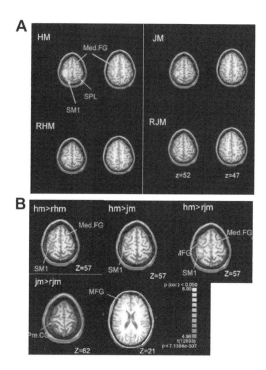

Figure 5.2. Areas of brain activity common to all or most of the experimental conditions. The network includes primary motor cortex, medial motor areas, the superior parietal lobule, and the lateral premotor cortex. See accompanying CD-ROM for color version and a table of significantly activated areas.

(Marion et al., 2003). However, the female tendency towards greater interhemispheric connectivity could adversely affect the development of lateralization of hemispheres. Conversely, lesser interhemispheric connectivity in males, coupled with a greater degree of hemispheric lateralization, may account for males' functional dependence on one hemisphere. This lateralization may also facilitate better performance in spatial motor tasks and unimanual coordination tasks (Marion et al., 2003). Women are increasingly dependent on anterior brain structures for spatial motor tasks, whereas men are more dependent on posterior brain areas. As a result of this dependence, women have increased synaptic proximity to motor regions while men have increased proximity to visual areas (Kimura, 1993). This may explain, in part, why women have traditionally excelled at such manual dexterity tasks, while men tend to outperform women in motor tasks that require enhanced spatial ability. Of course, factors such as previous experience and general level of competitiveness may confound sex-related differences in the performance of eye-hand coordination. Lastly, sex-related behavioral differences have been observed clinically in stroke patients. For example, in a study by Labiche et al. (2002), women were significantly more likely to present "nontraditional" symptoms during acute stroke when compared with men. These symptoms included pain and changes in levels of consciousness. In contrast, men were more likely to present "traditional" symptoms such as imbalance and hemiparesis. In summary, these various studies have documented how, for certain tasks requiring eye-hand coordination, task performance can differ between males and females. They suggest underlying neuroanatomical and neuroconnectivity bases behind such differences.

5.5.2 Does the *activity* in the brain reflect any of these sex-related differences?

Turning around the question of whether males and females perform skilled movements differently, we will now ask: for the same performance on a skilled, complex movement, are the brains of males and females acting differently? To address this question directly, we repeated the imaging experiment described above but using male subjects as well (Gorbet and Sergio, 2007). Recall that the first study used only female subjects. This approach was taken as a precautionary measure because Diana Gorbet – who performed this research – noticed in the pilot data that there appeared to be sex-related differences in the activity in motor-related areas of the brain. Previous functional imaging of the human brain has also revealed significant sex-related differences in processes that are vital to normal motor control. These processes include tactile discrimination (Sadato et al., 2000), mental rotation (Jordan et al., 2002; Weiss et al., 2003; Seurinck et al., 2004), and virtual navigation (Gron et al., 2000).

In this second study, we had 19 participants (10 male, mean age 26.8 ±3.4 years and 9 female, mean age 25.3 ±4.1 years) perform the visually guided reaching movements while imaging cortical activity using event-related BOLD fMRI. Our analyses focused again on the preparation of movement during an instructed delay period that occurred in each trial prior to the "go signal" that told subjects to generate the required motor output.

Male and female group data were first examined separately to get a sense of the overall cortical networks involved in preparing the different visual-to-motor transformations in both sexes. In general, patterns of activity evoked during the preparation of movement included many of the same regions in both the male and female groups (see Table 2 associated with this chapter on the accompanying CD-ROM). However, notable differences were apparent in areas throughout the cortex. To examine directly these putative differences, two different statistical comparisons of data collected from males and females were performed (Note 2 on CD-ROM). First, a whole-brain "fixed-effects" analysis contrasting male and female data in each experimental condition was performed. Regions containing clusters of voxels with significantly different BOLD signals for males versus females included the primary sensorimotor, premotor, medial motor, superior parietal and superior temporal cortices and the thalamus (Figure 5.3, and Table 3 on CD-ROM). To explore these differences further, we performed a region of interest (ROI) analysis. Clusters of significant activity observed in the fixed-effect analysis were used to guide construction of ROI for use in a "random-effects" comparison of the mean beta weights for males and females for each of the experimental conditions. The random effects ROI analysis revealed significant differences in the a number of regions (Table 4 on CD-ROM). Regions showing significant sex-related differences using both the fixed-effects and random-effects approaches included the

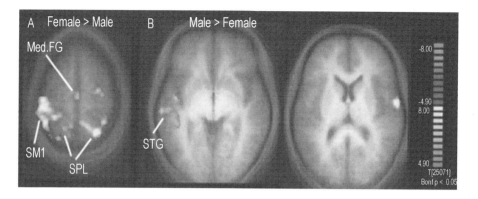

Figure 5.3. A partial illustration of the results of the whole brain fixed-effects comparison of male and female group data. Functional data is superimposed on a normalized, "averaged" brain constructed from all subjects. Bar represents corrected t values in significant voxels, p (cor) = 0.05. Med. FG indicates medial frontal gyrus; PM, premotor cortex; SM1, primary sensorimotor cortex; SPL, superior parietal lobule; STG, superior temporal gyrus. Images are shown using neurological convention (left = left). (A) Regions with significantly higher BOLD activity in females relative to males in the Joystick Movement (JM) condition (z = 61). (B) Regions with significantly higher BOLD activity in males relative to females in the Rotated Hand Movement (RHM) condition (z = -3 on left side of panel and z = 12 on right). See accompanying CD-ROM for color version.

left primary sensorimotor region, the right dorsal premotor cortex, the right superior parietal lobule and the left and right superior temporal gyri (Figure 4 on CD-ROM).

These data represent the first demonstration of sex-related differences in the cortical network used to produce visually guided limb movements. In general, the right dorsal premotor and superior parietal regions as well as the left sensorimotor cortex were more active in women than in men. Conversely, bilateral portions of the superior temporal gyri were significantly more active in men.

The implications of sex-related differences in a task as essential to daily life as visually guided movement are far-reaching in terms of a fundamental understanding of motor control. The regions in which sex-related differences were observed here are all known to be integral components of the control of sensory-guided movements. We ensured, through pre-screening, that none of our subjects had much experience with tasks requiring a joystick (e.g. "gaming"), and that they were all trained to the same extent. Thus, differences observed here are likely attributable to sex rather than experience or general ability. As a caveat, it is important to mention that the sex-related patterns of activity noted in the group results were not apparent in all individual subjects. For example, the activity in the right dorsal premotor and right superior parietal regions observed in the female group data was only apparent in approximately 70 – 80% of individual female subjects in conditions in which significant sex-related differences were observed. It is quite likely that individual variability contributed to this result, and this should be expected and taken into account during any examination of the human nervous system. Rather than having universal differences in cortical activity patterns for reaching, one might even speculate that these differences are related more to gender (a sociocultural construct) than to biological sex (a biological construct), although this idea is yet to be studied. Regardless, the fundamental assumption that cortical networks for visually guided movement are the same for men and women is no longer tenable.

In addition to being important in terms of fundamental neuroscientific knowledge, there are consequences in terms of our basic approach to certain clinical issues. For example, the sex-related differences observed here suggest that damage to similar regions of the brain in males and females could produce different motor symptoms. This possibility may explain clinical observations discussed above, whereby women are more likely to present nonmotor symptoms than men. Several studies have also indicated that women typically have a poorer functional outcome after stroke than men (Di Carlo et al., 2003; Roquer et al., 2003; Kapral et al., 2005). It may be that in women there is a greater potential for a delayed diagnosis of a condition in which timely treatment is critical to a favorable recovery. Lastly, an important feature of our findings is the presence of sex-related differences in brain activity that depend on the required visuomotor mapping. This indicates that researchers and clinicians must not only be aware of sex-related differences in visuomotor tasks, but also that the type of task performed can affect the nature of these differences.

Finally, there are methodological implications to these findings. Historically, our knowledge about brain function has been based on data from the "typical" 21-year-old, 70 kg male. Recently, the importance of including balanced data from both sexes has been recognized (Wizemann and Pardue, 2001). Our observations suggest that researchers must go a step further and examine data from males and females separately so as not to obscure functionally important sex-related differences. That is, studies hoping to disentangle the roles of brain regions involved in motor control should take sex-related differences into account. These differences could profoundly influence our understanding of how the human brain controls movement.

We have observed the activation of a frontoparietal network during visually guided reaching tasks, and the changes to this network for increasingly dissociated movements in males and females. Thus far our findings have been limited to actions performed by healthy young adults. We now consider how one's performance can change with age and with disease.

5.6 The effect of healthy aging on dissociated reaching tasks

Recall that the ability to perform a nonstandard, dissociated reaching task is not innate; for example, before a certain age it is quite difficult for a young child to use a computer mouse effectively. While some of this difficulty may have to do with the development of gross motor skills, the ability to inhibit a direct action – as is required for dissociated movements – calls for a well-developed frontal cortex. As anyone with a two-year-old can tell you, inhibitory behavior is not well-developed in young children, whose immature frontal lobes are at the mercy of a better developed limbic system. But what

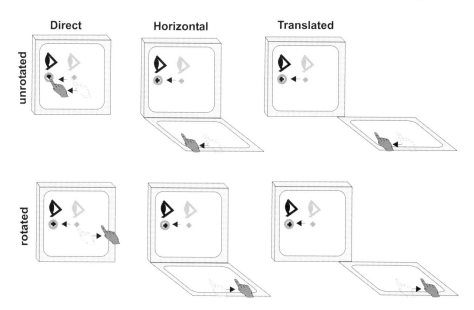

Figure 5.4. Task apparatus and experimental conditions, human behavioral studies. Left. Subjects make movements directly to targets on the touch screen placed directly over a vertically positioned monitor (Vertical condition) Middle. Subjects make movements using the touch screen placed horizontally in front of the computer (Horizontal condition) Right. Subjects make movements horizontally and to the right of the computer (Lateral "translated" condition). "Rotated conditions" follow the same three conditions with the visual feedback of cursor rotated 180° from hand position. Subjects were instructed to direct their eyes toward the target location.

about the performance at the other end of the spectrum? Can healthy aging affect performance of dissociated reaching tasks? Our immediate answer is "yes, to some degree."

There is a well-documented "psychomotor slowing" effect that comes with age. Several researchers have found a reduction in such things as movement speed and accuracy with age (Spirduso, 1980; Stelmach et al., 1987; Darling et al., 1989; Munoz et al., 1998; Seidler-Dobrin and Stelmach, 1998). Also, age brings a greater reliance on previously learned skills and vision in making corrective adjustments (Seidler-Dobrin and Stelmach, 1998). In addition, difficulties with complex visual scene processing have been observed in older adults (Sekuler et al., 2000; Ketcham et al., 2002; Seidler et al., 2002). These factors could, in theory, contribute to an overall degradation in motor performance as task complexity increases through the introduction of nonstandard mapping. However, there have been few studies directly comparing standard and nonstandard mapping between healthy younger and older adults. In our laboratory, we examined how motor performance changed as a function of age when the level of dissociation between vision and action was systematically increased.

The tasks were similar to those used in our neuroimaging experiments, although because these experiments were designed to be used in a clinical setting with time constraints (see ahead), the overall experiment was simplified somewhat. In this first behavioral study, we compared the performance of nine right-handed older adults (6 male, 3 female, mean age 69.1) and nine right-handed younger adults (2 males, 7 females, mean age 25.6). A laptop computer was used in conjunction with a clear touch-sensitive panel that was placed over the screen of the computer, in front of the keyboard, or lying flat and to the right of the computer (Figure 5.4). Subjects each slid a finger over the screen in order to displace a cursor between a central and a peripheral target. There were also two levels of visual feedback for each touch panel spatial location: (1) cursor reflected finger position, (2) cursor was 180° rotated from finger position. Note that only the condition in which the subject was sliding their finger directly over the vertically positioned computer monitor, with the cursor moving in the same direction, could be considered "standard mapping." The five other conditions required the use of nonstandard mapping rules for successful trial completion, with the "lateral rotated" condition having the greatest amount of dissociation between visual stimulus and motor action (Figure 5.4, lower right panel). Thus, unlike the imaging studies, no stylus or tool (e.g. joystick or mouse) was used to displace the cursor or move to the target. The behavioral task paradigm was similar to the imaging studies, except that the signal to move was the appearance of the peripheral target. Thus there was no instructed delay period. Subjects were given explicit instructions on how to complete the trials in each condition, and were asked to move as quickly and accurately as possible as soon as the peripheral target appeared ("go" signal). Also, they were instructed to focus on the screen and the cursor movement and not to look at their hand. We conducted a few familiarization trials at the start of each new condition, which typically did not exceed four trials.

We looked at a number of variables in comparing the performance of younger and older adults on our dissociated movement task. First, we simply counted the number of times they failed to complete a trial ("task completion error"), which could occur in several ways. They could fail to touch the central home target to start the trial, they could fail to hold their hand there until the peripheral target appeared, they could leave the central target too early (150 ms after central target extinction, suggesting that they were guessing the upcoming movement), they could leave the central target too late (we gave them 2000 ms to start moving), exceeding the time limit to reach the target (we gave them 4000 ms to move 8 cm), and failure to remain at the peripheral target for 1000 ms. We also assessed their movement trajectories. How straight were their movement paths between the central and peripheral targets? How variable were their hand paths? Did they ever reverse directions after starting a movement? Lastly we compared the movement timing between the younger and older adults in terms of reaction time and movement time.

We observed that both younger and older subjects showed a decline in performance when any level of nonstandard mapping was introduced (i.e. either a spatial plane location for the limb motion, or a visual feedback rotation, or both). This performance decline was manifested as increases in reaction time and movement time (Figure 5.5A, B). Across all conditions, our older adult group moved more slowly than their younger counterparts, based on a comparison across all three levels of spatial plane and two

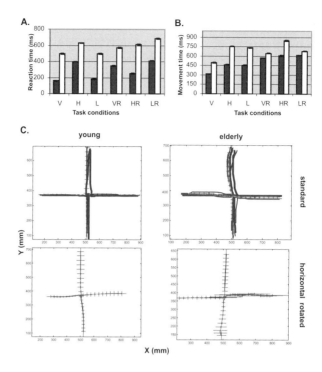

Figure 5.5. Movement planning and performance changes, young and elderly adults (A) Reaction time for all six conditions, (three spatial locations and two visual feedback conditions). R = cursor rotated 180° from hand movements and Vertical (V), Horizontal (H), and Lateral (L) represent spatial locations. Solid bars, young; open bars, elderly. (B) Movement time for all six conditions. For A and B, error bars represent the mean standard deviation across subjects. (C) Mean movement paths for two adults (one elderly, one young) in the standard task and in the horizontal rotated task. Individual paths are overlain for the standard condition. Movements have been divided into 10 equidistant sections, cross hatching represents the standard deviation at that point along the path. There was not a significant main effect of age or condition on path curvature (linearity ratio, $P = 0.05$). Paths for all conditions can be found in the accompanying CD-ROM.

levels of visual feedback compatibility. Further, task completion errors (i.e. failed trials) increased as the relationship between the guiding sensory input and required motor response became more complex, more so for the older group than for the younger group (Figure 5.5C). The decline in motor performance under all of the nonstandard mapping conditions may reflect additional processing by the brain to accommodate the arbitrary relationship between the visual target and the required limb movement.

We also observed group differences on cursor-feedback-rotated versus unrotated tasks, across all levels of the spatial plane conditions. This greater difficulty observed for the visuomotor adaptation conditions ("rotated feedback", Figure 5.5A, B) suggests that the neural substrate underlying the integration of cognitive information needed for these conditions may be, in part, distinct from that substrate processing the perceptual recalibration required for the plane change conditions. Specifically, reaction times and movement times were significantly longer in both participant groups when the visual feedback was altered, but not when the plane of limb motion was altered. These data support the notion of independent neural substrates for processing transformations requiring visuomotor adaptation compared with transformations requiring perceptual recalibration. Our ongoing single-unit recordings and patient studies will explore this idea further.

Notably, our older adults displayed only a modest increase in hand path curvature and trajectory variability relative to the younger subject group as task complexity increased (Figure 5.5C, two conditions; Figure 5 associated with this chapter on the CD-ROM, all conditions). That is, their actual movements, when completed, were not compromised. This is telling, in that it suggests their motor abilities were largely intact (although there was a small increase in variability, see figure); it was the processing of the cognitive information into a particular motor act that reduced their performance. Specifically, the dissonance associated with moving the limb in a direction opposite to both the eye motion and the cursor feedback engendered increased task errors and trajectory variability, likely a result of the increased cortical processing required for this situation.

Before concluding that our older subjects' degraded performance arose from a decline in CNS functioning, one must consider a simpler explanation: due to their advancing age, older adults cannot, in general, process and react to the information they are presented with at the same rate as younger adults (Ketcham et al., 2002; Seidler et al., 2002). However, other studies of arm movement performance (the most closely related for comparison with the task at hand) have found no differences in timing with age (Cooke et al., 1989). Nevertheless, increased movement variability observed in our older subjects could be related to changes in motor unit properties, improper control of phasic and tonic antagonist muscle activity (Darling et al., 1989), and the effects of both of these factors on muscle force outputs and joint torques (Galganski et al., 1993; Seidler-Dobrin and Stelmach, 1998). Age-related motor neuron death leaves a greater concentration of muscle fibers per motor unit, leading to a reduced control over fine force gradation. While such reduced control may account for the greater hand trajectory variability that we observed in the older adults, it is unable to account for all of the performance deficits that we observed. For instance, performance decline was observed between task conditions that were biomechanically identical, but required different levels of cognitive processing for completion (e.g. "horizontal" versus "horizontal-rotated" task conditions).

In this experiment, the neural processing load associated with using a different cortical network may underlie the increased variability observed in the nonstandard mapping conditions. The worsening performance with age may be related to a comprised communication among the network of areas involved in nonstandard mappings. It is known that older adults have difficulty with complex visual scene processing (Munoz et al., 1998; Sekuler et al., 2000). We suggest that this limitation may be expanded to include a difficulty with complex visuomotor associations as a consequence of dissociated feedback (Seidler-Dobrin and Stelmach, 1998), increased cognitive processing, and attentional requirements associated with nonstandard mapping tasks.

In our imaging studies discussed above, we observed the activation of additional areas of the brain as the required motor response became increasingly dissociated from its guiding sensory information. We suggested that such areas were involved in the extra processing required for complex sensory-to-motor transformations. Here we see that in healthy aging this extra processing may be compromised. We will now look at another group in which such processing may be further compromised: patients with Alzheimer's disease.

5.7 The effect of dementia on the performance of dissociated reaching tasks

In their seminal study, M.-Felice Ghilardi and her colleagues demonstrated that patients with Alzheimer's disease (AD) had difficulty performing an indirect visuomotor task which was very similar to the "indirect joystick movement" of our imaging studies (Ghilardi et al., 1999). In the joystick condition employed in our imaging study, we observed strong activations in the posterior parietal area, the precuneus, and the posterior cingulate. In fact, these are among the areas that degenerate in patients with AD. In the early stages of AD, the accumulation of amyloid deposits are normally restricted to the pyramidal layers of the subiculum and CA1, with minor or no accumulations observed in the hippocampal formation (Braak and Braak, 1991). Behaviorally, many individuals at this point may not experience any significant memory-related difficulties. However, a number of other brain regions can undergo larger amounts of Alzheimer's – related anatomical changes (Price et al., 1998), including large portions of the parietal and frontal lobes (Braak and Braak, 1991).

Behaviorally, previous studies have shown that AD patients were compromised when performing eye-hand coordination tasks under nonstandard mapping conditions. Discontinuous movement paths, prolonged movement times, and decreases in movement accuracy were all observed in AD patients who were instructed to move a cursor to targets on a monitor without vision of their limb. Their performance was affected both by the removal of continuous cursor position feedback and by the severity of the patients' disease and cognitive decline (Ghilardi et al., 1999, 2000b), suggesting that the functionally salient motor deficit in AD may involve visuomotor integration for coordinated action. Surprisingly, AD patients' skills were strongly compromised in relation to their mild diagnosis.

Given the early structural degradation in the parietal area, and the central role of parietofrontal networks in visuomotor skill, one might expect AD patients whose memory-based ratings indicate only a milder cognitive impairment to nonetheless demonstrate compromised abilities for movements that require the integration of cognitive information. To test this idea, we repeated our simplified experiment with Alzheimer's disease patients (Tippett and Sergio, 2006).

The performance of 12 neurologically healthy older adults (6 male, 6 female, mean age 71.2 ± 7.3) was compared with that of 14 patients with a diagnosis of probable AD (2 males, 12 females, mean age 79.7 ± 4.6). Neither group had extensive computer experience. With the introduction of nonstandard mapping conditions (i.e. either

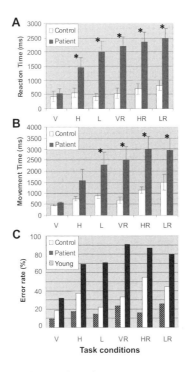

Figure 5.6. Movement planning and performance changes, elderly and Alzheimer's disease patients (A) Reaction time (RT) differences between AD patients and age-matched controls for all six task conditions (three spatial locations and two visual feedback conditions). R represents the cursor rotated $180°$ from hand movements and Vertical (V), Horizontal (H), and Lateral (L) represent spatial locations. (B) Movement time (MT) for all six conditions. (C) The total number of failed trials (errors) as a percentage of the total number of possible trials in each condition. Cross-hatched bars represent young adults (mean age 25.6), white bars represent older healthy adults (mean age 71.2), solid bars represent AD patients (mean age 79.7). Error bars represent standard error of the mean, asterisks (Mt and RT only) represent statistically significant differences ($p < 0.05$).

an altered spatial plane of limb motion relative to the plane of the viewing monitor, or a visual feedback rotation, or both), there was a systematic decline in movement performance in both groups (Figure 5.6). Further, substantial declines in performance were noted within the patient group but also within our control group. These performance deficits took the form of reduced rates of task completion (i.e. failed individuals trials) and increases in both reaction time (RT) and movement time (MT) (Figure 5.6A, B).

Relative to the age-matched controls, we saw a substantial increase in the number of failed trials in our AD patient group when they were doing the tasks that required either a visuomotor dissociation in terms of the spatial plane or visual feedback. Tasks that include both nonstandard components presented great difficulty for these patients, to the extent where on many occasions error rates of 100% were observed for some patients (Figure 5.6C). The relative proportion of error types made by the patient and control groups were similar. However, we did observe that the patient group had a greater number of failed trials due to not moving from the peripheral target of the previous trial back to the center "home" target for the next trial within five seconds. Also, the patient group had a greater number of failed trials caused by taking more than two seconds to leave the starting target to move out to the peripheral target upon the "go" signal. This suggests that they were unable to "task-switch." That is, they had the most difficulty when they had to conclude one trial and begin the next, or conclude one phase of the task (home target hold) and respond to a "go" signal. Such a difficulty may reflect reduced interactions between anatomically and functionally distinct frontal and parietal lobe systems engaged in the performance of different components of the task.

These error totals play a key role in distinguishing not only our healthy from our AD groups, but sub-groups within our patient population. It is easy to see that, when looking at the number of trials not completed by the patient group as a whole, there is a ceiling effect after only a few levels of nonstandard mapping have been added to the basic task (Figure 5.6C). We thus divided the patients into groups based on their Mini Mental State Exam (MMSE) scores. The MMSE is a standardized cognitive test for assessing mental state. The standard ratings are normally reported as the following: 25–29 is identified as questionable impairment, 20–25 mild impairment, 10–20 moderate impairment and 10 or less is considered severe impairment (Folstein et al., 1975). It is a paper and pencil test that takes only a few minutes to administer, and is far from the sophisticated battery of neuropsychological testing that one also does when working with these clinical populations. However, we chose to relate our error score to this test result as a conservative measure: if a significant relationship could come out of something this rough, it should also hold for the more extensive range of cognitive tests one uses. We were a bit surprised and pleased that indeed, a significant discrepancy in error rates was observed between patients who had a questionable impairment and those who had a mild to moderate impairment (Figure 5.7A). As AD patients cognitive rating score declined, their ability to complete movements that had any level of dissociation declined precipitously. For example, note that there was nearly a 10-fold increase in errors displayed by the mildly-impaired group compared with their questionably-impaired counterparts in the standard mapping condition (Figure 5.7A). Mild to moderately impaired individuals began with a 50% success rate, which deteriorated progressively when the spatial plane transformation was introduced. When these individuals were faced with both visual feedback and spatial change transformations, their error rates were nearly 100%. Two levels of visuomotor dissociation made the task nearly or completely impossible, even though their cognitive ratings were still in the upper range of the MMSE.

Especially noteworthy is the relative difficulty individuals with a mild/moderate cognitive impairment had in completing even the basic standard task, and the ceiling effect with respect to error counts as the task becomes increasingly complex. (Figure 5.7A). To explore this further, and determine the predictive strength of this MMSE/error totals relationship, we applied a curve linear measurement (log-linear regression) to the data (Tabachnick and Fidell, 1996). Using a log-linear regression fit, we determined that there was an observable relationship between the number of errors a subject produces and that individual's level of cognitive functioning (i.e. MMSE rat-

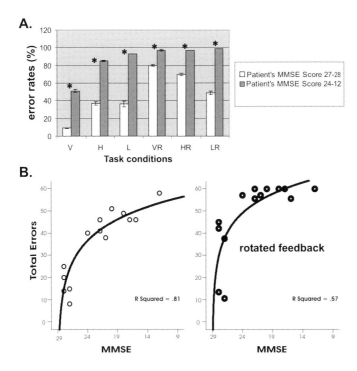

Figure 5.7. The relationship between cognitive rating and dissociated reaching performance in AD patients. (A) Percentage of errors for all six task conditions based on patients' cognitive ratings divided into two groups. Error bars represent standard error of the mean, * indicates $p < 0.05$. (B) Log-linear regression model representing the patient's level of cognitive impairment (MMSE) in relation to their errors (total number of failed trials across conditions). The left panel shows the relationship under conditions of veridical feedback. The right panel shows the relationship under conditions of rotated visual feedback.

ing) for both the nonrotated (V,H,L) and rotated (VR,HR,LR) conditions (Figure 5.7B). Importantly, this relationship occurs for the upper range of the MMSE, which suggests that AD is substantially affecting visuomotor performance even in its very early stages. It may be that regions of the brain that are affected early on in AD minimally affect what are traditionally considered cognitive abilities, but strongly affect the cortical networks required to process movements that require the integration of rule-based information. In fact, our task is of limited to no utility for those patients who are considered more severely impaired cognitively. Rather, it is sensitive quite early on in the disease's progression. We are currently in the process of examining adults who have been assessed as having Mild Cognitive Impairment (Salek et al., 2007) in order to see if the sensitivity of this visuomotor test can extend to a possible predementia stage. This type of skill testing could thus be useful for alerting clinicians about a potential AD diagnosis in its very early stages.

Lastly, we compared the actual movement performance between patient and control groups by comparing their mean hand paths to each target, for those trials that were successfully completed. Just as we found when we compared the younger and older adults, the patients demonstrated greater hand path variability. This variability became more pronounced as the relationship between visual cue and hand movement became more dissociated. Also similar to our younger-versus-older adult comparison, the deviation of the hand path from a straight line did not differ significantly between groups (Figure 6 associated with this chapter on the CD-ROM).

Thus, we again observed that if subjects were able to make successful movements to target locations, they then performed these movements using fairly straight hand paths. The neural machinery responsible for executing the actual movement, and the motor plant itself, does not seem to be a source of their task problems. Rather, the visuomotor integration is what is affected by the disease. This effect is progressive in nature as one goes from young, to older, to early-stage Alzheimer's disease (Figure 5.6C). The decline becomes exponential with a progression of disease. This decline in motor performance under all of the nonstandard mapping conditions may arise as a consequence of additional brain activity needed for processing the arbitrary relationship between the visual target and the required limb movement. The greater difficulty that we observed for the "rotated" visual feedback conditions suggests that the neural substrate that is responsible for the integration of cognitive information (which falls under the domain of "strategic control") may be, in part, distinct from the neural substrate responsible for the sensorimotor recalibration required for the plane change conditions.

The present behavioral study can only provide indirect evidence about the neural substrate affected by AD which underlies impaired visually guided movement. Nonetheless, the performance deficits observed in the present study may be related to early neuropathology in motor associate areas, and to the connections between them. AD is noted to be a global deficit affecting a multitude of cortical regions in the cerebral cortex. Structural deficits may not initially affect distinct cerebral regions. What may occur is an ineffective integration of the information that is transmitted from various regions (such as the motor cortices, the frontal lobe, and occipital areas) to a site in the cerebral cortex noted to be involved in visuomotor transformations: the posterior parietal cortex. It is to this part of the brain that we now turn our attention (pun fully intended).

5.7.1 Impaired posterior parietal cortex function in AD patients: evidence from nonstandard visuomotor integration deficits

The posterior parietal cortex (PPC) is an area involved in high-level cognitive functions involving action, intention for action, and the ability to generate early movement programs (Andersen and Buneo, 2002). One of the primary regional connections from the PPC is the frontal cortex, which is implicated in reaching, grasping, and oculomotor control (Goodale, 1993). These precentral areas are also involved in the integration of rule-based information into a motor act (Wise et al., 1996). Anatomical research has also indicated that the PPC is one of the primary regions involved in visuomotor function. Recent fMRI research has shown significant overlap of active regions in the posterior parietal cortex during eye and pointing movements (Medendorp et al., 2003). In addition, several additional neurophysiological and imaging studies have indicated that information regarding eye and hand position converge within the PPC (Oyachi and Ohtsuka, 1995; Kalaska, 1996; Rossetti et al., 2005).

In examining the performance of increasingly dissociated reaching movements by Alzheimer's disease patients, we found that they were slower to respond, had difficulty switching to a new phase of the task, and were not good at incorporating rule-based information into their movement plan. These performance problems may arise from a breakdown in the parietofrontal networks required to transform visual information into an appropriate pattern of limb muscle activity. That is, in addition to the frontal lobe areas known to be affected in AD patients, the PPC and the parietofrontal connections may also be compromised. Interestingly, one of the primary anatomical areas noted to be affected by AD in the early stages of the disease are regions within the parietal cortex (Braak and Braak, 1991), as well as corticocortical connections to the frontal lobe (Kitamura and Terashi, 1990; Braak and Braak, 1991; Ghilardi et al., 2000a; Pennisi et al., 2002). These regional deficits may cause early visuomotor disruptions before a significant area of perfusion is observed within cerebral regions primarily identified for cognitive/memory functioning.

Evidence for a reduced efficacy of parietal lobe function in AD patients comes mainly from the observation that certain patients display apraxia (Benke, 1993). There is no consensus, however, around the prevalence of apraxia in AD, and the stage of the disease in which it occurs (Crutch et al., 2007; Parakh et al., 2004). We approach this debate by asking whether a visuomotor integration task might provide a clearer sense of the functional integrity of the PPC in AD patients. Might our type of task provide evidence for the deterioration of PPC function, and parietofrontal network function, in this population?

To test for this putative PPC deterioration, we repeated our experiment using a condition designed to probe parietal function: a short-term spatial location memory task (Tippett et al., 2007). Studies have found that the PPC is involved in the storage of the short-term spatial location of objects (Moscovitch et al., 1995; Ricciardi et al., 2006). We asked a second group of patients with Alzheimer's disease (and a second group of age-matched controls) to repeat two of the six conditions: the standard task, and the horizontal task (i.e. there were no "rotated feedback" or "lateral screen place-ment" conditions). In addition to the usual reaction time task, we added a two-second delay between the presentation of the peripheral target and the disappearance of the central target (which served as the "go signal"). Thus, the participants were required to maintain in memory the spatial location of the peripheral target for two seconds.

We observed that the AD patients took significantly longer to plan and make a movement than the age-matched controls, expressed as a main effect of Group for both RT and MT measures. We also saw a significant main effect of Condition for both MT and RT. In addition, we again observed an increase in the number of failed trials across both patient and control groups when the mapping between vision and action became nonstandard. The addition of a memory component also increased the number of failed trials across both the patients and the age-matched control groups. However, we did indeed find a significantly greater number of failed trials in those adults suf-fering from Alzheimer's disease. The types of failures were mostly failing to return

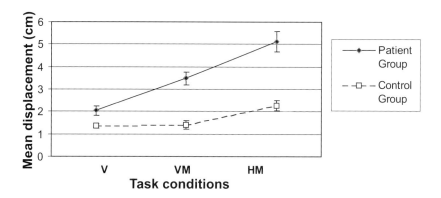

Figure 5.8. The effect of a delay period on dissociated reaching accuracy and precision in AD patients. The mean displacement from the center of the target (constant error) is shown for each condition. V, vertical touch screen placement (over monitor, standard task), no memory period; VM, vertical touch screen placement, memory delay; HM, horizontal touch screen placement, memory period.

to the center target after finishing a previous trial (a task switching problem, perhaps), failure to wait for the "go" signal before moving (suggesting that they had difficulty inhibiting their movements) and failure to start a movement following the "go" signal. We believe that these errors indicate difficulty in processing and integrating visually identified target locations, and in generating the appropriate motor response. Lastly, hand path formation, endpoint accuracy, and endpoint precision were affected by the addition of a memory delay. On many trials AD patients often made small, incomplete movements and had few completed trials to target positions, particularly on the vertical and horizontal memory conditions. With respect to their reaching accuracy, we observed no difference in endpoint accuracy (as measured by the constant error) between control and patient groups in the standard task with no memory delay. Thus, as we'd seen previously, AD patients' ability to reach to targets directly was not impaired. With the introduction of either a memory delay, or a spatial displacement and memory delay, the accuracy (constant error) worsened for the AD patients (Figure 5.8). Specifically, endpoint accuracy decreased in going from the standard to the standard-memory condition, and decreased further going from the standard-memory to the nonstandard memory condition. However, there was no significant difference in precision (variable error) between the standard-memory and dissociated-memory conditions (Figure 5.8, error bars); patients had difficulty in making precise movements with the introduction of any complexity, but these deficits were not additive.

Thus, patients once again struggled to reach to visual targets dissociated from the required final hand location, and this difficulty was exacerbated by the inclusion of a brief spatial memory component. We predicted that AD patients would experience great difficulty when confronted with a short-term memory task requiring a motor response. It has been shown by several researchers that motor performance deficits can often be observed in individuals with AD (Kluger et al., 1997; Ghilardi et al., 1999; Belanger et al., 2005; von Gunten et al., 2006); however an extensive search revealed no previous studies incorporating short-term visuomotor memory performance in individuals with AD. Visual short-term memory relies on a network of brain regions, including neurons in the PPC, that are essential for retaining the location of stimuli immediately following perception (Constantinidis and Steinmetz, 1996, 2005) and after a two second delay (Moscovitch et al., 1995). Here, we believe that the dissociated reaching difficulties experienced by AD patients following the introduction of a short-term memory component lend support to the idea that an impaired PPC is contributing to their motor dysfunction. Such visuomotor difficulties may not be solely attributable to deficits in planning, but rather to a breakdown in the parietofrontal network that we have characterized for the performance of dissociated reaching movements. The primary deficits observed in this study could be a result of information that is initially encoded in the PPC being transferred ineffectively (Belanger et al., 2005) to frontal regions, a network which is essential for understanding spatial relationships between the eye and hand (Ghilardi et al., 1995).

AD patients displayed a compromised ability to effectively complete certain visuomotor tasks. When asked to make decisions that required the immediate integration of vision and rule-based action, AD patients were less able to respond appropriately. Together, these studies emphasize the utility of using an increasingly dissociated reaching task to provide a sensitive measure of functional movement ability in neurological patients.

5.8 Cortical mechanisms for increasingly complex reaching movements: nonhuman primate studies

To summarize thus far, we have taken a few different methodological approaches to study the control of reaching movements that require the visuomotor integration of increasingly dissociated components. We find that the performance of such movements employ a parietofrontal network that calls in various activity-specific areas as needed. Whether one is a female or a male will change the exact anatomical substrate that comprises this network, and one's visuomotor behavior can deteriorate with age or more dramatically with disease. In order to address more directly how and where (and even when) the control of increasingly complex movements takes place, we need to study brain activity on a single-cell level. We have already reviewed a sample of nonhuman primate studies related to the issue of nonstandard mapping in eye-hand coordination. A consistent limitation in the task design of most studies that examine the neurophysiology of eye-hand coordination has been the incorporation of a visuomotor transformation in even the most "direct" task conditions. Often joysticks or other types of manipulanda are used, or there is a gain change between the movement and the visual stimulus being viewed by the animal. To distinguish the cortical mechanisms for integrating vision and motion from those cortical mechanisms for dissociated visually guided movements, we have to first examine the brain activity beginning at the most direct, standard level. We then must study how this brain activity changes as we advance systematically in movement complexity. This has been our guiding principle for the behavioral and imaging studies, and it holds for our single cell recording studies as well.

Before making sense of actual cell activity, it is important to establish that, behaviorally, we observe the same performance pattern for dissociated tasks in the nonhuman primate that has been observed in healthy humans. To this end, we have preceeded our neurophysiological studies of dissociated eye-hand coordination with some motor behavioral work. Recall that in previous human behavioral studies, changes in constant directional errors (Ghilardi et al., 1999), endpoint variability (Messier and Kalaska, 1997), path curvature (Goodbody and Wolpert, 1999), and motor learning rates (Clower and Boussaoud, 2000) could be seen when going from a standard to a nonstandard reaching task (as reviewed in the introduction). These data demonstrate nicely the effect of representational sensory input on movement planning variability, suggesting differential neural processing in these situations. We examined whether or not the same motor behavioral patterns could be observed in monkeys, as a precursor to the actual cell recording.

Two rhesus monkeys were trained on a task nearly identical to that used with the human behavioral work. The monkeys sat in a primate chair positioned at a table, into which a thin, custom-built 15 inch touch screen monitor (Touch Controls Inc, San Diego CA) was embedded. Thus in the monkey set-up, the touch screen was over their lap rather than vertically placed in front of them. A vertical 15 inch computer monitor was placed on the table, 40 cm away from the monkey's frontal plane, centered with its midline. All other aspects of the task were the same, however. The animals were required to slide their finger across the touch screen over their lap in order to displace a cursor from a central to a peripheral target. In one condition the targets were presented on the touch screen (standard condition), in the other they were presented on the vertical monitor in front of the animal (nonstandard condition).

We observed an effect of task both on the form of the trajectory and on the spatial distribution of endpoints. The task effects were similar for both animals. With respect to trajectory formation, the variability in the hand path was considerably greater in the situation where the animal was moving toward the peripheral target using representational, or indirectly aligned, visual information to guide the movement (Figure 5.9A), relative to that observed when the finger was moved between the directly-viewed targets. There was some heterogeneity in the trajectory variability at the different targets, regardless of task. In particular, movements to the leftward and rightward targets showed a greater range along the y-axis throughout the movement. Movements to the outward and inward targets (or upward and downward in the case of the indirect, vertical visual presentation) were less variable. Notably, this effect was accentuated in the indirect task relative to the direct task (Figure 5.9A). We divided the trajectories into equidistant segments and compared the standard deviation at each segment between the nonstandard and standard reaching conditions (see methods section on accompanying CD-ROM). The variance measured at the end of most segments (starting between 25% and 50% into the movement) was significantly larger in the nonstandard task compared with the same segment in the standard task. The standard deviation values themselves

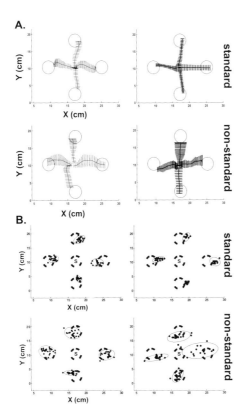

Figure 5.9. (A) Mean movement trajectories (n = 20 to each target) for directly viewed ("standard") and dissociated ("nonstandard") targets, both monkeys. The trajectories do not include final corrective movements. Trajectories are divided into 20 equal segments, with standard error bars shown at each segment end. Circles represent the size of the target viewed by the animal. (B) Individual initial endpoints for standard and nonstandard reach movements. Solid ellipse around each set of points is the 95% confidence interval as determined by a PCA analysis. Dotted circles represent the size of the target viewed by the animal. S indicates starting location.

were 1.8 to 19 times larger in the condition in which there was a spatial dissociation between the vision and the action, relative to the condition in which the animals were interacting directly (in this case, touching) with the viewed targets.

We also observed an effect of task on the spatial distribution of hand movement endpoints reached by the animal. In general, the dispersion of endpoints was significantly greater in the nonstandard task compared with the visually direct task (Figure 5.9B). Lastly, the 95% confidence ellipses in the dissociated condition are notably larger compared with the standard condition (Figure 5.9B). Across animals, the mean area was on average 3.4 times larger in the nonstandard task (mean across targets 16.9 versus 5.0 cm^2, Figure 7 on the accompanying CD-ROM).

In this study we observed in monkeys significant increases in both the variability of the path taken and the initial stopping point towards targets presented in a representational display compared with the targets appearing directly below the animal's hand. We have demonstrated that nonhuman primates can be used to study eye-hand movements guided by indirect, abstract information, a skill of basic importance to human function. The strong similarities in the observed behavioral patterns suggest a homologous functional organization such that, in both human and nonhuman primates, there are additional neural processing requirements to accommodate the more cognitively related nonstandard mapping task.

In general, increases in behavioral variability may be due to the greater attentional demands of the nonstandard task, the use of tools, and the greater processing demands associated with representational visual input. We base this supposition, in part, on the observed activation of the attention- and tool-related areas as movements become increasingly nonstandard, discussed above for our human imaging studies. Also, single-cell recordings in the parietal cortex have revealed neurons that are responsive to the manipulation of objects that are viewed on a video monitor; these cells are distinct from the neurons that are active during direct manipulation (Iriki et al., 1996, 2001). Precentrally, ventral premotor areas contain neurons thought to be related to the coding of representational objects and actions (e.g. an experimenter's hand performing an action versus animal's own hand (Rizzolatti et al., 2002). In addition, dorsal premotor neurons have been shown to have both attentional gaze-related and intentional limb-movement related activity to targets that are both directly presented and arbitrary in nature (Wise et al., 1992, 1996; Boussaoud and Wise, 1993; Boussaoud, 2001). Within the premotor area these effects appear to be preferentially encoded along a rostral-caudal gradient (Fujii et al., 2000; Boussaoud, 2001). All of these areas may be involved in the more complex visuomotor transformations needed for eye-hand coordination when the guiding sensory information is not in direct alignment with the required motor action. We are now in the process of confirming these ideas through multi-unit recording studies in awake behaving monkeys.

5.9   Conclusion

Moving a limb to interact with an object that is not in direct sensory alignment is a basic skill that we perform effortlessly every day. Yet this ability is not innate in humans and it can deteriorate with age and disease. In this chapter we have reviewed a number of studies that employed a variety of methodological approaches to examine the cortical mechanisms of vision for complex action. We have made the argument, using behavioral evidence, that the three basic types of nonstandard visuomotor compatibility discussed at the beginning of this chapter (arbitrary mapping, strategic control/visuomotor adaptation, and sensorimotor recalibration) are subserved by distinct neural mechanisms. In our opening schematic, we propose that different pathways underlie these functions: a parietal-prefrontal cortex pathway for processing the more arbitrary, rule-based type of information and a parietal-premotor cortex pathway for integrating and realigning the sensory and motor aspects of a task. Research in our laboratory and others characterizing empirically these functional neural arrangements continues to find evidence for these dissociable yet interdependent pathways. We hope that we have convinced you that the neural control of reaching when "what you see isn't where you get" involves a basic parietofrontal network of brain areas which can vary depending on both the level of dissociation of the task and the sex, age, and neurological health of the individual making the movement. In closing, we point you toward forthcoming work looking at the neurophysiology of dissociated movement control (Neagu et al., 2007), and the use of increasingly dissociated reaching tasks as a means to evaluate patients with specific types of neuropathological conditions such as mild cognitive impairment (Salek et al., 2007), Alzheimer's disease, acquired brain injury, and stroke. Importantly, we are evaluating the effects of experience on these brain networks (McCullough et al., 2006; Granek et al., 2007).

Meanwhile, back with our surgical patient: Miraculously (to you), your surgeon guided all those swirling knives and camera tubes most adeptly, despite the distant, angled monitor position. Yes! Experience saved the day!! "If only," you think wistfully, "my years of experience with this soccer ball were as successful." Leaving the science of dissociated reaching movements to the neuroscientists, you turn to face another season of recreational soccer glory.

Acknowledgments

The authors would like to thank Saihong Sun, Taiwo McGregor, John Currell, and Tyrone Lew for their technical expertise. We also acknowledge the assistance of J. Douglas Crawford, Mera Barr, and Xiaomu Ma with the neurophysiological studies discussed in this chapter. Lastly, we are grateful for the expert editorial assistance provided by Margaret Gibson. The original research reviewed in this chapter was funded by operating grants from the Canadian Institutes of Health Research.

References

Andersen, R. A. and Buneo, C. A. (2002). Intentional maps in posterior parietal cortex. *Ann. Rev. Neurosci.*, 25: 189–220.

Bedford, F. L. (1993). Perceptual and cognitive spatial learning. *J. Exp. Psychol.*, 19: 517–530.

Belanger, H. G., Wilder-Willis, K., Malloy, P., Salloway, S., Hamman, R. F. and Grigsby, J. (2005). Assessing motor and cognitive regulation in AD, MCI, and controls using the behavioral dyscontrol scale. *Arch. Clin. Neuropsychol.*, 20: 183–189.

Benke, T. (1993). Two forms of apraxia in Alzheimer's disease. *Cortex*, 29: 715–725.

Boussaoud, D. (2001). Attention versus intention in the primate premotor cortex. *NeuroImage*, 14: S40–545.

Boussaoud, D. and Bremmer, F. (1999). Gaze effects in the cerebral cortex: Reference frames for space coding and action. *Exp. Brain Res.*, 128: 170–180.

Boussaoud, D. and Wise, S. P. (1993). Primate frontal cortex: effects of stimulus and movement. *Exp. Brain Res.*, 95: 28–40.

Boussaoud, D., Jouffrais, C. and Bremmer, F. (1998). Eye position effects on the neuronal activity of dorsal premotor cortex in the macaque monkey. *J. Neurophysiol.*, 80: 1132–1150.

Braak, H. and Braak, E. (1991). Neuropathological stageing of Alzheimer-related changes. *Acta. Neuropathol.*, 82: 239–259.

Brasted, P. J. and Wise, S. P. (2004). Comparison of learning-related neuronal activity in the dorsal premotor cortex and striatum. *Eur. J. Neurosci.*, 19: 721–740.

Buch, E. R., Brasted, P. J. and Wise, S. P. (2006). Comparison of population activity in the dorsal premotor cortex and putamen during the learning of arbitrary visuomotor mappings. *Exp. Brain Res.*, 169: 69–84.

Canavan, A. G., Nixon, P. D. and Passingham, R. E. (1989). Motor learning in monkeys (macaca fascicularis) with lesions in motor thalamus. *Exp. Brain Res.*, 77: 113–126.

Carey, D. P., Coleman, R. J. and Della Sala, S. (1997). Magnetic misreaching. *Cortex*, 33: 639–652.

Clower, D. M. and Boussaoud, D. (2000). Selective use of perceptual recalibration versus visuomotor skill acquisition. *J. Neurophysiol.*, 84: 2703–2708.

Connolly, J. D., Goodale, M. A., DeSouza, J. F., Menon, R. S. and Vilis, T. (2000). A comparison of frontoparietal fMRI activation during anti-saccades and anti-pointing. *J. Neurophysiol.*, 84: 1645–1655.

Constantinidis, C. and Steinmetz, M. A. (2005). Posterior parietal cortex automatically encodes the location of salient stimuli. *J. Neurosci.*, 25: 233–238.

Constantinidis, C. and Steinmetz, M. A. (1996). Neuronal activity in posterior parietal area 7a during the delay periods of a spatial memory task. *J. Neurophysiol.*, 76: 1352–1355.

Cooke, J. D., Brown, S. H. and Cunningham, D. A. (1989). Kinematics of arm movements in elderly humans. *Neurobiol. Aging*, 10: 159–165.

Crammond, D. J. and Kalaska, J. F. (1994). Modulation of preparatory neuronal activity in dorsal premotor cortex due to stimulus-response compatibility. *J. Neurophysiol.*, 71: 1281–1284.

Crutch, S. J., Rossor, M. N. and Warrington, E. K. (2007). The quantitative assessment of apraxic deficits in Alzheimer's disease. *Cortex*, 43: 976–986.

Darling, W. G., Cooke, J. D. and Brown, S. H. (1989). Control of simple arm movements in elderly humans. *Neurobiol. Aging*, 10: 149–157.

Dassonville, P., Lewis, S. M., Foster, H. E. and Ashe, J. (1999). Choice and stimulus-response compatibility affect duration of response selection. *Cogn. Brain Res.*, 7: 235–240.

Davatzikos, C. and Resnick, S. M. (1998). Sex differences in anatomic measures of interhemispheric connectivity: correlations with cognition in women but not men. *Cereb. Cortex*, 8: 635–640.

Di Carlo, A., Lamassa, M., Baldereschi, M., Pracucci, G., Basile, A. M., Wolfe, C. D, Giroud, M., Rudd, A., Ghetti, A., Inzitari, D., European BIOMED Study of Stroke Care Group (2003). Sex differences in the clinical presentation, resource use, and 3-month outcome of acute stroke in europe: data from a multicenter multinational hospital-based registry. *Stroke*, 34: 1114–1119.

Eliassen, J. C., Souza, T. and Sanes, J. N. (2003). Experience-dependent activation patterns in human brain during visual-motor associative learning. *J. Neurosci.*, 23: 10540–10547.

Everling, S. and Munoz, D. P. (2000). Neuronal correlates for preparatory set associated with pro-saccades and anti-saccades in the primate frontal eye field. *J, Neurosci.*, 20: 387–400.

Folstein, M. F., Folstein, S. E. and McHugh, P. R. (1975). "Mini-mental state". A practical method for grading the cognitive state of patients for the clinician. *J. Psychiatr. Res.*, 12: 189–198.

Fozard, J. L., Vercryssen, M., Reynolds, S. L., Hancock, P. A. and Quilter, R. E. (1994). Age differences and changes in reaction time: the Baltimore longitudinal study of aging. *J. Gerontol.*, 49: P179–89.

Fujii, N., Mushiake, H. and Tanji, J. (2000). Rostrocaudal distinction of the dorsal premotor area based on oculomotor involvement. *J. Neurophysiol.*, 83: 1764–1769.

Galganski, M. E., Fuglevand, A. J. and Enoka, R. M. (1993). Reduced control of motor output in a human hand muscle of elderly subjects during submaximal contractions. *J. Neurophysiol.*, 69: 2108–2115.

Ghilardi, M. F., Alberoni, M., Marelli, S., Rossi, M., Franceschi, M., Ghez, C. and Fazio, F. (1999). Impaired movement control in Alzheimer's disease. *Neurosci. Lett.*, 260: 45–48.

Ghilardi, M. F., Alberoni, M., Rossi, M., Franceschi, M., Mariani, C. and Fazio, F. (2000a). Visual feedback has differential effects on reaching movements in Parkinson's and Alzheimer's disease. *Brain Res.*, 876: 112–123.

Ghilardi, M. F., Ghez, C., Dhawan, V., Moeller, J., Mentis, M., Nakamura, T., Antonini, A. and Eidelberg, D. (2000b). Patterns of regional brain activation associated with different forms of motor learning. *Brain Res.*, 871: 127–145.

Ghilardi, M. F., Gordon, J. and Ghez, C. (1995). Learning a visuomotor transformation in a local area of work space produces directional biases in other areas. *J. Neurophysiol.*, 73: 2535–2539.

Goodale, M. A. (1993). Visual pathways supporting perception and action in the primate cerebral cortex. *Curr. Opin. Neurobiol.*, 3: 578–585.

Goodbody, S. J. and Wolpert, D. M. (1999). The effect of visuomotor displacements on arm movement paths *Exp. Brain Res.*, 127. 213–223.

Gorbet, D. J. and Sergio, L. E. (2006). The behavioral consequences of spatially disso-ciating the direction of eye and hand movements. I. The effects of anti-pointing. *Soc. Neurosci. Abstr.*, 242.15.

Gorbet, D. J. and Sergio, L. E. (2007). Preliminary sex differences in human cortical BOLD fMRI activity during the preparation of increasingly complex visually guided movements. *Eur. J. Neurosci.*, 25: 1228–1239.

Gorbet, D. J., Staines, W. R. and Sergio, L. E. (2004). Brain mechanisms for preparing increasingly complex sensory to motor transformations. *NeuroImage*, 23: 1100–1111.

Grafton, S. T., Fagg, A. H. and Arbib, M. A. (1998). Dorsal premotor cortex and con-ditional movement selection: a PET functional mapping study. *J. Neurophysiol.*, 79: 1092–1097.

Granek, J. A., Gorbet, D. J. and Sergio, L. E. (2007). The effects of video-game expe-rience on the cortical networks for increasingly complex visuomotor tasks. *Soc. Neurosci. Abstr.*, 618.24.

Gron, G., Wunderlich, A. P., Spitzer, M., Tomczak, R. and Riepe, M. W. (2000). Brain activation during human navigation: gender-different neural networks as sub-strate of performance. *Nat. Neurosci.*, 3: 404–408.

Hadj-Bouziane, F., Meunier, M. and Boussaoud, D. (2003). Conditional visuo-motor learning in primates: a key role for the basal ganglia. *J. Physiol. (Paris)*, 97: 567–579.

Hanakawa, T., Honda, M., Zito, G., Dimyan, M. A. and Hallett, M. (2006). Brain activ-ity during visuomotor behavior triggered by arbitrary and spatially constrained cues: an fMRI study in humans. *Exp. Brain Res.*, 172: 275–282.

Henriques, D. Y., Klier, E. M., Smith, M. A., Lowy, D. and Crawford, J. D. (1998). Gaze-centered remapping of remembered visual space in an open-loop pointing task. *J. Neurosci.*, 18: 1583–1594.

Inoue, K., Kawashima, R., Sugiura, M., Ogawa, A., Schormann, T., Zilles, K. and Fukuda, H. (2001). Activation in the ipsilateral posterior parietal cortex during tool use: a PET study. *NeuroImage*, 14: 1469–1475.

Iriki, A., Tanaka, M. and Iwamura, Y. (1996). Coding of modified body schema during tool use by macaque postcentral neurones. *NeuroReport*, 7: 2325–2330.

Iriki, A., Tanaka, M., Obayashi, S. and Iwamura, Y. (2001). Self-images in the video monitor coded by monkey intraparietal neurons. *Neurosci. Res.*, 40: 163–173.

Johnson, H., Van Beers, R. J. and Haggard, P. (2002). Action and awareness in pointing tasks. *Exp. Brain Res.*, 146: 451–459.

Johnson, M. T., Coltz, J. D. and Ebner, T. J. (1999). Encoding of target direction and speed during visual instruction and arm tracking in dorsal premotor and primary motor cortical neurons. *Eur. J. Neurosci.*, 11: 4433–4445.

Jordan, K., Wustenberg, T., Heinze, H.-J., Peters, M. and Jancke, L. (2002). Women and men exhibit different cortical activation patterns during mental rotation tasks. *Neuropsychologia*, 40: 2397–2408.

Kalaska, J. F. (1996). Parietal cortex area 5 and visuomotor behavior. *Can. J. Physiol. Pharmacol.*, 74: 483–498.

Kapral, M. K., Fang, J., Hill, M. D., Silver, F., Richards, J., Jaigobin, C., Cheung, A. M. and Investigators of the Registry of the Canadian Stroke Network (2005). Sex differences in stroke care and outcomes: results from the Registry of the Canadian Stroke Network. *Stroke*, 36: 809–814.

Ketcham, C. J., Seidler, R. D., Van Gemmert, A. W,. and Stelmach, G. E. (2002). Age-related kinematic differences as influenced by task difficulty, target size, and movement amplitude. *J. Gerontol. B Psychol. Sci. Soc. Sci.*, 57: P54–64.

Kimura, D. (1993). *Neuromotor Mechanisms in Human Communication*. New York: Oxford University Press.

Kimura, D. and Harshman, R. A. (1984). Sex differences in brain organization for verbal and nonverbal functions. *Prog. Brain Res.*, 61: 423–441.

Kitamura, S. and Terashi, A. (1990). Measurements of cerebral blood flow and metabolism in patients with Alzheimer's disease. *Rinsho. Byori.*, 38: 494–498.

Kluger, A., Gianutsos, J. G., Golomb, J., Ferris, S. H., George, A. E., Franssen, E. and Reisberg, B. (1997). Patterns of motor impairement in normal aging, mild cognitive decline, and early alzheimer's disease. *J. Gerontol. B Psychol. Sci. Soc. Sci.*, 52: P28–39.

Labiche, L. A., Chan, W., Saldin, K. R. and Morgenstern, L. B. (2002). Sex and acute stroke presentation. *Ann. Emerg. Med.*, 40: 453–460.

Lackner, J. R. and Dizio, P. (1994). Rapid adaptation to coriolis force perturbations of arm trajectory. *J. Neurophysiol.*, 72: 299–313.

Lee, J. H. and van Donkelaar, P. (2006). The human dorsal premotor cortex generates on-line error corrections during sensorimotor adaptation. *J. Neurosci.*, 26: 3330–3334.

Ma, X., Gorbet, D. J. and Sergio, L. E. (2006). The behavioral consequences of spatially dissociating the direction of eye and hand movements. II. The effects of central fixation and anti-saccades. *Soc. Neurosci. Abstr.*, 242.16.

Marion, S. D., Kilian, S. C., Naramor, T. L. and Brown, W. S. (2003). Normal development of bimanual coordination: visuomotor and interhemispheric contributions. *Dev. Neuropsychol.*, 23: 399–421.

McCullough, K. L., Granek, J. A. and Sergio, L. E. (2006). Visuomotor skill performance asymmetries related to sex and athletic experience. *Soc. Neurosci. Abstr.*, 242.2.

Medendorp, W. P., Goltz, H. C., Vilis, T. and Crawford, J. D. (2003). Gaze-centered updating of visual space in human parietal cortex. *J. Neurosci.*, 23: 6209–6214.

Messier, J. and Kalaska, J. F. (1997). Differential effect of task conditions on errors of direction and extent of reaching movements. *Exp. Brain Res.*, 115: 469–478.

Mitz, A. R., Godschalk, M. and Wise, S. P. (1991). Learning-dependent neuronal activity in the premotor cortex: activity during the acquisition of conditional motor associations. *J. Neurosci.*, 11. 1855–1872.

Moscovitch, C., Kapur, S., Kohler, S. and Houle, S. (1995). Distinct neural correlates of visual long-term memory for spatial location and object identity: a positron emission tomography study in humans. *Proc. Natl. Acad. Sci. USA*, 92: 3721–3725.

Munoz, D. P. and Everling, S. (2004). Look away: the anti-saccade task and the voluntary control of eye movement. *Nat. Rev. Neurosci.*, 5: 218–228.

Munoz, D. P., Armstrong, I. T., Hampton, K. A. and Moore, K. D. (2003). Altered control of visual fixation and saccadic eye movements in attention-deficit hyperactivity disorder. *J. Neurophysiol.*, 90: 503–514.

Munoz, D. P., Broughton, J. R., Goldring, J. E. and Armstrong, I. T. (1998). Age-related performance of human subjects on saccadic eye movement tasks. *Exp. Brain Res.*, 121: 391–400.

Murray, E. A., Bussey, T. J. and Wise, S. P. (2000). Role of prefrontal cortex in a network for arbitrary visuomotor mapping. *Exp. Brain Res.*, 133: 114–129.

Neagu, B., Sayegh, P. F. and Sergio, L. E. (2007). Dorsal premotor activity during increasingly complex visuomotor tasks. *Soc. Neurosci Abstr.*, 818.16.

Neggers, S. F. and Bekkering, H. (2000). Ocular gaze is anchored to the target of an ongoing pointing movement. *J. Neurophysiol.*, 83: 639–651.

Neggers, S. F. and Bekkering, H. (2001). Gaze anchoring to a pointing target is present during the entire pointing movement and is driven by a nonvisual signal. *J. Neurophysiol.*, 86: 961–970.

Nixon, P. D., McDonald, K. R., Gough, P. M., Alexander, I. H. and Passingham, R. E. (2004). Cortico-basal ganglia pathways are essential for the recall of well-established visuomotor associations. *Eur. J. Neurosci.*, 20: 3165–3178.

Oyachi, H. and Ohtsuka, K. (1995). Transcranial magnetic stimulation of the posterior parietal cortex degrades accuracy of memory-guided saccades in humans. *Invest. Ophthalmol. Vis. Sci.*, 36: 1441–1449.

Parakh, R., Roy, E., Koo, E. and Black, S. (2004). Pantomime and imitation of limb gestures in relation to the severity of Alzheimer's disease. *Brain Cogn.*, 55: 272–274.

Passingham, R. E. (1988). Premotor cortex and preparation for movement. *Exp. Brain Res.*, 70: 590–596.

Pennisi, G., Alagona, G., Ferri, R., Greco, S., Santonocito, D., Pappalardo, A. and Bella, R. (2002). Motor cortex excitability in Alzheimer disease: one year follow-up study. *Neurosci. Lett.*, 329: 293–296.

Petrides, M. (1982). Motor conditional associative-learning after selective prefrontal lesions in the monkey. *Behav. Brain Res.*, 5: 407–413.

Petrides, M. (1997). Visuomotor conditional associative learning after frontal and temporal lesions in the human brain. *Neuropsychologia*, 35: 989–997.

Piaget, J. (1965). *The Construction of Reality in the Child*. New York: Basic Books, Inc.

Prablanc, C., Echallier, J. F., Komilis, E. and Jeannerod, M. (1979). Optimal response of eye and hand motor systems in pointing at a visual target. I. Spatio-temporal characteristics of eye and hand movements and their relationships when varying the amount of visual information. *Biol. Cybern.*, 35: 113–124.

Price, D. L., Tanzi, R. E., Borchelt, D. R. and Sisodia, S. S. (1998). Alzheimer's disease: genetic studies and transgenic models. *Ann. Rev. Genet.*, 32: 461–493.

Redding, G. M. and Wallace, B. (1996). Adaptive spatial alignment and strategic perceptual-motor control. *J. Exp. Psychol. Hum. Percept. Perform.*, 22: 379–394.

Redding, G. M., Rossetti, Y. and Wallace, B. (2005). Applications of prism adaptation: a tutorial in theory and method. *Neurosci. Biobehav. Rev.*, 29: 431–444.

Ricciardi, E., Bonino, D, Gentili, C., Sani, L., Pietrini, P. and Vecchi, T. (2006). Neural correlates of spatial working memory in humans: a functional magnetic resonance imaging study comparing visual and tactile processes. *Neuroscience*, 139: 339–349.

Rizzolatti, G., Fogassi, L. and Gallese, V. (2002). Motor and cognitive functions of the ventral premotor cortex. *Cur. Opin. Neurobiol.*, 12: 149–154.

Roalf, D., Lowery, N. and Turetsky, B. I. (2006). Behavioral and physiological findings of gender differences in global-local visual processing. *Brain Cogn.*, 60: 32–42.

Roquer, J., Campello, A. R. and Gomis, M. (2003). Sex differences in first-ever acute stroke. *Stroke*, 34: 1581–1585.

Rossetti, Y., Revol, P., McIntosh, R., Pisella, L., Rode, G., Danckert, J., Tilikete, C., Dijkerman, H. C., Boisson, D., Vighetto, A., Michel, F. and Milner, A. D. (2005). Visually guided reaching: bilateral posterior parietal lesions cause a switch from fast visuomotor to slow cognitive control. *Neuropsychologia*, 43: 162–177.

Sadato, N., Ibanez, V., Deiber, M. P. and Hallett, M. (2000). Gender difference in premotor activity during active tactile discrimination. *NeuroImage*, 11: 532–540.

Salek, Y., Anderson, N. D. and Sergio, L. E. (2007). Impaired visuomotor integration in adults with mild cognitive impairment. *Soc. Neurosci. Abstr.*, 281.23.

Scherberger, H., Goodale, M. A. and Andersen, R. A. (2003). Target selection for reaching and saccades share a similar behavioral reference frame in the macaque. *J. Neurophysiol.*, 89: 1456–1466.

Seidler, R. D., Alberts, J. L. and Stelmach, G. E. (2002). Changes in multi-joint performance with age. *Motor Control*, 6: 19–31.

Seidler-Dobrin, R. D. and Stelmach, G. E. (1998). Persistence in visual feedback control by the elderly. *Exp. Brain Res.*, 119: 467–474.

Sekuler, A. B., Bennett, P. J. and Mamelak, M. (2000). Effects of aging on the useful field of view. *Exp. Aging Res.*, 26: 103–120.

Sergio, L. E. and Kalaska, J. F. (2003). Systematic changes in motor cortex cell activity with arm posture during directional isometric force generation. *J. Neurophysiol.*, 89: 212–228.

Seurinck, R., Vingerhoets, G., de Lange, F. P. and Achten, E. (2004). Does egocentric mental rotation elicit sex differences? *NeuroImage*, 23: 1440–1449.

Shen, L. and Alexander, G. E. (1997). Preferential representation of instructed target location versus limb trajectory in dorsal premotor area. *J. Neurophysiol.*, 77: 1195–1212.

Spirduso, W. W. (1980). Physical fitness, aging, and psychomotor speed: a review. *J. Gerontol.*, 35: 850–865.

Stelmach, G. E., Goggin, N. L. and Garcia-Colera, A. (1987). Movement specification time with age. *Exp. Aging Res.*, 13: 39–46.

Tabachnick, B. G. and Fidell, L. S. (1996). *Using Multivariate Statistics*. New York, NY: Harper Collins College Publishers.

Tippett, W. J. and Sergio, L. E. (2006). Visuomotor integration is impaired in early stage Alzheimer's disease. *Brain Res.*, 1102: 92–102.

Tippett, W. J., Krajewski, A. and Sergio, L. E. (2007). Visuomotor integration is compromised in alzheimer's disease patients reaching for remembered targets. *Eur. Neurol.*, 58: 1–11.

Toni, I. and Passingham, R. E. (1999). Prefrontal-basal ganglia pathways are involved in the learning of arbitrary visuomotor associations: a PET study. *Exp. Brain Res.*, 127: 19–32.

Toni, I., Rushworth, M. F. and Passingham, R. E. (2001). Neural correlates of visuomotor associations. spatial rules compared with arbitrary rules. *Exp. Brain Res.*, 141: 359–369.

Vercher, J. L., Magenes, G., Prablanc, C. and Gauthier, G. M. (1994). Eye-head-hand coordination in pointing at visual targets: spatial and temporal analysis. *Exp. Brain Res.*, 99: 507–523.

von Gunten, A., Bouras, C., Kovari, E., Giannakopoulos, P. and Hof, P. R. (2006). Neural substrates of cognitive and behavioral deficits in atypical alzheimer's disease. *Brain Res. Rev.*.

Weiss, E., Siedentopf, C. M., Hofer, A., Deisenhammer, E. A., Hoptman, M. J., Kremser, C., Golaszewski, S., Felber, S., Fleischhacker, W. W. and Delazer, M. (2003). Sex differences in brain activation pattern during a visuospatial cognitive task: a functional magnetic resonance imaging study in healthy volunteers. *Neurosci. Lett.*, 344: 169–172.

Wise, S. P., di Pellegrino, G. and Boussaoud, D. (1992). Primate premotor cortex: dissociation of visuomotor from sensory signals. *J. Neurophysiol,*, 68: 969–972.

Wise, S. P., di Pellegrino, G. and Boussaoud, D. (1996). The premotor cortex and nonstandard sensorimotor mapping. *Can. J. Physiol. Pharmacol.*, 74: 469–482.

Wizemann, T. M. and Pardue, M. L. (2001). *Exploring the Biological Contributions to Human Health: Does Sex Matter?* Washington, DC: National Academy Press.

6 Neural mechanisms of self-movement: perception for navigation and spatial orientation

C. J. Duffy, D. J. Logan, M. J. Dubin and W. K. Page

As arboreal primates navigate through their jungle environment they are immersed in visual motion that they must distinguish from the movement of predators and prey. The variety of simultaneous stimuli in natural settings demands the active allocation of cortical capacity to processing self-movement cues versus other features. The flexibility of resource allocation is augmented by maintaining alternative navigational strategies based on the selective processing of various self-movement cues.

We recorded the activity of dorsal medial superior temporal (MSTd) cortical neurons in behaving monkeys. Optic flow patterns of visual motion that simulate observer self-movement were presented in a variety of behavioral contexts. The addition of visual object motion to optic flow creates dynamic interactions between neuronal responses to these stimuli that facilitate the selection of either landmark or environment based navigation.

Engaging the monkey in tasks that demand shifting between optic flow and object cues alters the strength and selectivity of MSTd neuronal responses to optic flow. The nature of these changes in neuronal responses is shaped by both the cues and the tasks. Engaging the monkey in actively steering its simulated self-movement alters optic flow responses depending on the monkey's learned strategy for steering: using local motion cues diminishes responses, using global pattern cues enhances them.

In sum, we find that MSTd neuronal responses to self-movement are influenced by the presence of competing cues and the demands of ongoing behavioral tasks. The control of alternative processing strategies may involve dynamic interactions between bottom-up and top-down mechanisms in cerebral cortex.

6.1　Introduction

The patterned visual motion of optic flow provides robust cues about the observer's heading of self-movement. The moving observer is also exposed to the visual motion of discrete objects. When those objects are earth-fixed, they are an important source of information about the heading of relative self-movement, as in navigation in relation to a recognized landmark. The independent movement of animate objects presents cues that conflict with the optic flow field, potentially enhancing the detection of animate objects. Thus, interactions between optic flow and object motion can facilitate self-movement perception for navigation and the recognition of animacy for the detection of predators and prey.

The observer cannot be viewed as a passive recipient of these signals, self-movement cues being inherently reafferent in nature, that is, a sensory input resulting from motor output. The reafferent nature of optic flow is evident in the impact of pursuit eye movements on the perception of heading from optic flow (Warren Jr. et al., 1987; Banks et al., 1991) and on MSTd neuronal responses to optic flow (Page et al., 1993; Bradley et al., 1996). In exploring the influence of an active observer on the processing of optic flow, one must consider the observer's active control of perceptual resources as well as the active control of the heading of the self-movement that generates optic flow.

In this review, we describe our recent experiments that characterize the responses of MSTd neurons to optic flow and object motion stimuli presented to simulate congruent self-movement cues or noncongruent cues to object animacy (Logan et al., 2006). These studies are joined to our findings regarding attentional influences on optic flow responses in MSTd neurons (Dubin and Duffy, 2007), and the impact of active steering on those responses (Page and Duffy, 2008).

6.2　Methods

6.2.1　Animal preparation

Monkeys were prepared for MSTd single neuron recording with established protocols, as detailed in recent papers (Logan et al., 2006; Page and Duffy, 2008). Single neuron responses were recorded from ten cerebral hemispheres of five rhesus monkeys. Surgery was performed under general anaesthesia to implant bilateral scleral search coils (Judge et al., 1980), a head holder, and bilateral recording cylinders. Postoperative analgesia was administered as judged appropriate by veterinary staff. All protocols used in these studies were approved by the University Committee on Animal Research and complied with Society for Neuroscience and Public Health Service Policy on the care of laboratory animals.

6.2.2   Visual motion stimuli

Stimuli were presented using a personal computer to drive a CRT projector (Electro-home ECP4100) to produce an image covering the central visual field ($90° \times 90°$). Optic flow stimuli made of 350 white dots ($0.19°$ at 2.61 cd/m^2) were presented on a dark background (0.18 cd/m^2) in patterns of dot motion (average speed of $40°$/s) that simulate the scene surrounding a moving observer. The dots were evenly distributed in a smoothed, random pattern in the first frame of each stimulus with lifetimes of 1–60 frames and speed proportionate to twice the sine of the angle from the observer's line of sight in centered fixation to that dot.

Object motion stimuli were an outline of dots forming three concentric circles traversed by four diameter lines. The object moved to simulate the image of an earth-fixed landmark as seen during relative observer movement. In simulating object motion in the frontoparallel plane, objects moved across the screen at $40°$/s. In simulating object motion in depth, object size ranged from $5°$ to $20°$ diameter.

Optic flow and object motion stimuli were presented separately and together. Same direction combined stimuli presented an object moving as an element of the superimposed optic flow field, as with earth-fixed objects. Opposite direction combined stimuli presented an object moving on a heading $180°$ offset from the heading in the superimposed optic flow. Optic flow and object motion stimuli are named for the corresponding directions of observer self-movement.

6.2.3   Single neuron recording

Tungsten microelectrodes (Microprobe, Inc.) were passed through a transdural guide tube (Crist et al., 1988) to record single neuron activity digitized using a dual window discriminator and stored with event markers on the REX experiment control system (Hays et al., 1982). MSTd neurons were identified by their physiologic characteristics: large receptive fields ($> 20° \times 20°$) containing the fixation point, direction-selective responses, preferring large moving patterns (Komatsu and Wurtz, 1988; Duffy and Wurtz, 1991). At the conclusion of experiments with a monkey, electrolytic marking lesions were placed bounding the recorded cortical sites. Histological analysis confirmed that these sites were in the anterior bank of the superior temporal sulcus in the area corresponding to the zone of heavy myelination associated with MSTd.

6.2.4   Preliminary data analysis

Spike records from 5–7 trials were combined in average poststimulus time histograms after spike convolution with 20 ms Gaussians. Average firing rates in identified response periods were used to quantify the impact of visual stimuli.

3-D tuning surfaces were derived using fits to Kent spherical distributions (Fisher et al., 1987) yielding unidirectional response profiles that ranged from nondirection selective spheres to symmetrically or asymmetrically elongated ellipsoids. These 3-D response profiles characterized directional strength, preferred direction, and goodness-of-fit measures for each stimulus type in each neuron. 3-D population responses were derived by combining preferred direction vectors across neurons (Georgopoulos et al., 1986).

We compared the heading directional profiles of behaviorally relevant and irrelevant stimuli by fitting response amplitude profiles with Gaussian curves across eight radial center of motion locations in optic flow (Matlab, Mathworks, Inc). Amplitude, baseline, tuning width, and preferred radial center of motion were all independent parameters in the Gaussian fit. F-ratios of summed residuals to the Gaussian versus linear fits yielded a goodness-of-fit measure to accept Gaussian fits with $p < 0.05$ (McAdams and Maunsell, 1999).

In the steering studies, response data was entered in to a mixed-model 2-way ANOVA having within-subjects effects of radial center of motion (eight locations) and task (active steering versus passive viewing) and having between-subjects effects of behavioral paradigms (local versus global tasks). We assessed the significance of effects using Greenhouse-Geisser corrected F values.

6.2.5   Anatomical distribution of neuronal responses

The plane of the superior temporal sulcus (STS) was determined from inspection of MRI images and histological sections for each hemisphere. Neuronal recording positions were confirmed to be in the plane of the STS and projected views of each hemisphere were oriented to that plane. Correlations of single neuron physiological parameters (peak response and directionality ratios for optic flow versus object motion) and anatomical position were measured. These correlations tested the distribution of each physiological parameter along a large number of axes in the plane of the STS.

Two further analytic approaches were used: (a) cluster analyses across the 2-D plane of the STS were used to identify any grouping in the distribution of optic flow and object motion peak responses, heading direction selectivities, and 3-D heading preferences; (b) the 2-D anatomical distances between pairs of neurons were linearly regressed against the physiological parameters yielding correlation coefficients and p-value measures of significant correlations.

6.3   Results

6.3.1   3-D heading representation from optic flow and object motion

Optic flow and object motion stimuli simulating 14 directions of self-movement were presented to assess MSTd neuronal representation of 3-D heading (details of this study were presented in Logan and Duffy, 2006). Single neuron responses showed selective responses to optic flow and object motion yielding coherent profiles of 3-D self-movement heading selectivity (Figure 6.1). Optic flow and object motion evoked similar response amplitudes with responses to optic flow being more sustained than those evoked by object motion. The longer responses to optic flow may reflect receptive field interactions with the complete coverage of the stimulus area by these stimuli versus object motion's transient crossing of the spatial extent of the display.

MSTd neuronal responses to optic flow and object motion simulating self-movement were plotted in 3-D polar coordinates oriented with reference to the monkey and hav-

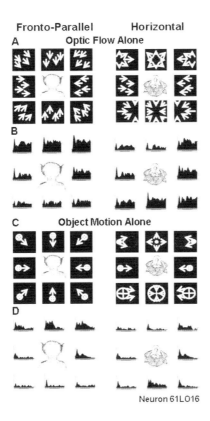

Figure 6.1. Optic flow and object motion stimuli used in these studies. This MSTd neuron responded to both optic flow and object motion stimuli simulating right-upward heading directions. (A) Optic flow stimuli simulating 14 directions of observer translational self-movement in the fronto-parallel plane (left) and horizontal ground plane (right). (B) Spike density histograms (SDHs) of an MSTd neuron's responses to optic flow stimuli showing preferences for headings in the right-upward heading directions. Responses are arranged to correspond to the stimuli depicted in (A). Vertical lines represent the 50 spikes/s firing rate, horizontal lines represent the 2 s stimulus duration, and histograms represent activity averaged over six to eight stimulus repetitions. (C) Object motion stimuli simulating 14 directions of relative translational self-movement in the frontoparallel plane (left) and horizontal ground plane (right). SDHs of the same MSTd neuron illustrated in (B) showing its responses to object motion stimuli with preferences for the right-upward heading directions.

ing each response plotted toward its direction of simulated self-movement at a distance from the origin in proportion to the evoked firing rate (Figure 6.2A). The optic flow and object motion responses were fit by generalized normal distributions in 3-D space (Kent distributions) with good fits ($r^2 > 0.6$) obtained for most optic flow (66%) and object motion (59%) responses (Figure 6.2B). These findings suggest that individual neurons can provide a veridical contribution to the representation of self-movement

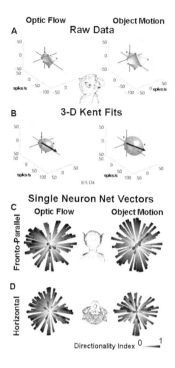

Figure 6.2. 3-D heading preferences for optic flow and object motion. (A) 3-D polar plots of average responses to 14 stimuli (asterisks) are displaced from the origin in the direction of the heading simulated. (B) 3-D Kent spherical fits to the responses show the neuron's preferred 3-D heading direction and the strength of that preference (bold arrow) while accommodating the flattening of the distributions on any plane in 3-D space. (C and D) The preferred heading of each neuron studied is shown as a radial cone viewing the fronto-parallel plane (C) and horizontal ground plane (D). The direction of the preferred heading cone indicates the preferred heading of that neuron and the length of the cone indicates the strength of that preference (directional index, DI). These distributions are not significantly different from 3-D uniformity; there is no significant unimodality or bimodality ($p > 0.05$) in the 3-D distributions (Fisher et al., 1987) for responses to optic flow (left) or object motion (right).

heading in 3-D space with similar heading preferences evident in responses to both optic flow and object motion.

We combined the heading direction response vectors of all neurons tested revealing a uniform distribution across all headings in 3-D space. Although inspection might suggest some clustering in this distribution, there is no significant unimodality or bimodality ($p > 0.05$), suggesting that single neuron heading preferences are not concentrated on any particular heading direction or plane, such as the forward heading or the ground plane (Figure 6.2C and D). Thus, MSTd's representation of self-movement is homogeneous and isotropic, encoding all possible heading directions across 3-D space.

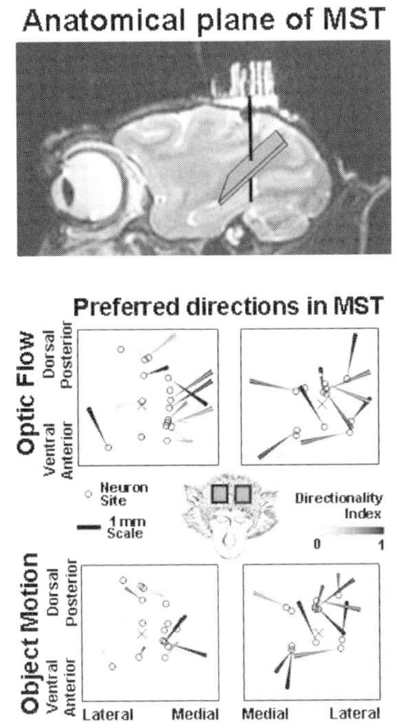

Anatomical plane of MST

Preferred directions in MST

Figure 6.3. Anatomic distribution of optic flow and object motion responses. (Upper) An MR image of the right cerebral hemisphere of the monkey in which the greatest number of neurons was studied. This image shows the position of the recording chamber and the plane of MSTd cortex on the anterior bank of the STS. (Lower) The distribution of single neuron (circles) net vectors across the plane defined by the cortical surface on the anterior bank of the STS, here shown for the left and right hemispheres of the monkey illustrated above. There is no areal separation of optic flow (top) and object motion (bottom) responses or a significant pattern of heading direction preferences across MSTd. The Xs mark the center of the recording chamber projected on to the plane of MSTd cortex and positioned on the coordinates (AP − 2mm, ML ±15 mm).

Although topographic mapping was not the goal of this study, we did search for a pattern in the anatomical distribution of neuronal response properties. The recording sites for all neurons were located in 3-D for each hemisphere in each monkey. These maps were rotated in 3-D space to match the anatomical plane formed by the superior temporal sulcus (STS) around the recording sites (Figure 6.3, upper). This created a representation of recording sites across MST cortex in the plane of the STS. In these monkeys, all recording sites were within the dorsal-anterior bank of the STS away from the curved surface of the sulcus.

The relative amplitude of optic flow and object motion responses was uniformly distributed across the three hemispheres of the two monkeys. Neither the relative responsiveness to optic flow or object motion, nor the strength or directional preferences of 3-D direction selectivity was systematically related to anatomical location.

We tested these distributions for significant biases by correlating relative responsiveness with location across the cortical surface along 360 different axes, including the directly anterior-posterior axis and the directly medial-lateral axis. No significant pattern was identified in any of the hemispheres (Figure 6.3, lower). We compared the distance between neurons with the difference in their 3-D direction preferences and again found no significant response relations in any of the hemispheres studied or in data combined across those hemispheres.

These data can not be considered definitive because extensive mapping studies were not conducted. Nevertheless, it is worth noting that we do not find evidence for a systematic topographic organization in MSTd cortex of response properties related to the representation of 3-D self-movement in these studies.

6.3.2   MSTd neuronal population responses to combined optic flow and object motion

During naturalistic self-movement we commonly view object motion superimposed on optic flow. We are regularly surrounded by the images of a variety of earth-fixed objects that move through our visual field as a feature in the optic flow. In addition, we also see animate objects moving independent of the optic flow field created by our own movements. In these studies, we superimposed object motion on optic flow in two stimulus sets to create a set of same direction combined stimuli simulating the addition of an earth-fixed object and a set of opposite direction combined stimuli simulating the independent movement of an animate object. We recorded interactions between optic flow and object motion in responses to combined stimuli that we compared with the responses evoked by optic flow and object motion presented alone.

Population vector analysis was used to compare MSTd's composite neural response across the four resulting stimulus conditions: optic flow alone, object motion alone, same direction combined stimuli, and opposite direction combined stimuli. This provides measures of the strength and accuracy of the population vector as relative indices of MSTd's heading estimation in response to each type of stimulus. MSTd's population response to each type of stimulus was derived summing the response of all neurons. First, each neuron's responses were fit with the 3-D Kent function so that all responses contributed to that neuron's net vector. This described each neuron's net vector by two values from the Kent fit: the net vector's direction in 3-D space describes the neuron's preferred direction and the net vector's magnitude describes the strength of that directional preference. We then combined the responses of all neurons to create a population response vector for each of the 14 optic flow heading directions under each of the four stimulus conditions.

Responses to the 14 heading directions yielded population net vectors with average resultant lengths that are 60% larger for optic flow than for object motion (260 versus 163 population spk/s = 1.60) ($F_{1, 16} = 30.65$, $p < 0.0001$) (Figure 6.4A and B). Since both optic flow and object motion vectors point radially outward from the unit sphere, they can support a veridical population estimate of heading direction, but optic flow yields a more robust signal than object motion. Same direction combined optic flow and object motion yielded population vector resultant lengths that are not significantly

Population Net Vector Responses

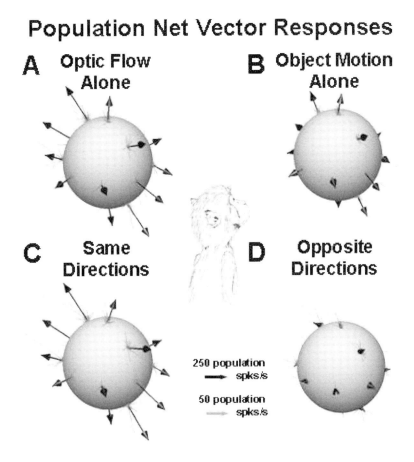

A Optic Flow Alone

B Object Motion Alone

C Same Directions

D Opposite Directions

250 population
spks/s

50 population
spks/s

Figure 6.4. Population net vectors indicate MSTd's heading estimate. Population net vectors (large black arrows) were derived from single neuron vectors ($n = 107$, small gray lines) for 14 directions and four stimulus types. Accurate population net vectors point directly outward from the spheres indicating the heading direction simulated by that stimulus. Population net vector resultant lengths are larger for optic flow alone (A, 260 spks/s) and matched direction combined stimuli (C, 272 spks/s) than for object motion alone (B, 164 spks/s) and opposite direction combined stimuli (D, 68 spks/s). Data in (D) is aligned to the heading simulated by the optic flow, opposite to the object motion direction.

different from those evoked by optic flow alone ($F_{1,16} = 0.41$, $p = 0.53$) (Figure 6.4C). In marked contrast, responses to opposite direction combined stimuli yield population vector resultant lengths that are much smaller than those evoked by optic flow alone ($F_{1,16} = 195$, $p < 0.0001$) (Figure 6.4D). These results suggest that the influence of object motion on optic flow in combined stimuli depends on the relative heading directions simulated by the combined stimuli. Same direction combined stimuli yield population responses like those obtained with optic flow alone. Opposite direction

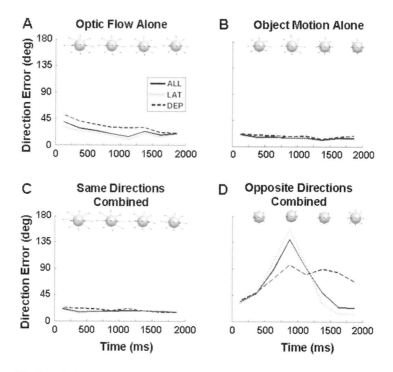

Figure 6.5. Population net vector error across headings for each condition. Ball plots (top) show amplitude and direction of population net vectors from four 500 ms intervals for each condition, as viewed from behind. Line graphs show population net vector heading errors (ordinates) averaged across stimulus heading directions for the eight 250 ms stimulus intervals (abscissa). Optic flow alone (A), object motion alone (B), and same direction combined stimuli (C) show similar patterns of averaged net vector heading error. (D) Opposite direction combined stimuli show significantly greater heading error as the object approaches central vision during the middle response intervals, especially for lateral movement in the frontoparallel plane (light dotted line), as opposed to movement in the horizontal, or depth plane (darker dashed line).

combined stimuli yield responses that are substantially more affected by the addition of object motion, generally yielding less robust net vectors.

We examined the impact of object motion interactions with optic flow across the 2 s period of combined stimulation. We derived population net vectors for eight 250 ms time intervals to compare the four stimulus conditions. We took the difference between the net vector direction evoked by each stimulus and the heading direction simulated by that stimulus and averaged the magnitude of that difference across all heading directions tested to derive an overall population direction error.

Optic flow alone yielded population net vectors having gradually decreasing error with respect to the simulated heading of self-movement during the first half of the 2 s stimuli (Figure 6.5A). Object motion alone yielded population net vectors having larger error with respect to the simulated heading of self-movement that gradually decreased throughout the 2 s stimulus period (Figure 6.5B). Same-direction combined stimuli yielded population net vector responses that were about as accurate as those evoked by optic flow alone (Figure 6.5C). Uniquely, opposite-direction combined stimuli yielded population net vectors having initially low error that increased throughout the first half of the stimuli to decrease during the second half (Figure 6.5d). These changes with opposite-direction combined stimuli represent increasing deviation from the self-movement heading simulated by the optic flow when the object moved in towards central vision (stimulus $\times$ time ANOVA all four conditions $F_{3,383} = 61.21$, $p < 0.016$; all post-hoc comparisons to opposite direction stimuli $p < 0.001$). When the object moved outward from central vision, in the course of lateral movement in the frontoparallel plane, heading error declined to resume its veridical representation of the simulated heading in optic flow (Figure 6.5D "LAT"). This effect was not seen when the object remained in central vision during movement in depth along the horizontal plane (Figure 6.5D "DEP").

6.3.3 Behavioral influences on MSTd neuronal responses to optic flow

The responses to optic flow and object motion demonstrate that MSTd neuronal responses can encode self-movement heading direction in 3-D space. Further, they suggest that dynamic interactions between optic flow and object motion responses create unique response properties that might support the behaviorally critical differentiation of earth-fixed objects versus animate objects. This raises the question of whether the subject's behavioral agenda might influence these responses. To address this issue we manipulated the behavioral relevance of optic flow stimuli in a series of four experiments, each of which included the direct comparison of responses to behaviorally relevant versus irrelevant optic flow (details of this study were presented in Dubin and Duffy, 2007).

In the first experiment, 27% (36/135) of MSTd neurons showed significant differences in their responses to optic flow that was presented as behaviorally relevant cues rather than behaviorally irrelevant cues in the context of an exogenous spatial cueing paradigm (Figure 6.6A, left). Relevant optic flow evoked larger responses than irrelevant optic flow with a magnitude difference of 21% ($p = 0.0006$) based on Gaussian amplitude measures. Relevant optic flow also evoked greater radial center selectivity than irrelevant optic flow with significantly narrower averaged tuning width for the radial center of relevant optic flow (difference of 32%, $p = 0.008$) based on Gaussian tuning width measures (Figure 6.6B, left). We also compared responses to irrelevant optic flow depending on whether it was preceded by a pre-cue that was near to, versus far from, the radial center in the subsequently presented irrelevant optic flow yielded a further remarkable effect (Figure 6.6A, right). This analysis revealed larger responses after pre-cues that were near the location of the subsequent radial center. The magnitude of these effects was comparable to the differences between responses to relevant and irrelevant optic flow. However, the near/far differences were not significant (radial center X near/far interaction $F_{7,450} = 1.0$, $p = 0.43$), likely because the near/far comparisons were based on half as many trials as the relevant/irrelevant comparisons.

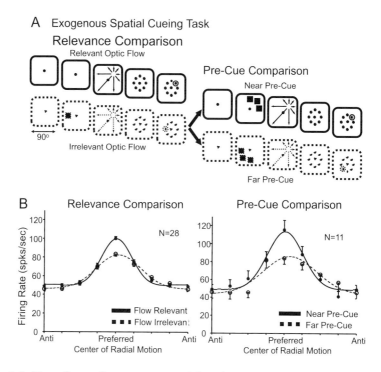

Figure 6.6. The effects of exogenous spatial cueing on neuronal responses. (A) Left: In relevant optic flow trials (red), centered fixation is followed by optic flow visual motion with one of eight eccentric radial centers-of-motion and then an eight spot array requiring a saccade to the remembered location of the radial center. In irrelevant optic flow trials (dashed boxes), a flashed square preceded the optic flow and a saccade was required to the remembered square location. Right: Pre-cue effects were seen in the irrelevant optic flow condition by comparing trials in which the pre-cue was nearby (solid line boxes) versus far from (dashed boxes) the radial center. (B) Left: Average tuning profiles of neurons with significant differences between responses to relevant (solid line) and irrelevant (dashed line) optic flow and with good fits in the relevant and irrelevant conditions. The responses of each neuron were normalized to the amplitude of its largest radial center response. These curves show a larger magnitude (21%) and narrower tuning curve width (32%) in response to relevant optic flow. Right: Average responses of neurons with significant pre-cue proximity effects and with good fits in the near (solid line) and far (dashed line) conditions. There are non-significantly larger responses and narrower tuning to optic flow following pre-cues that were nearer to the subsequent radial center. See CD-ROM for color version.

In the second experiment on behavioral influences on optic flow responses we tested the hypothesis that the larger and more selective responses to relevant versus irrelevant optic flow, seen in experiment 1, might reflect a direct visual effect of pre-cue stimuli presented in different parts of the visual field to mark a subsequent optic flow stimulus as being behaviorally irrelevant. To do so, we used an endogenous spatial cueing paradigm that presented differently shaped pre-cues at the center of the display to mark the subsequent stimulus as irrelevant. In the shape pre-cued trials, the shape of the pre-cue encoded a fixed, learned correspondence to that shape's location as a saccade target in the target array. As in the previously described exogenous spatial cueing experiment, relevant optic flow had one of eight radial centers followed by a target array requiring a saccade to the location of the preceding radial center with four orthogonal alternatives presented in each trial. Pre-cued trials flashed one of four shapes at the center of the screen, followed by behaviorally irrelevant optic flow. The four shapes were then presented in a fixed array, presenting the same familiar arrangement in all irrelevant optic flow trials, and prompting the monkey's saccade to the expected location of the specified target shape (Figure 6.7A).

Significant behavioral effects on optic flow responses were seen in 31% (27/86) of the neurons: in 17% (15/86), the relevance of the optic flow significantly altered the responses; in another 19% (16/86), the distance from the target location implied by the shape pre-cue to the radial center in the optic flow (far versus near) significantly affected the responses. Most MSTd neurons (87%, 27/31) with significant behavioral effects on optic flow responses also yielded significant Gaussian fits to tuning curves for the radial centers. Behavioral effects on the Gaussian fit parameters were in the same direction as those seen with exogenous spatial cueing of experiment 1: responses to relevant optic flow were larger than those to irrelevant optic flow (magnitude difference of 16%, $p = 0.004$) with relevant optic flow yielding greater radial center selectivity (tuning width difference of 18%, $p = 0.03$) (Figure 6.7B, left). The comparison of responses to irrelevant optic flow preceded by shape pre-cues that implied far versus near target locations again yielded somewhat smaller responses in the far pre-cue condition (Figure 6.7B, right), but again these effects did not attain statistical significance (interaction $F_{7, 1520} = 1.65, p = 0.12$).

Shifting from exogenous spatial cueing in experiment 1 to endogenous spatial cueing in experiment 2 resulted in smaller tuning width effects in relevance-irrelevance comparisons and smaller differences between near and far pre-cue trials. In experiment 3 we considered that the impact of pre-cue location, actual or implied, might be assessed by using nonspatial pre-cueing. We created a nonspatial variant of the endogenous cueing task by eliminating the shape pre-cue's learned correspondence to specific target locations. As in both the exogenous and endogenous spatial cueing experiments, relevant optic flow was followed by a target array requiring a saccade to the location of the preceding radial center with four orthogonal alternatives per trial. Pre-cued trials flashed one of four shapes at the center of the screen followed by irrelevant optic flow, and then the four pre-cue shapes in an arrangement that was randomized across trials. In these irrelevant optic flow trials, the monkey's task was to saccade to the shape that had preceded the optic flow. Each of the four shape target arrays appeared with equal probability, dissociating pre-cue shape from location (Figure 6.8A).

Nonspatial pre-cueing resulted in significant effects of behavioral relevance on optic flow responses in 23% (20/88) of the neurons. Most of those neurons (60%, 12/20) also yielded significant Gaussian fits to tuning curves for optic flow. Relevant optic flow evoked larger responses than the irrelevant optic flow (magnitude difference of 25%, $p = 0.002$) without a significant change in radial center selectivity (tuning width difference of 2%, $p = 0.45$) (Figure 6.8B). Since cue location information was not

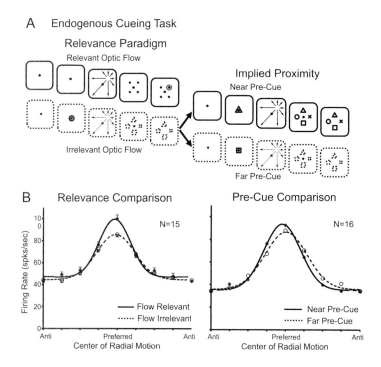

Figure 6.7. The effects of endogenous spatial cueing on neuronal responses. (A) Left: In relevant optic flow trials (solid line boxes), centered fixation is followed by optic flow with one of eight radial centers and then a saccade to the remembered location of the radial center. Four-spot arrays of either cardinal or diagonal targets (diagonal shown) included the radial center used in a given trial so that both relevant and irrelevant trials were four-alternative forced choices. In irrelevant optic flow trials (dashed boxes), a flashed shape (a circle, square, triangle or "x") preceded the irrelevant optic flow and a saccade was required to that shape within an array of targets presented after the optic flow. The four target shapes were always in the same arrangement in this endogenous spatial cueing paradigm. Right: Effects of implied pre-cue proximity were seen in the irrelevant optic flow condition by comparing trials in which the expected pre-cue target location was nearby (solid line boxes) versus far from (dashed boxes) the radial center in the subsequent optic flow. (B) Average tuning profiles of neurons with significant effects of optic flow relevance and with good fits in the relevant and irrelevant conditions. Left: As with exogenous spatial cueing (Figure 6.6B), relevant optic flow (solid line) evoked larger responses (16%) and narrower tuning (18%) than evoked by irrelevant optic flow (dashed line). Right: Average tuning profiles of neurons with significant pre-cue proximity effects and with good fits in the near (solid line) and far (dashed line) conditions. In contrast to the exogenous spatial cueing task (Figure 6.6C), there was no significant difference between averaged responses to optic flow preceded by pre-cues that implied target positions that were near versus far from the radial center.

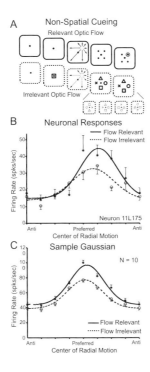

Figure 6.8. The effects of nonspatial endogenous cueing on neuronal responses. (A) In relevant optic flow trials (solid line boxes), centered fixation is followed by optic flow visual motion with one of eight radial centers and then a four-spot array requiring a saccade to the remembered location of the radial center. In irrelevant optic flow trials (dashed boxes), a flashed shape (a circle, square, triangle or "x") preceded the irrelevant optic flow and a saccade was required to that shape within an array of targets presented after the optic flow. In contrast to the endogenous spatial cueing task, the four shape targets were presented in one of four randomly selected arrangements, removing the spatial information in the shape pre-cue. (B) Single neuron responses (mean ± SEM) to optic flow with Gaussian fits to relevant (solid line) and irrelevant (dashed line) optic flow showing larger responses to relevant than irrelevant optic flow. (C) Average tuning profiles of neurons with significant effects of optic flow relevance and with good fits in the relevant and irrelevant conditions. As with exogenous and endogenous spatial cueing, relevant optic flow (solid line) evoked larger responses (25%) than irrelevant optic flow (dashed line). However, there was no significant difference in the width of these tuning curves.

available during optic flow stimulation, no basis for near-far effects was present. Thus, the lack of spatial information in the pre-cue stimuli prevented significant tuning width effect in the comparison of responses to relevant and irrelevant optic flow, suggesting that the spatial information in the pre-cue is required for the tuning width effects.

These three experiments suggest that pre-cueing decreases the size of neuronal responses to subsequent optic flow. In the fourth experiment we tested whether pre-cueing effects might be reversed by manipulating the behavioral significance of the pre-cue. That is, can pre-cues be manipulated so that they increase the size and selectivity of optic flow responses? To do so, we presented a pre-cue that indicated that the subsequent optic flow was behaviorally relevant; that is, it must be used to guide the eye movement response. In these trials, the behaviorally relevant optic flow was preceded by a pre-cue optic flow stimulus. The use of optic flow, rather than a shape, as the spatial pre-cue in relevant optic flow trials avoided confusion with the shape pre-cues presented in irrelevant optic flow trials. The pre-cue optic flow in relevant optic flow trials randomly presented either the same or the opposite radial center as in the subsequent, behaviorally relevant, optic flow (Figure 6.9A).

This relevance cueing experiment yielded 43% (43/101) of the neurons with significant differences between responses to the relevant and irrelevant optic flow, the highest percentage in all of these studies. Most of these neurons (51%, 22/43) also had significant Gaussian fits to tuning curves for the radial center of the optic flow. There were no significant differences between the responses to optic flow presented as a pre-cue before relevant optic flow, nor to responses to the irrelevant optic flow presented in the shaped pre-cued trials, neither of which required a behavioral response. In contrast, responses to relevant optic flow were substantially larger than responses to the shape pre-cued irrelevant optic flow. Averaged responses to pre-cue optic flow were not significantly larger (3%, $p = 0.28$) than responses to irrelevant optic flow in shape pre-cued trials, but the pre-cue optic flow did show significantly narrower tuning width (35%, $p = 0.006$) (Figure 6.9B). This narrowing of tuning width for the radial center in optic flow was not associated with a difference in responses to the relevant optic flow that followed same versus opposite radial centers in the pre-cue versus relevant optic flow comparison (Figure 6.9C).

These four studies suggest that a behaviorally relevant pre-cue can lead to either smaller or larger optic flow responses depending on the associated behavioral contingencies. Optic flow evokes larger and more selective responses when it must be used to guide behavior. Behaviorally irrelevant optic flow yields larger and more selective responses when the pre-cue that marks it as irrelevant happens to be near the subsequent radial center of optic flow.

6.3.4 The influences of dynamic motor control on optic flow responses

We tested whether engaging the monkey in an active steering task, one in which it controlled the simulated heading direction, altered MSTd neuronal responses to optic flow (details of this study were presented in Page and Duffy, 2008). All trials began with optic flow appearing with a radial center of motion at one of eight eccentric positions. In active steering trials, the monkey used a joystick to move the radial center of motion toward the centered fixation point (Figure 6.10). In passive viewing trials, the monkey released the joystick and viewed a replay of the optic flow seen during active steering.

To our surprise, we found that passive viewing yielded larger responses than active steering (Figure 6.11). After subtracting the baseline activity, recorded during fixation before stimulus onset, responsive neurons showed an average of 77% larger peak

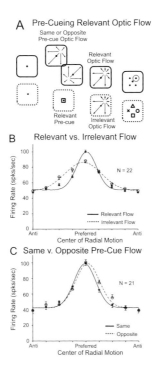

Figure 6.9. The effects of spatial cueing of relevant optic flow on neuronal responses. (A) In relevant optic flow trials (solid line boxes), centered fixation is followed by optic flow with one of eight radial centers and then the random selection of a second optic flow with either the same radial center or the radial center on the opposite side of the fixation point. The irrelevant optic flow trials (blue) are the same as those in the non-spatial paradigm (Figure 6.8A). Averaged responses to the spatial cueing of relevant optic flow. (B) Average responses of neurons with significant differences between tuning curves to relevant (solid line) versus irrelevant (dashed line) optic flow and with good fits in the relevant and irrelevant conditions. There is both substantially larger magnitude (15%) and substantially narrower tuning width (45%) with relevant (solid line) versus irrelevant (dashed line) optic flow. (C) Average responses of neurons with significant differences between tuning curves to relevant versus irrelevant optic flow and with good fits in the same and opposite conditions. Comparison of responses to relevant optic flow when it was preceded by pre-cue optic flow having the same (solid line) versus the opposite (dashed line) radial center. There are no significant differences of magnitude or tuning width between these response profiles. See CD-ROM for color version.

responses in passive viewing trials compared with active steering trials in the 500–1000 ms stimulus interval.

Finding smaller optic flow responses during active steering prompted us to consider how the monkeys might be performing the steering by optic flow task. In particular, whether the smaller responses during active steering might reflect the monkeys using

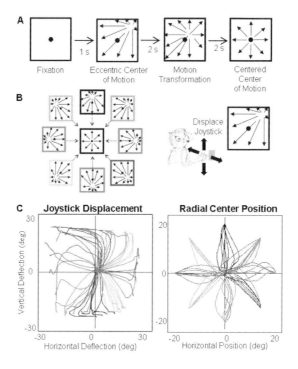

Figure 6.10. Behavioral paradigm for comparing optic-flow responses during active steering and passive viewing. (A–B) Following centered fixation 1 of 8 eccentric radial center of motion, optic-flow stimulus was actively moved to the center of the screen or the same visual stimuli were replayed during passive viewing. The monkey maintained centered fixation in all trials. In active-steering trials, the monkey used horizontal and vertical joystick displacement to control the movement of the radial center of motion. (C) Left: Averaged traces from trials recorded in six studies showing the joystick deflection during the first 1s of active steering. Joystick deflection added a vector of corresponding direction and magnitude to alter the simulated heading in the optic-flow display. Right: Corresponding screen positions of the radial center of motion over the complete 4-s stimulus. See CD-ROM for color version.

local motion cues in the optic flow rather than the global pattern of optic flow for which MSTd neurons are specialized. We tested this hypothesis by changing the stimuli presented during the active steering task in a manner that ambiguated local motion cues in the optic flow by randomly interleaving trials presenting inward or outward radial patterns. Interleaved inward and outward optic flow makes local motion ambiguous. For example, leftward pericentral local motion is seen with outward optic flow having a right-sided center of motion (Figure 6.12A, left) and with inward optic flow having a left-sided center of motion (Figure 6.12B, left).

When we first presented interleaved inward and outward radial motion stimuli, both monkeys made 100% errors in inward optic flow trials, uniformly moving the joystick in the opposite direction required to move the center of motion toward the fixation

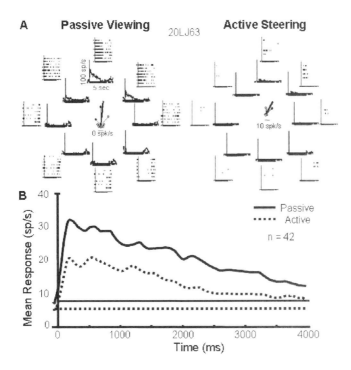

Figure 6.11. MSTd neuronal responses to optic flow during active steering and passive viewing. (A) Spike raster plots (outer ring), spike-density histograms (SDHs, inner ring), and polar plots (center) of responses to the eight centers of motion stimuli in passive-viewing (left) and active-steering (right) trials for one MSTd neuron. Horizontal bars indicate the 4-s stimulus period along with 500 ms pre- and post-stimulus intervals. (B) Responses to preferred radial center of motion stimuli averaged across all neurons in the passive-viewing (blue line) and active-steering (active line) trials. Passive viewing trials yielded larger responses than active steering with decreasing response amplitude in both test conditions as the radial center of motion deviated from its eccentric position to the center of the screen. Dashed lines indicate average baseline activity level. See CD-ROM for color version.

point. We then retrained the monkeys to use the global radial motion cues in optic flow (Figure 6.12C). After retraining with interleaved inward and outward radial optic flow, emphasizing steering by the global pattern of motion, the monkeys showed longer (t-test, $p = 0.004$) average joystick response latencies (297 ± 14 ms) than in the preceding study (273 ± 10 ms).

We repeated recording MSTd neuronal responses to optic flow using interleaved active steering and passive viewing trials with interleaved inward and outward radial motion under both conditions. To compare these results with those of the previous study we used only outward radial trials in the analysis of the neuronal responses to optic flow. In these studies, many MSTd neurons showed substantially stronger optic flow responses during active steering trials (Figure 6.13). Most neurons (78%, 31/40)

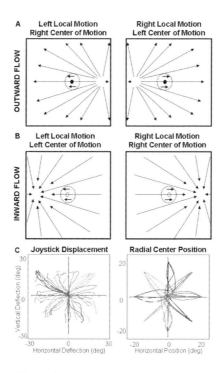

Figure 6.12. Stimuli and behavioral responses in active-steering trials presented after retraining to use the global pattern of visual motion in optic flow. (A and B). Global pattern of optic flow uniquely specifies the radial center of motion in outward (A) or inward (B) radial stimuli. Local motion around the centered fixation point is ambiguous with respect to the location of the radial center of motion in interleaved outward and inward optic flow. (C) Analog traces of the first 1s of the monkey's 2-D joystick deflections (left) and of the 4 s of radial center of motion stimulus presentation (right) for each center of motion stimulus (colors as in Figure 6.10C) averaged across the trials in six separate studies. See CD-ROM for color version.

showed significant responses ($p < 0.05$) to radial optic flow in either the active or passive condition, or both. After subtracting baseline activity, these neurons showed an average of 159% larger peak responses (500 ± 1000 ms after stimulus onset) during active steering versus passive viewing, the opposite of the previous result in which the monkey might have used only local motion cues.

We directly compared neuronal responses obtained in the active steering and passive viewing conditions for neurons recorded before (n = 42) and after (n = 31) we retrained the monkeys to use the global pattern of visual motion. A two-way ANOVA of averaged neuronal firing rates during the second 500 ms of each stimulus (500–1000 ms after stimulus onset) had a between-subjects variable of local versus global condition (before and after retraining) and repeated measures variables of active steering versus passive viewing and of the eight initial radial center of motion locations (simulated heading directions). We found significant interactions between active steering versus

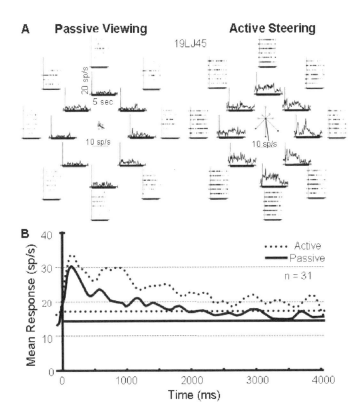

Figure 6.13. Active steering evokes larger responses than passive viewing when using the global pattern of optic flow for steering. (A) Responses of a single MSTd neuron to outward radial optic flow (format as in Figure 6.11A) in passive-viewing (left) and active-steering (right) trials after the monkeys were trained on interleaved inward and outward radial optic flow. This neuron shows larger responses in the active-steering trials than in the passive-viewing trials. (B) Responses to preferred outward radial center of motion stimuli after retraining averaged across all neurons in the passive-viewing (solid line) and active-steering (dashed line) trials. Active-steering trials yielded larger responses than passive-viewing trials, again with decreasing response amplitude as the radial center of motion approaches the center of the screen. Dashed lines indicate average baseline activity level.

passive viewing across the local (before retraining) versus global (after retraining) conditions ($F_{1,71} = 5.67$, $p = 0.02$).

Comparing Gaussian fits with the radial center of motion tuning curves, averaged across neurons in the active and passive trials, revealed other effects of these changes in experimental conditions. In this first study the Gaussian parameters (active vs. passive: mean $\pm$ confidence interval, p value from t-test) yielded higher amplitude (15.6 ± 0.10 vs. 19.1 ± 0.08 spks/s, $p = 0.0001$) and baseline (8.5 ± 0.07 vs. 9.4 ± 0.06 spks/s, $p = 0.039$) measures in the passive condition, with non-significantly broader tuning

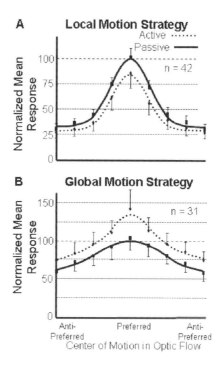

Figure 6.14. Averaged firing rate across all neurons in the passive-viewing (solid line) and active-steering (dashed line) trials during the 500 to 1000 ms interval after optic flow onset. (A) Gaussian fits to center of motion response curve for passive and active trials from the first study averaged across neurons with significant differences between active and passive trials (n = 31). (B) Gaussian fits to center of motion tuning curves from the second study averaged across neurons with significant differences between active and passive trials shows larger responses in the active-steering condition.

width in passive trials (0.95 ± 0.09 vs. 1.04 ± 0.07 spks/s, $p = 0.16$). The preferred heading did not change across conditions (Figure 6.14A).

In the second study, after retraining with interleaved inward and outward radial optic flow, the Gaussian fits showed a nonsignificantly larger amplitude during active steering (11.8 ± 0.23 vs. 10.1 ± 0.31 spks/s, $p = 0.067$) with a significantly larger baseline during active steering (17.4 ± 0.07 vs. 11.4 ± 0.14 spks/s, $p < 0.0001$) and a significantly sharper tuning width in active steering trials (1.12 ± 0.20 vs. 2.04 ± 0.18 spks/s, $p = 0.0002$). Again, the preferred heading across conditions did not change appreciably (Figure 6.14B).

These findings support the view that training the monkeys to use the global pattern of motion significantly changed the relationship between responses to radial optic flow during active steering and passive viewing. Using local motion, the passive viewing trials yielded significantly stronger responses with significant amplitude and baseline effects. Using global patterns, the active steering trials yielded significantly stronger responses with significant tuning width and baseline effects.

6.4 Discussion

Cortical area MSTd occupies a central position in the dorsal extrastriate visual pathway (Mishkin et al., 1983; Ungerleider and Desimone, 1986) containing neurons that respond to optic flow (Tanaka et al., 1986; Tanaka and Saito, 1989; Duffy and Wurtz, 1991; Orban et al., 1992; Graziano et al., 1994) with selectivity for the simulated heading of self-movement (Duffy and Wurtz, 1995; Lappe et al., 1996).

6.4.1 3-D self-movement perception

We find that MSTd neurons access self-movement cues in both optic flow and object motion, with similar preferred 3-D heading directions in response to both types of stimuli. The isotropic distribution of single neuron preferred headings in 3-D space suggest that a balanced neuronal population might facilitate unbiased heading estimation. In the context of a distributed representation of 3-D headings in MSTd it might be considered surprising that we do not find evidence for a topographic organization of heading preferences. Microstimulation has demonstrated that local activation can result in systematic changes in the perception of simulated headings (Britten and van Wezel, 1998). However, those findings can be interpreted as suggesting local homogeneity that does not demand the existence of a large-scale patterned arrangement of neuronal properties across an area.

MSTd's neuronal population responses to optic flow are not substantially altered by the addition of object motion that simulates the same heading direction. This is consistent with the finding that same direction optic flow and object motion does not substantially alter human heading estimation (Royden and Hildreth, 1996). A different circumstance arises with object motion that does not match that simulated in superimposed optic flow, which induces dramatic changes in population estimation of heading from the superimposed optic flow. This too is consistent with human psychophysical findings of superimposed animate objects disrupting heading estimation (Royden and Hildreth, 1996; Royden, 2002). Thus, our studies suggest that MSTd receptive fields form a neural infrastructure that may shape perceptual performance characteristics with respect to self-movement perception and the detection of independently moving objects.

6.4.2 Behavioral relevance enhances optic flow responses

We manipulated the behavioral relevance of optic flow stimuli in four behavioral paradigms: (1) Exogenous spatial pre-cueing of irrelevant optic flow by a spot flashed at one of eight locations yielded responses to subsequently presented optic flow that were 21% smaller than the responses evoked by relevant optic flow in 27% of the neurons. (2) Endogenous spatial pre-cueing of irrelevant optic flow by centrally placed shapes indicating the location of target stimuli yielded responses that were 16% smaller than those evoked by relevant optic flow in 31% of the neurons. (3) Nonspatial precueing of irrelevant optic flow by shape stimuli indicating the shape of target stimuli yielded responses that were 25% smaller than those evoked by relevant optic flow in 23% of the neurons. (4) The nonspatial pre-cueing of irrelevant optic flow combined with the spatial pre-cueing of relevant optic flow yielded a net effect of 15% larger responses to relevant optic flow in 43% of the neurons. These findings led us to conclude that behaviorally relevant optic flow yields larger responses than behaviorally irrelevant optic flow, regardless of how the relevance of the optic flow is signaled.

Studies of dorsal (Bushnell et al., 1981) and ventral (Fuster and Jervey, 1982; Reynolds et al., 1999) stream neurons have linked the behavioral relevance of stimuli within a neuron's receptive field to spatial attention. Attentional modulation may enhance MT and MST neuronal responses to local motion (Treue and Maunsell, 1996) in a manner consistent with multiplicative gain effects without changes in the selectivity of the responses (Treue and Martinez-Trujillo, 1999). Such gain effects might underlie the response amplitude changes in our studies when behavioral relevance focuses attention on optic flow.

The sharpening of heading tuning effects for behaviorally relevant optic flow successively declined from 32% narrower tuning with exogenous spatial cueing, to 18% with endogenous spatial cueing, to only a 1% effect with nonspatial cueing. This suggest that tuning effects are linked to the strength of spatial information in the pre-cues, effects that may be mediated by a stored representation of the pre-cued location on optic flow heading selectivity. The remembered pre-cue location could interact with MSTd neurons to enhance responses encoding radial centers near that location or suppress responses to radial centers far from that location. This is consistent with the near-far pre-cue proximity effects seen in the exogenous and endogenous pre-cueing experiments that resulted in significant tuning width effects. Top-down response modulation by a stored representation of the pre-cued location might have different effects than competing stimuli which do not show effects of stimulus proximity (Seidemann and Newsome, 1999).

Combining the nonspatial paradigm with the addition of an optic flow pre-cue in the behaviorally relevant optic flow trials enhanced the narrowing of heading tuning for the optic flow pre-cue by 35% and for relevant optic flow by 45%. This may be because the random presentation of valid and invalid pre-cues increases the spatial demands of the task to result in substantially narrower tuning curves. In the current context, the main point is that alterations in the behaviorally relevant trials can result in the same types of tuning effects as seen in the other experiments with alterations in the behaviorally irrelevant trials.

All four studies of behavioral influences on optic flow responses suggest that response magnitude and tuning width effects are independent. In the first three studies magnitude increases of 21%, 16%, and 25% were seen with width decreases of 32%, 18%, and 2%; this shows no systematic relationship. In the fourth study, the spatial pre-cueing of relevant optic flow resulted in magnitude increases of 3% for pre-cue optic flow and of 15% for relevant optic flow with decreases in tuning width of 35% and 45%. Thus, neither the direction nor the size of magnitude effects were linked to tuning width effects, even in responses from the same neurons with comparisons from within the same trials.

The effects of behavioral relevance on the amplitude of optic flow responses showed relevant optic flow evoking larger responses than irrelevant optic flow in all four experiments. This may reflect the activation of a neuronal population devoted to a particular task in a manner consistent with the multiplicative gain control of responses (Treue and Maunsell, 1996), in this case activating MST when the task requires optic flow heading discrimination. In contrast, task effects on tuning width for the heading of self-movement in optic flow were linked to spatial information in the competing task: exogenous spatial cues evoked stronger tuning effects than endogenous spatial cues, which evoked stronger effects than non-spatial cues. This may reflect the differential activation of neurons within a population to represent a particular stimulus attribute, possibly by engaging local competitive interactions within that population (Reynolds et al., 1999), in this case favoring MST neurons devoted to a particular heading direction.

Thus, behavioral context induces amplitude and tuning effects in MST related to demands placed on optic flow analysis and the spatial attributes of the task. The dissociable effects of behavior on response amplitude and tuning are consistent with separate top-down influences on MST that are responsible for interareal activation linked to response amplitude modulation and intraareal activation linked to tuning width modulation.

6.4.3   Task effects on optic flow analysis

We engaged trained monkeys in an active steering task that required them to use optic flow to guide manual responses. Finding smaller neuronal responses during active steering was unexpected, especially in the context of the many studies demonstrating increased visual cortical neuronal activity during attentive fixation to visual stimuli (Lynch et al., 1977; Bushnell et al., 1981; Moran and Desimone, 1985) and heightened neuronal excitability when attention was focused on the receptive field of neurons being studied either in area MSTd or adjacent MT cortex (Treue and Maunsell, 1996; Seidemann and Newsome, 1999; Cook and Maunsell, 2002).

We considered the hypothesis that MSTd neuronal responses to optic flow were reduced because the monkey was not using the global pattern of optic flow to guide its steering behavior, possibly relying on local motion cues instead. Our previous psychophysical work had suggested that interleaving inward and outward optic flow stimuli forces observers to use the global pattern of motion to make decisions about the simulated heading direction (O'Brien et al., 2001). We reasoned that if the monkey had learned to ignore the global pattern of optic flow, in favor of a reliance on local motion cues, then the presentation of inward and outward patterns would present ambiguous stimuli: right center of motion outward flow contains the same central local motion as left center of motion inward flow. Initially, the monkeys consistently made errors suggesting that they were using local motion cues. After retraining the monkeys so that they would use global motion, we repeated the neurophysiological studies and found that the effects of active steering had been reversed; active steering now enhanced neuronal responses instead of suppressing them.

These observations support the view that learned stimulus-response associations can alter the relationship between neuronal activity and behavioral tasks. Specifically, MSTd neuronal responses to identical optic flow stimuli depend on the monkeys' perceptual strategy for using visual information to control steering. However, these data were not recorded in the same neurons so we could not resolve whether local and global strategies might change the effects of active steering in individual neurons or might engage different groups of neurons.

Differences in neuronal activity during local motion and radial pattern steering might reflect receptive field organization interactions with attentional mechanisms. Optic flow's simultaneous stimulation of the central and peripheral visual field might promote competitive interactions between neurons having different receptive field structures (Moran and Desimone, 1985; Spitzer et al., 1988; Reynolds et al., 1999). Competitive interactions in MSTd might be modulated by top-down signals that tip the balance in favor of a particular segment of the receptive field. A related phenomenon, or at least an apt analogy, might be seen in the effects of frontal micro-stimulation on receptive field specific activation of V4 neurons, an effect that is thought of as being linked to spatial attention (Armstrong et al., 2006). Such mechanisms might contribute to activating MSTd neurons with receptive fields overlapping the attended segment of the visual field.

Acknowledgments

We gratefully acknowledge the assistance of William Vaughn, Jennifer Postle and Sherry Estes in this research and artwork by Teresa Steffenella. We thank Drs. Roberto Fernandez, Michael T. Froehler, and Voyko Kavcic as well as William Vaughn for comments on the manuscript. This work was supported by EY10287 from the NEI to cjd. Address correspondence to Dr. Charles Duffy, Dept. of Neurology, Univ. of Rochester Medical Center, Rochester, New York, 14642–0673.

References

Banks, M. S., Sekuler, A. B. and Anderson, S. J. (1991). Peripheral spatial vision: limits imposed by optics, photoreceptors, and receptor pooling. *J. Opt. Soc. Am. A*, 8: 1775–1787.

Bradley, D. C., Maxwell, M., Andersen, R. A., Banks, M. S. and Shenoy, K. V. (1996). Mechanisms of heading perception in primate visual cortex. *Science*, 273: 1544–1549.

Britten, K. H. and van Wezel, R. J. (1998). Electrical microstimulation of cortical area MST biases heading perception in monkeys. *Nature Neurosci.*, 1: 59–63.

Bushnell, M. C., Goldberg, M. E. and Robinson, D. L. (1981). Behavioral enhancement of visual responses in monkey cerebral cortex. I. Modulation in posterior parietal cortex related to selective visual attention. *J. Neurophysiol.*, 46: 755–772.

Cook, E. P. and Maunsell, J. H. (2002). Attentional modulation of behavioral performance and neuronal responses in middle temporal and ventral intraparietal areas of macaque monkey. *J. Neurosci.*, 22: 1994–2004.

Crist, C. F., Yamasaki, D. S., Komatsu, H. and Wurtz, R. H. (1988). A grid system and a microsyringe for single cell recordings. *J. Neurosci. Meth.*, 26: 117–122.

Dubin, M. J. and Duffy, C. J. (2007). Behavioral influences on cortical neuronal responses to optic flow. *Cereb. Cortex*, 17: 1722–1732.

Duffy, C. J. and Wurtz, R. H. (1991). Sensitivity of MST neurons to optic flow stimuli. I. A continuum of response selectivity to large-field stimuli. *J. Neurophysiol.*, 65: 1329–1345.

Duffy, C. J. and Wurtz, R. H. (1995). Response of monkey MST neurons to optic flow stimuli with shifted centers of motion. *J. Neurosci.*, 15: 5192–5208.

Fisher, N. I., Lewis, T. and Embleton, B. J. J. (1987). *Statistical Analysis of Spherical Data*. Cambridge, UK: Cambridge University Press.

Fuster, J. M. and Jervey, J. P. (1982). Neuronal firing in the inferotemporal cortex of the monkey in a visual memory task. *J. Neurosci.*, 2: 361–375.

Georgopoulos, A. P., Schwartz, A. B. and Kettner, R. E. (1986). Neuronal population coding of movement direction. *Science*, 233: 1416–1419.

Graziano, M. S. A., Andersen, R. A. and Snowden, R. J. (1994). Tuning of MST neurons to spiral motion. *J. Neurosci.*, 14: 54–67.

Hays, A. V., Richmond, B. J. and Optican, L. M. (1982). A UNIX-based multiple process system for real-time data acquisition and control. *WESCON Conference Proceedings*, 2: 1–10.

Judge, S. J., Richmond, B. J. and Chu, F. C. (1980). Implantation of magnetic search coils for measurement of eye position: an improved method. *Vision Res.*, 20: 535–538.

Komatsu, H. and Wurtz, R. H. (1988). Relation of cortical areas MT and MST to pursuit eye movements. I. Localization and visual properties of neurons. *J. Neurophysiol.*, 60: 580–603.

Lappe, M., Bremmer, F., Pekel, M., Thiele, A. Hoffmann, K. P. (1996). Optic flow processing in monkey STS: a theoretical and experimental approach. *J. Neurosci.*, 16: 6265–6285.

Logan, D. J. and Duffy, C. J. (2006). Cortical area MSTd combines visual cues to represent 3-D self-movement. *Cereb. Cortex*, 16: 1494–1507.

Lynch, J. C., Mountcastle, V. B., Talbot, W. H. and Yin, T. C. (1977). Parietal lobe mechanisms for directed visual attention. *J. Neurophysiol.*, 40: 362–389.

McAdams, C. J. and Maunsell, J. H. (1999). Effects of attention on orientation-tuning functions of single neurons in macaque cortical area V4. *J. Neurosci.*, 19: 431–441.

Mishkin, M., Ungerleider, L. G. and Macko, K. A. (1983). Object vision and spatial vision: two cortical pathways. *Trends Neurosci.*, 6: 414–417.

Moran, J. and Desimone, R. (1985). Selective attention gates visual processing in the extrastriate cortex. *Science*, 229: 782–784.

O'Brien, H. L., Tetewsky, S., Avery, L. M., Cushman, L. A., Makous, W. and Duffy, C. J. (2001). Visual mechanisms of spatial disorientation in alzheimer's disease Cereb. Cortex, 11: 1083–1092.

Orban, G. A., Lagae, L., Verri, A., Raiguel, S., Xiao, D., Maes, H. and Torre, V. (1992). First-order analysis of optical flow in monkey brain. *Proc. Nat. Acad. Sci.*, 89: 2595–2599.

Page, W. K. and Duffy, C. J. (2008). Cortical neuronal responses to optic flow are shaped by visual strategies for steering. *Cereb. Cortex*, 18: 727–739.

Page, W. K., King, W. M., Merigan, W. H. and Maunsell, J. H. R. (1993). Magnocellular or parvocellular lesions in the lateral geniculate nucleus of monkeys cause minor deficits of smooth pursuit eye movements. *Vision Res.*, 34: 223–239.

Reynolds, J. H., Chelazzi, L. Desimone, R. (1999). Competitive mechanisms subserve attention in macaque areas V2 and V4. *J. Neurosci.*, 19: 1736–1753.

Royden, C. S. (2002). Computing heading in the presence of moving objects: a model that uses motion-opponent operators. *Vision Res.*, 62: 3043–3058.

Royden, C. S. and Hildreth, E. C. (1996). Human heading judgments in the presence of moving objects. *Percept. Psychophys.*, 58: 836–856.

Seidemann, E. and Newsome, W. T. (1999). Effect of spatial attention on the responses of area MT neurons. *J. Neurophysiol.*, 81: 1783–1794.

Spitzer, H., Desimone, R. and Moran, J. (1988). Increased attention enhances both behavioral and neuronal performance. *Science*, 240: 338–340.

Tanaka, K. and Saito, H. (1989). Analysis of motion of the visual field by direction, expansion/contraction, and rotation cells clustered in the dorsal part of the medial superior temporal area of the macaque monkey. *J. Neurophysiol.*, 62: 626–641.

Tanaka, K., Hikosaka, K., Saito, H., Yukie, M., Fukada, Y. and Iwai, E. (1986). Analysis of local and wide-field movements in the superior temporal visual areas of the macaque monkey. *J. Neurosci.*, 6: 134–144.

Treue, S. and Martinez-Trujillo, J. C. (1999). Feature-based attention influences motion processing gain in macaque visual cortex. *Nature*, 399: 575–579.

Treue, S. and Maunsell, J. H. (1996). Attentional modulation of visual motion processing in cortical areas MT and MST. *Nature*, 382: 539–541.

Ungerleider, L. G. and Desimone, R. (1986). Projections to the superior temporal sulcus from the central and peripheral field representations of V1 and V2. *J. Comp. Neurol.*, 248: 147–163.

Warren Jr., W. H., Kim, E. E. and Husney, R. (1987). The way the ball bounces: visual and auditory perception of elasticity and control of the bounce pass. *Perception*, 16: 309–336.

Part II

Ventral stream

7 Differential development of the human ventral stream

K. Grill-Spector and
G. Golarai

The human visual cortex has been extensively studied in adults. More than a dozen visual areas have been identified based on their retinotopic organization[1] and functional selectivity[2] (Grill-Spector and Malach, 2004; Wandell et al., 2005). Visual cortex includes a hierarchy of regions, beginning with early visual areas, which are delineated based on their retinotopic organization, and then ascends into high-level visual cortex which displays weaker retinotopy (Grill-Spector et al., 1998; Levy et al., 2001) and higher stimulus selectivity such as selective responses to objects, faces and places (Malach et al., 1995; Kanwisher et al., 1997; Epstein and Kanwisher, 1998). Functional magnetic resonance imaging (fMRI) studies in adults reveal that these retinotopic maps and selective regions can be reliably detected within individual subjects and are remarkably consistent across people in their spatial characteristics. However, several key questions remain. It is unknown how the selectivity of visual regions comes about, when the visual cortex reaches maturity and what the relation is between cortical maturation and proficiency in various visual tasks.

Retinotopic map – A topographic map in which two adjacent points on the retina (or the visual field, if the subject maintains fixation) map into adjacent points on the cortex. The human visual cortex contains multiple retinotopic maps. For example, each of the lower visual areas V1, V2, V3, V3a and hV4 contains a hemifield representation in each hemisphere. Thus, each of these areas contains a topographic map of the entire visual field.

Selectivity – Differential responses to specific visual stimuli. Selective regions as measured with fMRI refer to cortical regions that respond significantly more to some stimuli over other stimuli, usually determined via a statistical criterion.

Cortical Mechanisms of Vision, ed. M. Jenkin and L. R. Harris. Published by Cambridge University Press.

7.1 Behavioral investigations of the development of perception

Behavioral measurements have established that the visual system continues to develop for several years postnatally. Although the largest changes occur in the first year of life, some aspects of vision require many years of visual experience to reach an adult-like state. Until age 6 or 7 there are significant improvements in visual proficiency in tasks involving second-order motion (Ellemberg et al., 2004), form-from-motion (Parrish et al., 2005), grating acuity discrimination (Ellemberg et al., 1999), and orientation discrimination (Lewis et al., 2007).

More striking, a significant body of research has documented the particularly slow development of face perception and recognition memory[3] which reportedly reach the adult level only around age 16. Although there is evidence that newborn infants preferentially attend to faces (Johnson et al., 1991), it is well documented that face recognition undergoes a prolonged development before reaching the adult level (Ellis, 1975; Carey, 1992; Mondloch et al., 2003). Face recognition memory dramatically increases between 6 and 16 years of age. Among children aged 6–14 face recognition memory consistently ranges from 50 to 70% of the adult level, with slow gains after age 16 (Carey, 1981). Even in matching tasks, which eliminate memory demands, performance improves dramatically between 4 and 11 years of age (Bruce et al., 2000; Mondloch et al., 2003).

What is much less agreed upon is whether or not there is a qualitative difference in the way that children and adults recognize faces. One extensively studied marker of "expertise" is the face inversion effect (FIE,[4] Yin, 1969). Inversion is thought to disrupt holistic processing of faces.[5] (However, a recent computational model showed that the FIE can occur in a hierarchical architecture with nonlinear summation and without explicit holistic computations Jiang et al., 2006.) In their original study Carey and Diamond (1977) reported no FIE in children in contrast to adults. Therefore, they proposed a developmental model involving a qualitative difference between children and adults' face processing, where children process face information in a more piecemeal manner than adults who process faces holistically. However, in their subsequent studies Carey and Diamond (1994) found the FIE in young children. More recently other investigators found the FIE in children as young as 4 or 5 (Mondloch et al., 2002; Pellicano and Rhodes, 2003; Sangrigoli and de Schonen, 2004). Additional evidence for holistic processing of faces in children include reports of children's better recognition of

---

[3]Recognition memory – Describes a behavioral paradigm consisting of a study phase and test phase. In the study phase a subject is shown a sequence of stimuli. Later (minutes or days) the subject participates in the test phase and is shown some stimuli which he/she saw during the study phase and some stimuli which are new. The subject's task is to report on each test stimulus whether it is old (seen it before) or new (has not seen it before).

[4]FIE – Face Inversion Effect. Recognition of faces is disproportionally impaired for inverted faces. The FIE is thought to impair both holistic and configural processing of faces.

[5]Holistic processing of faces – Reflects the idea that the perception of the whole is more than the perception of the sum of its parts. Tasks showing holistic processing of faces report that the recognition memory for a face part (e.g. Harry's nose) in isolation is worse than when it is in a face. In other words, recognition of a face part is affected by the context (i.e. if it is part of a face or disjointed from a face).

Stimuli:
900 ms/image

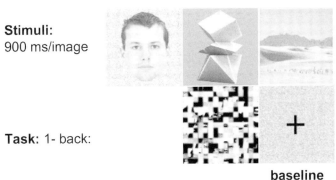

Task: 1- back:

baseline

Figure 7.1. Experimental Design. Twenty children (7–11 years old), ten adolescents (12–16 years old) and 15 adults (18–35 years old) participated in this study. During fMRI subjects viewed 60 grayscale photographic images of faces, abstract sculptures (objects), indoor and outdoor scenes, and textures (created by randomly scrambling object pictures into 225, 8 × 8 pixel squares). Each stimulus type was presented during five pseudo-randomly ordered blocks. Blocks were 14 s long followed by 14 s of fixation. Images were presented at 1 s intervals, each for 970 ms, followed by a 30 ms fixation baseline. Each image was presented only once, except for two random images per block, which were presented twice in succession. Subjects were instructed to fixate on each image and press a button using their right index finger whenever they detected identical images appearing successively (a one-back task).

face parts when presented within a face than in isolation (Pellicano and Rhodes, 2003) and evidence that children's performance on composite faces is similar to adults (de Heering et al., 2007). Taken together, there is substantial evidence for holistic processing of faces in children, suggesting that the development of face processing involves quantitative, rather than qualitative changes.

Another debate surrounds differences in configural processing of faces[6] across development. One hypothesis suggests that children are particularly impaired at configural processing, but not feature processing (Mondloch et al., 2002). However, others provide evidence for configural processing of faces even in 4 year olds (McKone and Boyer, 2006).

---

[6]Configural processing of faces – Processing of the second-order relation between face parts, such as spacing between eyes or spacing between the mouth and nose.

7.2 Developmental neuroimaging is critical for revealing the neural changes underlying the development of perception

Behavioral studies have revealed important clues regarding the developmental time course of visual processes in humans. However, we know very little about how brain changes during development relate to behavioral improvements in perception. Neuroimaging methods are critical for understanding the neural substrates of this development. Developmental neuroimaging studies allow tracking changes in brain anatomy with MRI (Giedd et al., 1999; Gogtay et al., 2004; Sowell et al., 2004), brain function with fMRI, and connectivity using DTI[7] (Dougherty et al., 2005). These methods are noninvasive and permit repeated scanning of the same individual over time. Longitudinal studies may allow more precise measurements of anatomical and functional maturation than cross-sectional studies (Giedd et al., 1999).

A substantial body of neuroscience research in animals has revealed the role of experience in shaping cortical function during critical periods of development (Wiesel and Hubel, 1965; Shatz and Stryker, 1978; Antonini and Stryker, 1993; Dragoi et al., 2001) and several forms of cortical plasticity following prolonged experience in adulthood (Logothetis et al., 1995; Kobatake et al., 1998; Baker et al., 2002; Sigala and Logothetis, 2002; Rainer et al., 2004; Freedman et al., 2006). This research has emphasized the role of visual experience in combination with genetic factors in the development and plasticity of the visual cortex. However, much less is known about the neural correlates of development in human ventral stream and whether there are critical temporal windows for development.

Recently, several laboratories used fMRI in children and adolescents to study the development of visual cortex including retinotopic organization in early visual cortex (Conner et al., 2004), contrast sensitivity in MT, V3a and V1 (Ben-Shachar et al., 2007), functional organization of high-level visual areas involved in face processing (Gathers et al., 2004; Aylward et al., 2005; Golarai et al., 2007; Passarotti et al., 2007; Scherf et al., 2007), place processing (Golarai et al., 2007; Scherf et al., 2007) and object processing (Golarai et al., 2007; Scherf et al., 2007). Results of these studies suggest that retinotopic maps in V1, V2, V3, V3a and contrast sensitivity in MT reach an adult-like state by age 7. In contrast, face (Gathers et al., 2004; Aylward et al., 2005; Golarai et al., 2007; Passarotti et al., 2007; Scherf et al., 2007) and place-selective cortex (Golarai et al., 2007) follow a much slower developmental trajectory and continue to mature after age 7, in correlation with age dependent improvements in recognition memory for faces (Golarai et al., 2007) and places (Golarai et al., 2007) and increased specialization in processing faces (Passarotti et al., 2007).

---

[7]DTI - Diffusion Tensor Imaging is a magnetic resonance imaging technique that enables the measurement of the restricted diffusion of water in tissue. DTI is used to measure the isotropy of water diffusion due to white matter structures. Therefore, it is used to measure and visualize fiber tracks.

7.3 fMRI measurements of the development of the human ventral stream

When considering the development of the ventral stream we hypothesize that functional specialization emerges slowly during childhood with accumulated experience. The emerging functional specialization during development may manifest in several ways with fMRI. One possibility is that the spatial extent of selective regions changes across development (e.g. the size of face-selective regions may be smaller in children than adults). This change in spatial extent may be coupled with an increase in the number of selective neurons and/or an increase in their selectivity. Another possibility is that the spatial extent of selective regions is similar across children and adults, but experience changes the magnitude of response (e.g. the size of face-selective regions is similar across children and adults, but the response to faces is higher in adults than children). A third alternative is that development changes the distributed pattern of responses across visual cortex regardless of the size or the mean response amplitude of selective regions. In adults, the distributed responses across the ventral stream to different object categories are known to be reliable and distinct (Haxby et al., 2001). However, these distributed responses may be less distinct and/or reliable in children.

Here we describe experiments in which we characterized the development of cortical specialization for faces, places, and objects using a combination of fMRI and behavioral methods with children (ages 7 – 11), adolescents (ages 12 – 16), and adults (Golarai et al., 2007) see Figure 7.1. Face, place, and object-selective cortex in the ventral stream were defined independently in each subject. We examined the influence of age on the spatial extent, magnitude, and selectivity of activations in the ventral stream. We then related cortical development to the development of recognition memory for faces, objects, and scenes in the same subjects. Importantly, when comparing adult and child data we controlled for nonspecific age-related fMRI confounds. This control is essential when comparing fMRI data across age groups (Huettel et al., 2001; Thomason et al., 2005).

7.4 Methodological issues in developmental neuroimaging

Finding differences in responses or extent of activations across development requires attention to several methodological issues (Gaillard et al., 2001; Poldrack et al., 2002; Thomason et al., 2005). Specifically, we examined whether nonspecific age-related factors may manifest in differential fMRI responses across age groups. We considered both structural differences and BOLD-related confounds.

7.5   No changes in the anatomical size of the fusiform and parahippocampal gyrus

The brain reaches a relatively stable volume by age 5 (Caviness et al., 1996; Reiss et al., 1996). However, the relative volumes of gray and white matter change well into early adulthood, following region-specific temporal trajectories across the brain. Pre-adolescence increases in cortical gray matter (due to synaptogenesis) are followed by gray matter loss (due to synaptic pruning) during adolescence, maturing first in early sensory-motor cortex and last in associational and prefrontal cortices (Gogtay et al., 2004; Sowell et al., 2004). Simultaneously, white matter volume increases until adulthood (Giedd et al., 1999). These structural changes may introduce confounds in the interpretation of results based on group analyses that involve spatial transformation of individual subject data to an adult template brain (e.g. Gathers et al., 2004; Aylward et al., 2005; Scherf et al., 2007). To circumvent this potential confound, we defined regions of interest (ROIs) on an individual subject basis. Furthermore, we examined whether there were volume differences in the anatomical size of the fusiform gyrus and parahippocampal gyrus from ages 7 and up. We found no significant differences across age groups in the size of the fusiform or parahippocampal gyrus, with a trend towards larger regional volumes in children (Golarai et al., 2007).

7.6   BOLD-related confounds across age groups

Many fMRI analyses are based on a general linear model (GLM) on which statistical thresholding is applied. Greater motion, higher variance of the BOLD responses and worse fit of the GLM model (reflected by the larger residual error of the GLM, %Res) in children than adults can compromise the detection of significant activations in children. We examined each of these factors in turn.

First, children may have difficulty staying still during the scan. To reduce motion during scan we supported each subject's head with foam pads and a "bite bar." However, children's total motion during the scan tended to be higher than adults' even with head support (Golarai et al., 2007) as shown in Figure 7.2a.

We next examined whether there are age-dependent changes in the variance of the BOLD signal during the fixation baseline period (%CV BOLD) and whether there are age-related differences in the residual error of the GLM (%Res). These factors showed (a nonsignificant) trend towards being higher in children than adults (Figure 7.2b, c). Overall, these measurements suggest that there are nonspecific age related differences between groups that may affect detectability of fMRI activations. Therefore, it is critical to control these factors in order to assess any between-group differences in activitations.

To control for nonspecific between-group differences, we measured %Res in anatomically defined ROIs of the parahippocampal gyrus and fusiform gyrus and repeated analyses on a subset of subjects which excluded children with the highest %Res and adults with the lowest %Res. This allowed us to equate age groups across motion, BOLD-variance and %Res. In this subset of subjects (including 10 children, 9 adolescents and 13 adults) there were no significant differences in motion, fluctuations during baseline or residual GLM error (Figure 7.2, open bars). All analyses presented

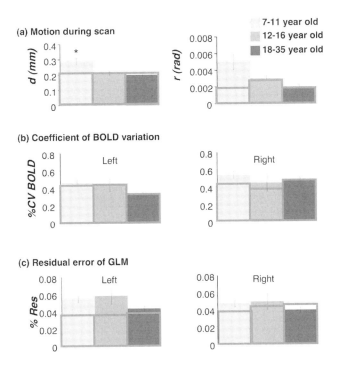

Figure 7.2. Matching BOLD-related confounds across agegroups. Filled bars, measurements of BOLD-related confounds across all subjects (20 children, 10 adolescents and 15 adults). Asterisk indicates significant difference from adults ($p < 0.04$). Open bars: same measurements after removing children with highest %Res and adults with least %Res (the subset of subjects includes 10 children, 9 adolescents and 13 adults). In this subset of subjects differences were not significantly different across groups in any of the comparisons. (a) Translation during scan: $d = \sqrt{x^2 + y^2 + z^2}$; rotation during scan: $r =$ pitch $+$ roll $+$ yaw. (b) Coefficient of variation of the BOLD response during baseline: %CV BOLD $= 100\frac{1}{N}\sum_{i=1}^{N}\sigma_i/\mu_i$. (c) Variance of the residual error of the GLM: %Res $= 100\frac{1}{N}\sqrt{\sum_{i=1}^{N}\text{ResMs}(i)/\text{MeanAmp}}$. %CV BOLD and %Res were calculated over an anatomical ROI of the mid fusiform gyrus.

here were conducted first using all subjects, and then repeated on the subset of subjects that were matched for BOLD-related confounds across age groups, to validate that between group effects were not driven by BOLD-related confounds.

7.7 Face, place and object-selective cortex in children and adults

We examined the influence of age on the spatial extent, magnitude, and selectivity of activations to faces, places and objects in the ventral stream, while controlling for possible age-related fMRI confounds (Figure 7.2).

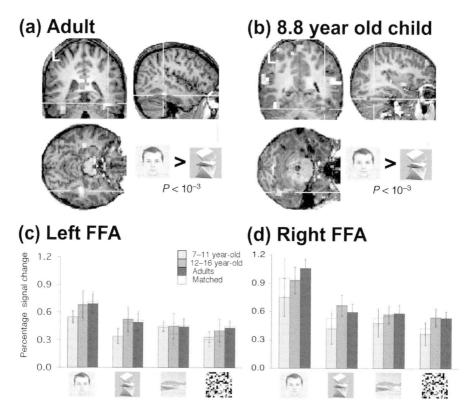

Figure 7.3. Face-selective regions in children, adolescents and adults. (a) The FFA was defined as the cluster of contiguous face-selective voxels in each subject's mid fusiform gyrus that responded more strongly to faces than objects ($p < 10^{-3}$, uncorrected). Crosshairs point to the right FFA in coronal, sagittal and horizontal views from a representative adult subject. (b) Same as (a) but from a representative 8.8-years-old child. (c, d) Shaded bars indicate percent BOLD signals relative to the fixation baseline for each image category and age group and include 20 children, 10 adolescents and 15 adults. Open bars indicate responses for the subset of subjects that were matched for BOLD-related confounds and include 10 children, 9 adolescents and 13 adults. Error bars indicate SEM across subjects. There were no significant differences in response amplitudes across age groups. (Adapted from Golarai et al., 2007.)

We detected in all age groups face-, place- and object-selective ventral stream activations in individual subjects. Face-selective activations were found in the fusiform gyrus (FFA) and along the posterior edge of the superior temporal sulcus (Figure 7.3). Place-selective activations were located more medially, overlapping the parahippocampal gyrus (PPA, Figure 7.4) and retrosplenial cortex. Object-selective regions (the lateral occipital complex, LOC, Figure 7.7) were found in lateral and ventral occipitotemporal regions, and were located posterior and lateral to face-selective fusiform ac-

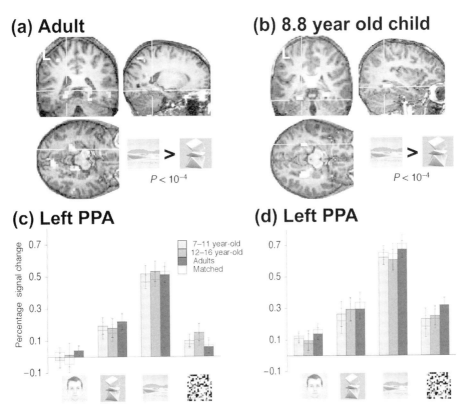

Figure 7.4. Place-selective regions in children, adolescents and adults. (a) The PPA was defined in each parahippocampal gyrus as the cluster of contiguous place-selective voxels that responded more to places than objects ($p < 10^{-5}$ uncorrected). Cross hairs point to the left PPA in activation maps from the same representative adult subject as in Figure 7.3. (b) Analogous to (a), but from the same 8.8 year-old child as in Figure 7.3. (c, d) Percent BOLD signals relative to the fixation baseline for each image category and age group. Shaded bar graphs represent data of all subjects, including 20 children, 10 adolescents and 15 adults. Open bars represent data from a subset of subjects who were matched for BOLD-related confounds (Figure 7.2) and include 10 children, 9 adolescents and 13 adults. Error bars indicate SEM across subjects. There were no significant differences in response across age groups. (Adapted from Golarai et al., 2007.)

tivations. Response amplitudes in face-, object- and place-selective ROIs were similar across age groups (Figures 7.3, 7.4, 7.7). Thus, there were no significant differences across age groups in the magnitude of responses in functionally defined face-, place- and object-selective regions.

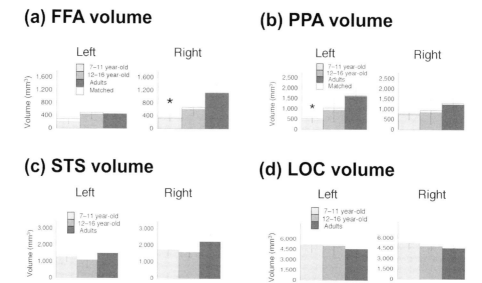

Figure 7.5. Volume of the FFA, PPA, STS and LOC across children, adolescents and adults. ROI sizes were calculated on subjects' 3-D volume. Gray bars indicate average volume across all subjects which include 20 children, 10 adolescents and 15 adults. Open bars indicate the average volumes for the subset of subjects that were matched for BOLD-related confounds (Figure 7.2) and include 10 children, 9 adolescents and 13 adults. Error bars indicate SEM across subjects. Asterisks indicate significantly smaller volume than adults, $p < 0.05$. (Adapted from Golarai et al., 2007.)

7.8   Differential development of the human ventral stream

We found evidence for prolonged development of the left PPA (lPPA) and right FFA (rFFA), which manifested as an expansion in the spatial extent of these regions across development. The rFFA and lPPA were significantly larger in adults than in children ages 7–11, with an intermediate size of these regions in adolescents (ages 12–16, Figure 7.5a, b). Notably, children's rFFA was about a third of the adult size (Figure 7.5a), but still evident in 85% of child subjects. These developmental changes could not be explained by smaller anatomical cortical volumes of the fusiform gyrus or parahippocampal gyrus, which were similar across children and adults (Golarai et al., 2007). Notably, results remained the same when we repeated analyses on the subset of subjects (10 children, 9 adolescents and 13 adults) that were matched for BOLD-related confounds (Figure 7.5, open bars). Overall, these data provide strong evidence that face- and place-selective cortices undergo a prolonged development that is not completed by age 11.

7.9   Expansion of selectivity into adjacent cortex

How does selectivity change across development in the FFA, PPA and adjacent cortex? One possibility is that the emerging selectivity to faces (or places) in the immature regions is due to increased responses to faces (or places) around the initial "hot spot." A second possibility is that it reflects decreased responses to objects. A third possibility is that responses are generally lower for all categories in the penumbral region in children, rather than reflecting a change in selectivity.

To examine these possibilities we measured the response amplitudes and selectivity in face- and place-selective ROIs and their neighboring voxels (Figure 7.6). Response amplitudes in the child FFA (Figure 7.3c, d) and PPA (Figure 7.4c, d) were similar to adults' suggesting adult-like response amplitudes in children's face- and place-selective cortex. Furthermore, face selectivity in the nascent rFFA and place selectivity in the nascent lPPA were similar to adult's selectivity (Figure 7.6a, b). However, penumbral regions that surrounded children's rFFA were characterized by adult-like responses to objects, but lower responses to faces, resulting in no selectivity for faces (Figure 7.6c). Similarly, penumbral regions that surrounded the lPPA showed adult-like responses to objects, and lower responses to places, exhibiting significantly lesser place selectivity in the penumbra (Figure 7.6d). Overall, developmental changes were accompanied by increases in the response to faces (or places) in the penumbral regions and no change in the response to objects. This resulted in increased selectivity to faces (or places) and spatial expansion of selective regions into adjacent cortex.

The neural correlates of these developmental changes in the penumbral regions of the rFFA or lPPA in children are unknown, and may involve sharpening of the neural tuning to faces or places, increases in the number of face- or place-selective neurons, or specific increases in the magnitude of responses to faces or places.

7.10   No developmental changes in the size of the LOC or the STS face-selective region after age seven

In contrast to the development of rFFA and lPPA, we found that the spatial extent of the object-selective lateral occipital complex (LOC) that responded more strongly to objects than scrambled objects ($p < 10^{-5}$, voxel level) was not significantly different across children, adolescents and adults (Figure 7.5d). Activation amplitudes to objects, faces and places in the LOC also did not differ across ages (Figure 7.7). Thus, LOC reaches adult-like volume and responses by age 7. These findings suggest that the human ventral stream undergoes a differential development process, whereby the LOC develops before the face- or place-selective regions of the rFFA and lPPA, which increase in size at least through age 11.

The differential time course of development across high-level visual cortex appeared to vary across regions (fusiform vs. superior temporal cortex, STS), not just categories (faces or places vs. objects). We defined a face-selective region in each subject's STS (faces > objects, $p < 10^{-3}$, voxel-level; Figure 7.3). There were no significant differences in the volume of the STS face-selective region across children, adolescents and adults (Figure 7.5c). Thus, in children (ages 7-11), we found a dissociation

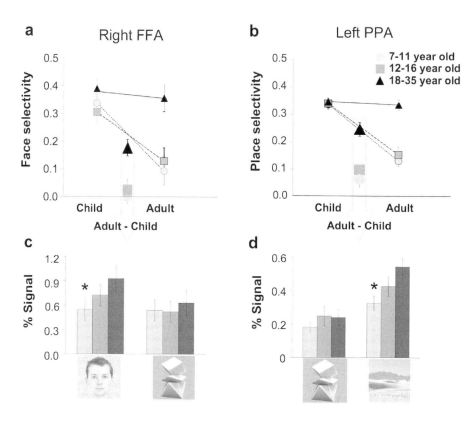

Figure 7.6. Selectivity of rFFA and lPPA across children, adolescents and adults. Face selectivity: (face−object)/ (face+object) across three ROIs: "child rFFA," "adult rFFA" and the penumbral region between these ROIs. In children and adolescents the "child ROI" reflects the subject-specific rFFA ROI. The "adult ROI" reflects an ROI centered on the subject-specific ROI and grown to the size of the average adult rFFA ROI by adding adjacent voxels. "adult–child ROI" reflects the penumbral region between these two ROIs. For adults we started from the subject-specific rFFA ROI to create the "adult ROI" and decreased its size by eliminating voxels from the edge of the ROI, till it reached the volume of the average child rFFA volume. The region between these ROIs is indicated as "adult - child". (b) Place selectivity: (place−object)/ (place+object) in a sequence of ROIs starting from subject-specific lPPA ROI. Same conventions as in (a). (c) Average BOLD response to faces and objects in the region between child and adult ROI (adult–child ROI). Light gray, 7–11 year olds; medium gray, 12–16 year olds; black, 18–35 year olds. (d) Average BOLD response to places and objects in the region between adult and child lPPA. Same conventions as (c). Data in this figure include 10 children, 9 adolescents and 13 adult subjects that were matched for BOLD-related confounds (Figure 7.2). Error bars indicate SEM across subjects.

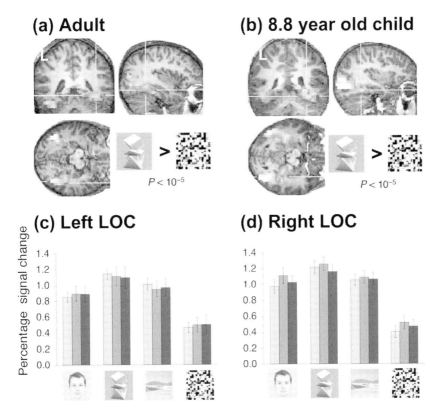

Figure 7.7. Object-selective regions in children, adolescents and adults. (a) The LOC was defined as a cluster of contiguously activated voxels that responded more to objects than textures in each subject's lateral occipital cortex ($p < 10^{-5}$, uncorrected). Crosshairs indicate the right LOC from the same representative adult subject in Figure 7.3. (b) Analogous to (a), but from the same 8.8-year-old child in Figure 7.3. (c, d) Average BOLD signals in the LOC for each age group and category and include 20 children, 10 adolescents and 15 adults. Conventions same as Figure 7.3 and 7.4. (Adapted from Golarai et al., 2007.)

between the smaller volume of rFFA and the adult-like volumes and responses of face-selective regions in lFFA and bilateral STS (Figure 7.5).

7.11 Correlation between differential cortical development and recognition memory performance

Several studies in adults have shown that the FFA is involved in face perception (Tong et al., 1998; Grill-Spector et al., 2004) and recognition (Grill-Spector et al., 2004) and

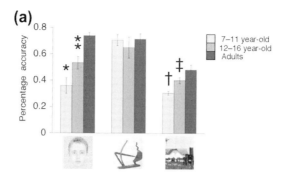

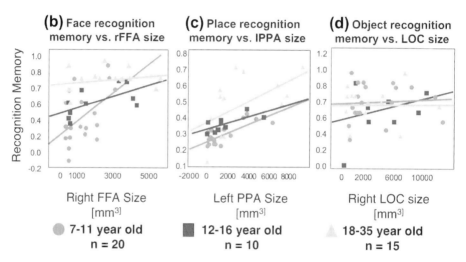

Figure 7.8. Recognition memory vs. size of FFA, PPA, and LOC. (a) Recognition memory accuracy = (hit − false alarm)/total for different categories across age groups. Recognition memory for faces was significantly better in adults than children ($*p <$ 0.0001) or adolescents ($**p < 0.03$). Adolescents' memory for faces was better than children's ($**p < 0.03$). Recognition memory for places was better in adults than in children ($†p < 0.0001$). Adolescents' memory for places was better than children's ($‡p < 0.01$). Recognition accuracy for objects was not different across age groups. Error bars indicate SEM. (b) Recognition memory for faces vs. FFA size; correlations are significant within children and adolescents ($r > 0.49$, $p < 0.03$), but not adults. (c) Recognition memory of places vs. PPA size. Correlations are significant within each age group ($r > 0.59$, $p < 0.03$). (d) Recognition memory for objects vs. LOC size. No correlations were significant ($p > 0.4$). (Adapted from Golarai et al., 2007.)

that the PPA is involved in perceiving (Tong et al., 1998) and remembering scenes (Brewer et al., 1998). Therefore, we examined whether there are behavioral consequences to the development of the rFFA and lPPA.

The same subjects who participated in fMRI scans also participated in a behavioral study which was conducted outside the scanner. During the behavioral study of recognition memory, subjects were shown a sequence of pictures. About 15 minutes later they were shown another sequence of pictures (half of which had seen before and half were new images from the same categories). Subjects were asked to report on each picture whether or not they had seen it previously. Consistent with previous studies, adults' face recognition memory was higher than children and adolescents (Figure 7.8a). Adults' place recognition memory was also higher than both children's and adolescents' (Figure 7.8a). There were no differences across age groups in object recognition memory.

Notably, we found that face-recognition memory was significantly correlated with age and rFFA size, but not with the size of any other ROIs. When considering each age group separately, face-recognition memory and rFFA size were significantly correlated in children and adolescents (Figure 7.8b), but not in adults (perhaps due to their higher and less variable performance). Place-recognition memory was significantly correlated with age and lPPA size (Figure 7.8c), but not with the size of other ROIs. In contrast, we found no developmental improvement in object-recognition memory. Further, LOC size was not correlated with object recognition memory in any of the age groups (Figure 7.8d). These findings support the hypothesis that during childhood and adolescence recognition memory improvements for faces and places are related to age-dependent increases in the size of the rFFA and lPPA, respectively.

7.12 Implications of the differential development of visual cortex

Our data suggest differential development trajectories across the human ventral stream in correlation with changes in recognition memory ability. First, our findings indicate that the entire visual ventral stream is not developing at the same rate. Second, some regions show a prolonged development well into adolescence. Third, the development of rFFA and lPPA is correlated with improvements in face and place recognition memory, respectively.

The reasons for different rates of development across high-level visual cortex are unknown. One possibility is that the type of representation and computations in rFFA and lPPA require more time and experience to mature than those in LOC or STS. Second, rFFA and lPPA may retain more plasticity (even in adulthood) than LOC and STS. Indeed, some studies suggest that even in adulthood FFA responses are modulated by expertise (Gauthier et al., 1999, 2000). Third, different neural mechanisms may underlie experience-dependent changes in LOC than FFA or PPA. For example, developmental changes in LOC may involve changes in distributed response patterns (Op de Beeck et al., 2006), whereas FFA and PPA development may involve changes in the number of selective neurons or their tuning.

These findings suggest the hypothesis that the differential development across visual regions underlies developmental improvements in performance of specific visual tasks. Thus, the slower development of rFFA maybe a limiting factor in the development of face perception and memory. In contrast, the more rapid development of

STS relative to the rFFA may imply that functions associated with the STS (such as processing of gaze direction and socially communicative cues; Allison et al., 2000; Hoffman and Haxby, 2000) develop more rapidly than functions associated with the FFA (such as face recognition). Further research on the development of the ventral stream in relation to specific improvements in behavioral proficiency is needed to test this hypothesis.

Consistent with this hypothesis, a similar link between cortical development and functional maturation may be evident in early visual cortex. For example, adult-like retinotopic maps in early visual cortex of 7-year-old children (Conner et al., 2004) may be associated with adult-like visual acuity in 6-7 year-olds. Similarly, adult-like responses in children's MT (Ben-Shachar et al., 2007) may be related to adult-like processing of global motion in 4-5 year-olds (Parrish et al., 2005). However, future research is necessary to determine the time course of the development of early visual cortex, and its relation to proficiency in visual tasks. Another open question is whether or not the prior maturation of early visual cortex is a prerequisite for the later development of high-level ventral stream regions.

7.13   Conclusions

Our study provides strong evidence for a prolonged developmental process in which the spatial extent of face-selective cortex in the fusiform gyrus and place-selective cortex in the parahippocampal gyrus continue to grow well into adolescence in correlation with improved proficiency in face and place recognition, respectively. The prolonged development of rFFA and lPPA sharply contrasts with adult-like spatial extent and responses of the LOC and face-selective STS regions by age 7. These developmental differences are unlikely to be due to nonspecific age-related differences across groups such as anatomical differences and differences in BOLD-related confounds.

Future studies are necessary for understanding the temporal characteristics of the development of visual cortex more generally, and the relation between cortical development and the development of visual abilities. Future research directions will include longitudinal studies, measurements of the maturation of connectivity (Dougherty et al., 2005), the development of distributed response patterns (Haxby et al., 2001), and changes in selectivity that may be manifested in more sensitive paradigms such as fMRI-adaptation (Grill-Spector and Malach, 2001) and high-resolution fMRI (Grill-Spector et al., 2006). Finally, future experiments in humans and animals will be critical for revealing the neural mechanisms underlying the development of visual cortex.

Acknowledgments

This research was founded by NIH grant 1R21EY017741, NSF grant BCS-0617688 and Klingenstein Fellowship to KGS.

References

Allison, T., Puce, A. and McCarthy, G. (2000). Social perception from visual cues: role of the STS region. *Trends Cogn. Sci.*, 4: 267–278.

Antonini, A. and Stryker, M. P. (1993). Rapid remodeling of axonal arbors in the visual cortex. *Science*, 260: 1819–1821.

Aylward, E. H., Park, J. E., Field, K. M., Parsons, A. C., Richards, T. L., Cramer, S. C. and Meltzoff, A. N. (2005). Brain activation during face perception: evidence of a developmental change. *J. Cog. Neuro. Sci.*, 17: 308–319.

Baker, C. I., Behrmann, M. and Olson, C. R. (2002). Impact of learning on representation of parts and wholes in monkey inferotemporal cortex. *Nat. Neurosci.*, 5: 1210–1216.

Ben-Shachar, M., Dougherty, R. F., Deutsch, G. K. and Wandell, B. A. (2007). Contrast responsivity in MT+ correlates with phonological awareness and reading measures in children. *NeuroImage*, 37: 1396–1406.

Brewer, J. B., Zhao, Z., Desmond, J. E., Glover, G. H. and Gabrieli, J. D. (1998). Making memories: brain activity that predicts how well visual experience will be remembered. *Science*, 281: 1185–1187.

Bruce, V., Campbell, R. N., Doherty-Sneddon, G., Import, A., Langton, S., McAuley, S. and Wright, R. (2000). Testing face processing skills in children. *Br. J. Develop. Psych.*, 18: 319–333.

Carey, S. (1981). Development of face perception. In G. Davies, H. Ellis and J. Shephard (eds.) *Perceiving and Remembering Faces*. New York: Academic Press, pp. 9–38.

Carey, S. (1992). Becoming a face expert. *Phil. Trans. Roy. Soc. Lond.*, 335: 95–103.

Carey, S. and Diamond, R. (1977). From piecemeal to configurational representation of faces. *Science*, 195: 312–314.

Carey, S. and Diamond, R. (1994) Are faces perceived as configurations more by adults than by children? *Visual Cog.*, 1: 253–274.

Caviness Jr., V. S., Kennedy, D. N., Richelme, C., Rademacher, J. and Filipek, P. A. (1996). The human brain age 7-11 years: a volumetric analysis based on magnetic resonance images. *Cereb. Cortex*, 6: 726–736.

Conner, I. P., Sharma, S., Lemieux, S. K. and Mendola, J. D. (2004). Retinotopic organization in children measured with fMRI. *J. Vision*, 4: 509–523.

de Heering, A., Houthuys, S. and Rossion, B. (2007). Holistic face processing is mature at 4 years of age: evidence from the composite face effect. *J. Exp. Child Psych.*, 96: 57–70.

Dougherty, R. F., Ben-Shachar, M., Deutsch, G. K., Potanina, P., Bammer, R. and Wandell, B. A. (2005). Occipital-callosal pathways in children: validation and atlas development. diffusivity predicts phonological skills in children. *Ann. NY Acad. Sci.*, 1064: 98–112.

Dragoi, V., Rivadulla, C. and Sur, M. (2001). Foci of orientation plasticity in visual cortex. *Nature*, 411: 80–86.

Ellemberg, D., Lewis, T. L., Dirks, M., Maurer, D., Ledgeway, T., Guillemot, J. P. and Lepore, F. (2004). Putting order into the development of sensitivity to global motion. *Vision Res.*, 44: 2403–2411.

Ellemberg, D., Lewis, T. L., Liu, C. H. and Maurer, D. (1999). Development of spatial and temporal vision during childhood. *Vision Res.*, 39: 2325–2333.

Ellis, H. D. (1975). Recognizing faces. *Br. J. Psychol.*, 66: 409–426.

Epstein, R. and Kanwisher, N. (1998). A cortical representation of the local visual environment. *Nature*, 392: 598–601.

Freedman, D. J., Riesenhuber, M., Poggio, T. and Miller, E. K. (2006). Experience-dependent sharpening of visual shape selectivity in inferior temporal cortex. *Cereb. Cortex*, 16: 1631–1644.

Gaillard, W. D., Grandin, C. B. and Xu, B. (2001). Developmental aspects of pediatric fMRI: considerations for image acquisition, analysis, and interpretation. *NeuroImage*, 13: 239–249.

Gathers, A. D., Bhatt, R., Corbly, C. R., Farley, A. B. and Joseph, J. E. (2004) .Developmental shifts in cortical loci for face and object recognition. *NeuroReport*, 15: 1549–1553.

Gauthier, I., Skudlarski, P., Gore, J. C. and Anderson, A. W. (2000). Expertise for cars and birds recruits brain areas involved in face recognition. *Nat. Neurosci.*, 3: 191–197.

Gauthier I., Tarr, M. J., Anderson, A. W., Skudlarski, P. and Gore, J. C. (1999). Activation of the middle fusiform 'face area' increases with expertise in recognizing novel objects. *Nat. Neurosci.*, 2: 568–573.

Giedd, J. N., Blumenthal, J., Jeffries, N. O., Castellanos, F. X., Liu, H., Zijdenbos, A., Paus, T., Evans, A. C. and Rapoport, J. L. (1999). Brain development during childhood and adolescence: a longitudinal MRI study. *Nat. Neurosci.*, 2: 861–863.

Gogtay, N., Giedd, J. N., Lusk, L., Hayashi, K. M., Greenstein, D., Vaituzis, A. C., Nugent 3rd, T. F., Herman, D. H., Clasen, L. S., Toga, A. W., Rapoport, J. L. and Thompson, P. M. (2004). Dynamic mapping of human cortical development during childhood through early adulthood. *Proc. Natl. Acad. Sci. USA*, 101: 8174–8179.

Golarai, G., Ghahremani, D. G., Whitfield-Gabrieli, S., Reiss, A., Eberhardt, J. L., Gabrieli, J. D. and Grill-Spector, K. (2007). Differential development of high-level visual cortex correlates with category-specific recognition memory. *Nat. Neurosci.*, 10: 512–522.

Grill-Spector, K. and Malach, R. (2001). fMR-adaptation: a tool for studying the functional properties of human cortical neurons. *Acta Psychol. (Amst.)*, 107: 293–321.

Grill-Spector, K. and Malach, R. (2004). The human visual cortex. *Ann. Rev. Neurosci.*, 27: 649–677.

Grill-Spector, K, Knouf, N. and Kanwisher, N. (2004). The fusiform face area subserves face perception, not generic within-category identification. *Nat. Neurosci.*, 7: 555–562.

Grill-Spector, K., Kushnir, T., Hendler, T., Edelman, S., Itzchak, Y. and Malach, R. (1998). A sequence of object-processing stages revealed by fMRI in the human occipital lobe. *Hum. Brain Mapp.*, 6: 316–328.

Grill-Spector, K., Sayres, R. and Ress, D. (2006). High-resolution imaging reveals highly selective nonface clusters in the fusiform face area. *Nat. Neurosci.*, 9: 1177–1185.

Haxby, J. V., Gobbini, M. I., Furey, M. L., Ishai, A., Schouten, J. L. and Pietrini, P. (2001). Distributed and overlapping representations of faces and objects in ventral temporal cortex. *Science*, 293: 2425–2430.

Hoffman, E. A. and Haxby, J. V. (2000). Distinct representations of eye gaze and identity in the distributed human neural system for face perception. *Nat. Neurosci.*, 3: 80–84.

Huettel, S. A., Singerman, J. D. and McCarthy, G. (2001). The effects of aging upon the hemodynamic response measured by functional MRI. *NeuroImage*, 13: 161–175.

Jiang, X., Rosen, E., Zeffiro, T., Vanmeter, J., Blanz, V. and Riesenhuber, M. (2006). Evaluation of a shape-based model of human face discrimination using FMRI and behavioral techniques. *Neuron*, 50: 1590-172.

Johnson, M. H., Dziurawiec, S., Ellis, H. and Morton, J. (1991). Newborns' preferential tracking of face-like stimuli and its subsequent decline. *Cognition*, 40: 1–19.

Kanwisher, N., McDermott, J. and Chun, M. M. (1997). The fusiform face area: a module in human extrastriate cortex specialized for face perception. *J. Neurosci.*, 17: 4302–4311.

Kobatake, E., Wang, G. and Tanaka, K. (1998). Effects of shape-discrimination training on the selectivity of inferotemporal cells in adult monkeys. *J. Neurophysiol.*, 80: 324–330.

Levy, I., Hasson, U., Avidan, G., Hendler, T. and Malach, R. (2001). Center-periphery organization of human object areas. *Nat. Neurosci.*, 4: 533–539.

Lewis, T. L., Kingdon, A., Ellemberg, D. and Maurer, D. (2007). Orientation discrimination in 5-year-olds and adults tested with luminance-modulated and contrast-modulated gratings. *J. Vision*, 7: 9.

Logothetis, N. K., Pauls, J. and Poggio, T. (1995). Shape representation in the inferior temporal cortex of monkeys. *Curr. Biol.*, 5: 552–563.

Malach, R., Reppas, J. B., Benson, R. R., Kwong, K. K., Jiang, H,, Kennedy, W. A., Ledden, P. J., Brady, T. J., Rosen, B. R. and Tootell, R. B. (1995). Object-related activity revealed by functional magnetic resonance imaging in human occipital cortex. *Proc. Natl. Acad. Sci. USA*, 92: 8135–8139.

McKone, E. and Boyer, B. L. (2006). Sensitivity of 4-year-olds to featural and second-order relational changes in face distinctiveness. *J. Exp. Child Psychol.*, 94: 134–162.

Mondloch, C. J., Geldart, S., Maurer, D. and Le Grand, R. (2003). Developmental changes in face processing skills. *J. Exp. Child Psychol.*, 86: 67–84.

Mondloch, C. J., Le Grand, R. and Maurer, D. (2002). Configural face processing develops more slowly than featural face processing. *Perception*, 31: 553–566.

Op de Beeck, H. P., Baker, C. I., DiCarlo, J. J. and Kanwisher, N. G. (2006). Discrimination training alters object representations in human extrastriate cortex. *J. Neurosci.*, 26: 13025–13036.

Parrish, E. E., Giaschi, D. E., Boden, C. and Dougherty, R. (2005). The maturation of form and motion perception in school age children. *Vision Res.*, 45: 827–837.

Passarotti, A. M., Smith, J., DeLano, M. and Huang, J. (2007). Developmental differences in the neural bases of the face inversion effect show progressive tuning of face-selective regions to the upright orientation. *NeuroImage*, 34: 1708–1722.

Pellicano, E. and Rhodes, G. (2003). Holistic processing of faces in preschool children and adults. *Psychol. Sci.*, 14: 618–622.

Poldrack, R. A., Pare-Blagoev, E. J. and Grant, P. E. (2002). Pediatric functional magnetic resonance imaging: progress and challenges. *Top. Magn. Reson. Imaging.* 13: 61–70.

Rainer, G., Lee, H. and Logothetis, N. K. (2004). The effect of learning on the function of monkey extrastriate visual cortex. *PLoS. Biol.*, 2: E44.

Reiss, A. L., Abrams, M. T., Singer, H. S., Ross, J. L. and Denckla, M. B. (1996). Brain development, gender and IQ in children. A volumetric imaging study. *Brain*, 119 (Pt 5): 1763–1774.

Sangrigoli, S. and de Schonen, S. (2004). Effect of visual experience on face processing: a developmental study of inversion and non-native effects. *Dev. Sci.*, 7: 74–87.

Scherf, K. S., Behrmann, M., Humphreys, K. and Luna, B. (2007). Visual category-selectivity for faces, places and objects emerges along different developmental trajectories. *Dev. Sci.*, 10: F15–30.

Shatz, C. J. and Stryker, M. P. (1978). Ocular dominance in layer IV of the cat's visual cortex and the effects of monocular deprivation. *J. Physiol.*, 281: 267–283.

Sigala, N. and Logothetis, N. K. (2002). Visual categorization shapes feature selectivity in the primate temporal cortex. *Nature*, 415: 318–320.

Sowell, E. R., Thompson, P. M., Leonard, C. M., Welcome, S. E., Kan, E. and Toga, A. W. (2004). Longitudinal mapping of cortical thickness and brain growth in normal children. *J. Neurosci.*, 24: 8223–8231.

Thomason, M. E., Burrows, B. E., Gabrieli, J. D. and Glover, G. H. (2005). Breath holding reveals differences in fMRI BOLD signal in children and adults. *NeuroImage*, 25: 824–837.

Tong, F., Nakayama, K., Vaughan, J. T. and Kanwisher, N. (1998). Binocular rivalry and visual awareness in human extrastriate cortex. *Neuron*, 21: 753–759.

Wandell, B. A., Brewer, A. A. and Dougherty, R. F. (2005). Visual field map clusters in human cortex. *Phil. Trans. Roy. Soc. (Lond.) B*, 360: 693–707.

Wiesel, T. N. and Hubel, D. H. (1965). Extent of recovery from the effects of visual deprivation in kittens. *J. Neurophysiol.*, 28: 1060–1072.

Yin, R. K. (1969). Looking at upside-down faces. *J. Exp. Psychol.*, 81: 141–145.

8 Clarifying the functional neuroanatomy of face perception by single case neuroimaging studies of acquired prosopagnosia

B. Rossion

In this chapter I review the neuroimaging studies carried out over the past few years on a brain-damaged patient presenting a face-selective recognition deficit (acquired prosopagnosia), the patient PS. These studies show that (1) in rare cases such as PS, a right inferior occipital lesion damaging the occipital face area (OFA) but sparing the adjacent nonface preferential area of the ventral lateral occipital complex (vLOC) can lead to prosopagnosia without object agnosia; (2) preferential responses to faces in the fusiform gyrus (fusiform face area, FFA) can be observed despite a lesion encompassing the lower-level ipsilateral OFA, suggesting that there is a direct pathway in the normal brain from early visual cortices to the FFA to categorize face stimuli at the basic level; (3) while categorization of the stimulus as a face can be preserved behaviorally and in the FFA response, fMR-adaptation studies show that individual representations of faces are not extracted properly in the FFA following acquired prosopagnosia. Based on these observations, I suggest a reformulation of current hierarchical neurofunctional models of face identity processing. Initial categorization of the visual stimulus as a face could take place in the right FFA following direct striate/extrastriate inputs, bypassing the OFA. This first representation would then be refined to achieve a full individual face representation, a process that depends critically on reentrant interactions with lower-level visual areas, mainly of the right hemisphere (OFA). Altogether, the studies reviewed here illustrate how combining functional imaging and lesion studies in a

Cortical Mechanisms of Vision, ed. M. Jenkin and L. R. Harris. Published by Cambridge University Press.
© Cambridge University Press 2009.

single-case approach can greatly contribute to our understanding of the neuroanatomy of face processing in the human brain.

8.1 Introduction

Today the question of how the human brain perceives and recognizes faces is widely investigated, in particular by means of functional neuroimaging studies of the healthy brain. Since the earliest studies in this field using positron emission tomography (PET, Sergent et al., 1992) and functional magnetic resonance imaging (fMRI, Puce et al., 1995), they aim at (1) localizing the brain areas involved in face processing, (2) characterizing the nature of face representations and processes in these areas, and (3) clarifying how these regions interact with each other while we process faces.

In this chapter, I would like to illustrate how functional neuroimaging single case studies of brain-damaged patients suffering from face recognition impairments, prosopagnosia, may help to reach these goals, beyond the information provided solely by neuroimaging studies of the healthy brain. After briefly reviewing the contributions of neuroimaging studies of face processing in the normal brain, I will present the functional neuroimaging studies carried out over the past five years by my colleagues and me on a remarkable case of acquired prosopagnosia, the patient PS (Rossion et al., 2003). In this chapter I hope to convince the reader that such neurofunctional investigations of single cases of brain-damaged prosopagnosic patients can be an extremely rich source of information to draw our map of the functional neuroanatomy of face processing in the human brain.

8.2 Neuroimaging studies of face perception in the healthy brain

Justine Sergent and her colleagues (1992) initiated the neuroimaging studies of face processing in the healthy brain using PET. These studies confirmed the right hemispheric dominance in processing faces that had been long reported by lesion analyses of cases of prosopagnosia (Hécaen and Angelergues, 1962) and divided visual field studies (Levy et al., 1972). These studies also confirmed the involvement of the fusiform and parahippocampal gyri during face processing, two areas that had been identified as being critical for face processing from lesion studies (Meadows, 1974; Damasio et al., 1982). Subsequent research using fMRI concentrated on the visual areas responding more to faces than pictures of other objects, irrespective of the task (e.g. Puce et al., 1995) and singled out a functional area of a few mm^3 in size, showing the strongest preferential response to faces, in the lateral part of the right middle fusiform gyrus, the FFA (Kanwisher et al., 1997; McCarthy et al., 1997). As demonstrated by many subsequent studies, the right FFA is in fact only one of three bilateral spots of preferential activations to faces over other object categories that are systematically observed in the human visual system, the others being localized posteriorly in the inferior occipital cortex (occipital face area, OFA, e.g. Gauthier et al., 2000b), and in the posterior part of the superior temporal sulcus (pSTS; e.g. Puce et al., 1998) (Figure 8.1A). While these areas respond also to many object categories (e.g. Avidan et al., 2002; Grill-Spector et al., 2006a), they are the only visual areas that consistently show a preference for face stimuli in fMRI. According to Haxby and colleagues (2000), these three areas form the "core" system for face perception, providing inputs to an extended system, that is, to temporal and prefrontal regions involved in emotional and semantic processing associated with person recognition (Figure 8.1b). These areas, which are bilateral but present a strong right hemispheric dominance on average (e.g. Kanwisher et al., 1997; Rossion et al., 2000; see Figure 8.1A), are defined functionally (faces vs. object categories; or vs. scrambled faces, preserving all low-level visual features of face stimuli): they are located outside of the retinotopic visual cortex and their borders are not defined anatomically (Halgren et al., 1999). They also present a large interindividual variability in terms of location, spatial extent, and hemispheric dominance (see Rossion et al., 2003).

Many studies have shown that these areas, in particular the FFA and OFA, are involved in discriminating individual face exemplars. The strongest evidence for this individual face coding comes from so-called fMRI adaptation studies, in which the neural response to a given stimulus is reduced when it is repeated (Grill-Spector and Malach, 2001; Grill-Spector et al., 2006b). If this adaptation is released when two different stimuli are presented repeatedly as compared with the repetition of the exact same stimulus, then one can assume that the populations of neurons in this area can differentiate the two stimuli. Release from adaptation to face identity (i.e. face A followed by face B vs. face A followed by face A) is found in all three functional areas, in particular in the OFA and FFA, strongly supporting their role in representing individual faces (e.g. Gauthier et al., 2000b; Eger et al., 2004; Schiltz et al., 2006; Gilaie-Dotan and Malach, 2007; for pSTS evidence, see Winston et al., 2004).

Even though the preferential response to faces of these areas is undisputed, it has been shown that the FFA also responds differently to distinct object categories (e.g. Haxby et al., 2001; Grill-Spector et al., 2006a), and can show increased activation to nonface objects of expertise (e.g. car pictures in car experts, Gauthier et al., 2000a). This indicates that the popular "face area" tag is incorrect and quite unfortunate, and suggests that the FFA is not a module for face perception: it carries out certain perceptual processes that are most important – perhaps critical – for faces but these processes can potentially be applied to other nonface object stimuli following expertise training, even in adulthood.

Most recent fMRI studies performed in the normal brain have attempted to clarify the nature of the face representations and processes in these areas (e.g. Eger et al., 2004; Winston et al., 2004; Fang et al., 2007; Chen et al., 2007). Directly related to some aspects of face perception that are highly documented by behavioral evidence (Sergent, 1984; Young et al., 1987), it has been shown for instance that in the "face areas," in particular in the right FFA, the perception of a facial feature is dependent of the presence and location of the other features ("holistic face representation," Schiltz and Rossion, 2006). Other studies have shown that the FFA is highly sensitive to inversion of individual faces (Yovel and Kanwisher, 2005; Mazard et al., 2006), in line with behavioral observations (Yin, 1969); and that faces are represented in this area with respect to a central tendency or prototype (Loffler et al., 2005) as is also described behaviorally (Rhodes et al., 1987; Valentine, 1991).

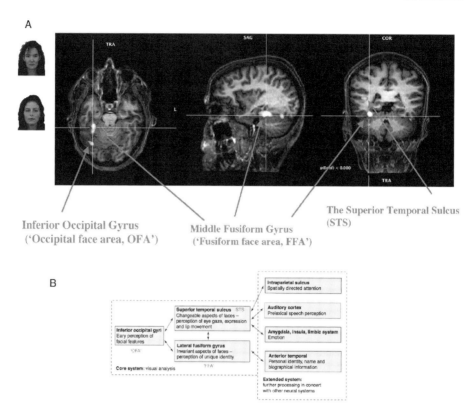

Figure 8.1. (A) The three functional areas forming the core system of face perception in the normal human brain (Haxby et al., 2000). These areas respond more to faces than any other object categories. They are illustrated here in the right hemisphere, in a single normal brain, during a functional face localizer contrast (faces vs. objects). (B) The three visual areas incorporated in a "core" system of face perception in the normal human brain as proposed by Haxby et al. (2000), and connected to brain areas in the temporal, parietal, and prefrontal lobes devoted to complex person recognition functions. (Figure adapted from Haxby et al., 2000, with permission.)

In summary, in a relatively short amount of time, functional neuroimaging studies of the normal brain have offered a relatively precise neuroanatomical map of face perception. However, the precise function(s) of the "face areas" with respect to face perception are still hotly debated, and their critical role in face perception, as well as their functional interactions, remain largely unknown.

8.3   Understanding how the human brain processes faces by combining lesion studies and functional neuroimaging

By itself, functional neuroimaging in the healthy brain is unable to indicate whether the areas activated during the presentation of face stimuli are necessary for their successful perception. To clarify this question, the identification of the localization of the lesions causing prosopagnosia may be of fundamental importance. The first cases of acquired prosopagnosia – that is, the inability to recognize faces despite intact intellectual function and preserved low-level visual processes – were described in the nineteenth century (Wigan, 1844; Quaglino and Borelli, 1867) and the term prosopagnosia (from the Greek "prosopon", for face and "a-gnosia", without knowledge) was introduced by Bodamer in 1947 (see Ellis and Florence, 1990). The majority of cases of prosopagnosia are due to (right) posterior cerebral artery infarcts (see Goldsmith and Liu, 2001) and the major complaint of these patients is in recognizing previously seen (i.e. familiar) faces and in learning new faces. However, as far as acquired prosopagnosia is concerned, even so-called associative prosopagnosic patients appear to have deficits at perceiving correctly an individual face. Hence, they fail at matching different pictures of unfamiliar faces, or when they succeed they use extremely slow and painstaking procedures (Levine and Calvanio, 1989; Davidoff and Landis, 1990; Farah, 1990; Delvenne et al., 2004; Bukach et al., 2006). Thus, while it is clearly acknowledged that low-level sensory deficits cannot explain prosopagnosia (Ettlinger, 1956; De Haan et al., 1995) and that there is a great amount of variability in terms of functional impairments among prosopagnosic patients (e.g. Schweich and Bruyer, 1993; Sergent and Signoret, 1992), I will refer in this chapter to prosopagnosia as a deficit of face perception, which is inevitably associated with the inability to recognize faces. While prosopagnosic patients can usually classify a visual stimulus as a face (face detection), they have difficulties in deriving a full percept of an individual face.

In principle, lesion analyses of prosopagnosia should be of great interest to understanding the neural basis of face perception. However, relying on this lesion method (i.e. correlating neuroanatomical data and clinical symptoms, Damasio and Damasio, 1989) as a means to establish the neuroanatomical basis of prosopagnosia is associated with a number of weaknesses, most notably a lack of precision due to the extent and variability of functional and anatomical impairments of the patients (e.g. Sergent et al., 1992). Another difficulty is that brain regions which may appear structurally intact and thus not considered to be critically associated with the impaired function(s) in a prosopagnosic patient may in fact be functionally depressed because they do not receive normal inputs from lesioned regions (diaschisis, see Price and Friston, 2002a). An illustration of this phenomenon was provided early on by Sergent and Signoret (1992), who reported a case of prosopagnosia with no structural damage to the right parahippocampal gyrus. Yet, a PET measurement of the patient's brain indicated a functional depression of this region, presumably because this area was deprived of normal inputs from other lesioned parts of the cortex. Thus, any attempt at correlating behavioral deficits of the patient due to the hypofunction of the hippocampal gyrus with visible structural damage would have been flawed. However, this observation

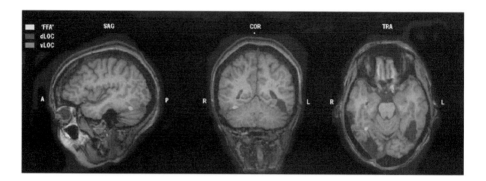

Figure 8.2. Localization of PS's lesions with respect to the right FFA and LOC complex (vLOC, ventral part; dLOC, dorsal part). Note that the lesion that is instrumental in causing the prosopagnosic deficit in the right hemisphere, encompassing the right OFA, is very close to the vLOC region. It is likely that in most cases of prosopagnosia following right posterior damage, both the OFA and vLOC are damaged, causing impairments for both face and object recognition.

highlights a potential interest in studying brain-damaged prosopagnosic patients with functional neuroimaging: such studies may not only improve the accuracy of associations between function and brain localizations, but they may also offer a powerful tool to investigate the relationship(s) between brain areas identified in the normal brain, and to test hypotheses regarding their functional connectivity (see Price et al., 2001; Price and Friston, 2002a). For instance, if the OFA is truly the front-end of the core face perception system, as suggested by Haxby and colleagues (2000), then a lesion to this area should prevent the flow of information to higher visual areas such as the FFA and the pSTS. In fact, this is precisely the opportunity to test this hypothesis that was offered to my colleagues and me a couple of years ago when we met the patient PS, a particularly interesting case of acquired prosopagnosia.

8.3.1   PS, a case of acquired pure prosopagnosia

The case of the patient PS has been described in detail in several publications over the past few years (Rossion et al., 2003; Caldara et al., 2005; Schiltz et al., 2006; Sorger et al., 2007; Dricot et al., 2008) and I will thus concentrate here on the main aspects of her neuropsychological profile. PS is a right-handed female born in 1950 who sustained a severe closed-head injury (she was hit by a bus) in 1992 which left her with damaged brain tissue in the lateral part of the occipital and temporal lobes, bilaterally, as well as in the anterior part of the left cerebellum. Her largest lesion extends from the posterior part of the right inferior occipital gyrus to the posterior fusiform gyrus. The left hemisphere lesion is more anterior and covers a large part of the middle fusiform gyrus (Figure 8.2). The exact localization of the lesions and their relationships to the prosopagnosic deficit have been described and discussed in detail (Sorger et al., 2007).

Several years after her accident, following spontaneous recovery and neuropsychological reeducation training, PS still presents a massive prosopagnosia, being unable to recognize both famous people and familiar people from their faces. Her deficit at face recognition is particularly severe, PS reporting several instances of failure to recognize extremely familiar persons from their face in real life situations (her daughter, her husband, close friends, etc.). This pattern is commonly reported by brain-damaged cases of acquired prosopagnosia and it contrasts with the excellent person recognition abilities of PS from people's voices for instance, but also from other visual cues such as the clothes, the gait, size and posture of familiar individuals.

Behavioral investigations carried out several years after PS's accident (i.e. from 2000 onward, see Rossion et al., 2003) have largely confirmed her prosopagnosia. For instance, she could classify as famous only 14 people's photographs out of 60 that she knows very well by their name, and she could identify only four of them. She is impaired at old/new face recognition tests on unfamiliar faces, and also at matching different pictures of unfamiliar faces either presented on the same or different viewing conditions (viewpoint, lighting changes, etc.). Her score at the Benton face discrimination test (Benton and Van Allen, 1968) is extremely low (27/54)[1] and she is particularly slowed down at this test and at other computer tests requiring to match/discriminate individual faces (Rossion et al., 2003; Schiltz et al., 2006). Hence, she is clearly unable to derive a full perceptual representation of an individual face. Yet PS is not impaired or slowed down at categorizing a face as a face, even in impoverished contexts requiring an integration of features at the basic level (e.g. Mooney faces), or in detecting a face stimulus in a visual scene presented briefly (Busigny and Rossion, in preparation).

Unlike most other cases of prosopagnosia, PS does not complain at all of object recognition difficulties. Her recognition of the colorized Snodgrass and Vanderwart's object set (Rossion and Pourtois, 2004) is perfect and fast and she performs in the normal range at matching pictures of common or novel objects (Rossion et al., 2003; Schiltz et al., 2006). This preserved function is also found in subordinate categorization and fine-grained discriminations (Rossion et al., 2003; Schiltz et al., 2006).

To determine the nature of PS's facial representations, we tested her by means of a response classification method revealing facial information randomly across spatial locations of the face (the bubbles technique, Gosselin and Schyns, 2001; for the origin of this random aperture method to isolate diagnostic face information, see Haig, 1985). In this study (Caldara et al., 2005) the patient PS had to learn 10 photographs of individual faces (2–3 hours of learning and frequent refreshers) and then to identify these faces individually during thousands of trials. On every single trial the face photograph was revealed through a number of apertures ("bubbles") randomly located on the face. Performance of the patient was maintained at 75% by increasing or decreasing the number of bubbles throughout the experiment, collecting images corresponding to correct and incorrect responses (Gosselin and Schyns, 2001). Unsurprisingly, PS required a much larger amount of bubbles (i.e. information) to perform the task at the same level as normal participants. More interestingly, response classification images,

---

[1] A more recent testing (2006) showed a much better score (39/54), even though it was still below normal range, but with extremely slow response times (37 min ± 34 secs to complete the test, mean age-matched control: 6 min ± 77 secs: Busigny and Rossion, in preparation).

contrasting correct and incorrect trials, showed that the patient did not use information located on the eyes area at all, relying almost exclusively on the lower part of the face for correct face identification (mouth and lower external contours; see Figure 8.3). In contrast, normal participants relied primarily on the eyes area of the face, with a preference for the right eye (i.e. left visual field; see also Gosselin and Schyns, 2001). These observations of a massive impairment at extracting diagnosticity from the face's eye region may be a characteristic feature of prosopagnosia, as indicated by the recent observations of difficulties at discriminating pictures of unfamiliar faces differing by the eyes but not the mouth in another brain-damaged case of prosopagnosia (Bukach et al., 2006). Most recently, we have showed that PS's failure to extract and represent diagnostic information on the eyes of faces extends to the identification of personally familiar faces (Ramon and Rossion, 2007). Eye movement recordings during familiar face identification also show a dominance of the number of fixations to the mouth area of the face relative to the fixations on the eyes (Orban de Xivry et al., in revision) in contrast with typical viewers' eye movement patterns (Figure 8.3). We are currently exploring the nature of this bias towards the mouth at the expense of the eyes in prosopagnosia and its functional significance (see Caldara et al., 2005; Ramon and Rossion, 2007), but in this chapter I will concentrate on the neural basis of PS's prosopagnosia.

8.3.2   The necessary role of the right OFA for face perception

Where are PS's brain lesions located relative to the areas that respond preferentially to faces (Figure 8.1)? Her largest lesion is located in the right hemisphere and concerns a substantial part of the inferior occipital cortex (Figure 8.2; see also Sorger et al., 2007). Based on the well-known right hemispheric prevalence in causing prosopagnosia and the absence of preferential response to faces in the vicinity of the right inferior occipital lesion for PS (Rossion et al., 2003), we hypothesized that the absence of right OFA activation was instrumental in causing PS's face perception impairment. This observation was later supported by a report showing that the site of maximal overlap of lesion localization in several cases of prosopagnosia concerns exactly the lateral part of the right inferior occipital cortex, where the right OFA is usually located (Bouvier and Engel, 2006). Hence, even though a complementary role of the left hemisphere in face processing functions should never be neglected (Sergent, 1988) and may possibly account in part for PS's face perception impairment (see Sorger et al., 2007), there is now converging evidence that the lateral part of the right inferior occipital cortex, including the OFA, is a necessary component of the intact face perception system.

8.3.3   Why so few cases of pure prosopagnosia?   Insights from neuroimaging

As indicated above, PS can be defined as a pure case of prosopagnosia, an impairment at face recognition without object recognition difficulties. Very few of such cases have been reported previously (e.g. De Renzi, 1986; De Renzi and di Pellegrino, 1998; Henke et al., 1998; Sergent and Signoret, 1992) and it is fair to say that they were not investigated thoroughly for object recognition so that the issue of a deficit restricted to the category of faces has remained largely debated in the literature (e.g. Damasio et al., 1982; Gauthier et al., 1999). I have no doubts that other such cases of pure acquired prosopagnosia, although extremely rare, will be reported with adequate testing in the literature in the years to come and will clarify this issue once and for ever. Yet, it remains that the large majority of prosopagnosic patients present deficit for both face and object recognition (e.g., Damasio et al., 1982; Farah, 1990; Clarke et al., 1997; Gauthier et al., 1999; Barton et al., 2002; Bouvier and Engel, 2006). Why is it the case? Here the functional neuroimaging studies of the patient PS provide some interesting clues.

In normal viewers there is an area in the lateral occipital complex (LOC, Figure 8.2) showing greater fMRI response to pictures of objects (including faces) than scrambled objects (Malach et al., 1995) which does not show systematic larger responses to certain object categories than others. It is located anteriorly to retinotopic visual areas extending in two anatomically segregated subregions both ventrally (vLOC) on the lateral bank of the fusiform gyrus and dorsally (dLOC) (Figure 8.2). These areas, in particular the vLOC, have been directly correlated with object perception (e.g. Avidan et al., 2002; Grill-Spector et al., 2000; James et al., 2000). The role of the vLOC in the discrimination of individual object exemplars has also been supported by fMRI-adaptation studies showing a larger response in this region to novel objects than to repeated objects (Grill-Spector et al., 1999; Avidan et al., 2002; Sayres and Grill-Spector, 2006).

Interestingly, in PS's brain, fMRI studies show a right vLOC area of normal size and height of signal, lying just next to the lesion that damaged the right OFA (Figure 8.2; see Sorger et al., 2007). One intriguing possibility is that the sparing of the right vLOC may be critical in accounting for PS's preserved object recognition and discrimination abilities. However, given the proximity of the right vLOC and OFA, it is likely that many acquired cases of prosopagnosia, in particular the patients who suffer from a right posterior artery infarct, will have *both* the OFA and at least a substantial section of the vLOC damaged by the lesion. For instance, the patient DF (Milner et al., 1991) is massively impaired at face and object recognition following lesions of the main part of the OFA *and* the vLOC in both hemispheres (James et al., 2003).

These observations suggest that prosopagnosia is most often associated with object recognition deficits (visual agnosia) because of right inferior occipital and occipitotemporal lesions damaging both the vLOC and part of the OFA/FFA complex (Figure 8.2). However, a lesion of the right OFA sparing the right vLOC, as in the case of PS, may lead to an isolated deficit at face perception. This observation will need complementary evidence from other brain-damaged cases but it has the merit of offering a tenable anatomical solution to this long debate regarding the very existence of acquired prosopagnosia with normal object recognition (e.g. Ellis and Young, 1989): in most cases, a right hemisphere lesion damaging the OFA will also encompass a substantial part of the vLOC of the same hemisphere, causing object perception impairments. In addition, neuropsychological evidence also indicates that object perception is less lateralized than face perception, with cases of visual agnosia generally presenting bilateral lesions (Farah, 1990). Hence, a unilateral right hemispheric lesion damaging the right OFA and the vLOC but sparing the homologous areas of the left hemisphere may cause prosopagnosia but leave object perception less impaired or even unimpaired. In

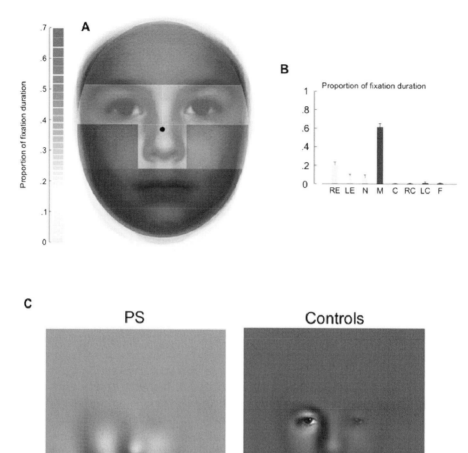

Figure 8.3. (A) Representation of the different regions scanned by PS during her identification task of familiar faces, showing the massive dominance of the mouth over all
other areas of the face. Note that the eyes are fixated also, showing that PS does not
avoid looking at this region of the face spontaneously. However, the eye region appears
to carry less diagnostic information for PS. The regions are superimposed on the average picture from all children's faces used in the experiment (Orban de Xivry et al., in
press). The color of each scoring regions corresponds to the proportion of fixation duration yielded by the color bar on the left of the panel. The black dot corresponds to the
fixation point displayed just before the picture. (B) Histogram of the interchild mean
($\pm$ 0.95 confidence interval) proportion of fixation duration for each scoring region.
RE, Right Eye; LE, Left Eye; N, Nose; M, Mouth; C, Chin; RC, Right Cheek; LC, Left
Cheek; F, Forehead. (C) Classification images for PS and controls obtained following
her identification task on learned faces presented through bubbles apertures (Caldara
et al., 2005). In contrast to controls, PS relied heavily on the mouth to recognize the
faces. She also needed many more apertures than control participants to perform the
task at the same level (see Caldara et al., 2005). See CD-ROM for color version.

other words, while there may be multiple pathways for normal object perception and recognition (e.g. Humphreys and Riddoch, 1984) face perception appears to rely on expert processes and more specialized areas, located largely in the right hemisphere. This lack of degeneracy (Edelman, 1978; Tononi et al., 1999) in the visual system for face perception may be a negative consequence of our expert processing skills for this category.

8.3.4   FFA without OFA, evidence for a direct pathway for basic face categorization

The previous section has underscored the important role that fMRI (compared with conventional structural MRI) can play in revealing the functional integrity of brain regions that might be potentially damaged in prosopagnosic patients. However, the case of the patient PS has proved most interesting when asking questions about the functional connectivity between visual areas responding preferentially to faces.

While the right posterior lesion of PS's brain damaged the territory of the OFA, we noticed that the middle and anterior sections of the fusiform gyrus, exactly where the right FFA is usually disclosed in normal participants when comparing the response to faces and objects (Figure 8.1), was intact in PS's brain. This pattern of damaged and spared brain tissue in a case of prosopagnosia offered us a unique opportunity to test one of the key features of the neuro-functional model proposed by Haxby et al. (2000): the hypothesis that the OFA is the front end of the system, providing the early inputs to higher visual areas such as the FFA and pSTS (Figure 8.1B). If this simple hierarchical model was correct, the destruction of the right OFA should have prevented face preferential activation in higher visual areas of the FFA and pSTS.

However, in contrast to the model, our first fMRI investigation of the patient PS (Rossion et al., 2003), using a simple face localizer experiment, showed a very clear preferential activation for faces in the middle fusiform gyrus (i.e. right FFA) in the absence of any face preferential activation around the lesioned area of the right inferior occipital cortex (i.e. no right OFA) (Figure 8.4). Hence, we found that the right middle fusiform gyrus may show a larger response for faces than objects (FFA), without getting any inputs from the ipsilateral OFA!

This observation suggests that in the normal brain the FFA may potentially be activated preferentially for faces through a direct pathway initially independent from the face preferential activation observed in the posteriorly located area in the inferior occipital cortex; that is, the OFA. This initial proposal (Rossion et al., 2003) has been reinforced by a number of subsequent observations:

- The activation of the right FFA for the patient PS has been replicated countless times, in different laboratories, with four different scanners (1.5T and 3T) and different acquisition parameters (block design or event-related paradigms) (Rossion et al., 2003; Schiltz et al., 2006; Sorger et al., 2007; Dricot et al., 2008). It is extremely robust.

- Compared with normal participants in our experiments, the FFA of the patient PS is in the normal range in terms of size and localization (see Rossion et al., 2003; Sorger et al., 2007).

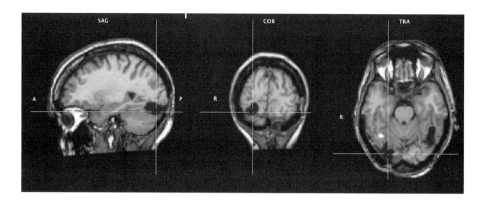

Figure 8.4. PS's main lesion, thought to be instrumental in causing her prosopagnosia, concerns the right inferior occipital cortex and posterior part of the fusiform gyrus (cursor), encompassing the OFA. This lesion does not prevent a preferential activation for faces in the right middle fusiform gyrus (FFA; here as the result of a combined analysis of six functional localizer runs, contrasting faces and object pictures in a face localizer contrast, see Sorger et al., 2007 for details).

- The amplitude difference between faces and objects is in the normal range for PS's FFA (Rossion et al., 2003), even though it can be in the lower range in some experiments, perhaps because of an absence of release from identity adaptation in her FFA (see below).

- The FFA activation in the patient PS's brain is observed whether the patient is impaired at performing the task (e.g. one back face matching task) or can perform the task normally (e.g. color detection task; see Rossion et al., 2003; Schiltz et al., 2006; Dricot et al., 2008).

- Besides the right FFA activation, the right pSTS also shows preferential activation for faces, in the absence of OFA inputs (Figure 8.5) (Sorger et al., 2007).

- PS's right FFA activation does not appear to originate from face preferential inputs coming from the OFA of the left hemisphere (e.g. through transcallosal connections): it is larger and peaks earlier for contralateral than ipsilateral face stimulation (Figure 8.6).

- Finally and most importantly, the FFA activation with no evidence for OFA activation has been also observed in another case of (prosop)agnosia due to bilateral damage to the inferior occipital cortex, the patient DF (Steeves et al., 2006). This is an important observation for two reasons. First, the damaged area that is common for both PS and DF is the right OFA, supporting the critical role of this region. Second, the left OFA is damaged in DF's brain, ruling out a contribution of the other hemisphere to the right FFA.

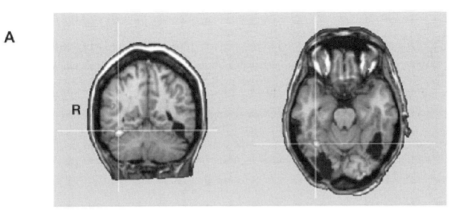

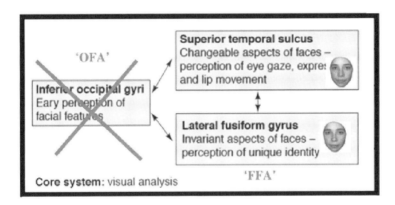

Figure 8.5. (A) Face preferential activations in the patient PS's brain on coronal and transversal views. The cursor is located on the right FFA activation. Note the pSTS activation on the coronal view, and the left OFA activation on the transversal view (see Sorger et al., 2007 for details). Lateralization experiments, as well as Granger causality mapping suggest that the left OFA activation originates from the right FFA activation (see text). (B) Schematic representation of PS's right hemisphere lesion on the neuro-functional model of face processing proposed by Haxby and colleagues (2000). PS's lesion damaged the cortical territory of the right OFA, and there is no evidence of face preferential activation around that area. This does not prevent face preferential activation to arise in both the right FFA and pSTS of the same hemisphere, suggesting that the onset of these anterior activations is independent of normal activation in the right OFA, against a simple hierarchical feedforward model of face processing.

Overall, these observations of a right FFA activation without ipsilateral OFA in two brain damaged cases suggests that, in the normal brain, the FFA may potentially be activated preferentially for faces independently of inputs coming from the posteriorly located area, the OFA, in contrast to the initial proposal of a simple hierarchical feed-forward model of face perception (Haxby et al., 2000). That is, both the OFA and the FFA are activated in parallel in the normal brain, independently from each other, such that a lesion to one of the areas does not prevent the face preferential activation in the other area. Alternatively, and more intriguingly, the FFA may be activated before any putative contribution from the OFA, and the functional relationship between the two areas goes in the other direction (FFA to OFA), at least for the initial face preferential response. That is, the onset of OFA activation in the normal brain may originate from FFA input. If the second hypothesis is correct, then a patient with a right FFA lesion should not present any OFA activation. This is precisely what we recently observed with the (prosop)agnosic patient NS reported earlier (Delvenne et al., 2004): while the territory of the right OFA appears structurally intact in this patient's brain activation pattern, and shows a large response to visual stimuli, there was no evidence of a preferential response to faces in this posterior location, in the absence of a right FFA (Figure 8.7). However, contrary to the observations of an FFA activation made with the patient PS, this can be considered as a null result and should be treated with caution before converging evidence is found.

To clarify further the source of the preferential activation for faces in the fusiform gyrus of the patient PS, we have recently applied Granger Causality Mapping (GCM) (Roebroeck et al., 2005) to a face localizer experiment of the patient PS. This has led to two interesting observations. First, we found that the right FFA activation for faces was influenced posteriorly only by a region of the ipsilateral primary visual cortex (V1, see Figure 8.8; Dricot et al., in preparation). This finding suggests a relationship between V1 and the right middle fusiform gyrus, possibly accounting for the FFA activation in PS's brain. It is in agreement with the evidence of direct projections from V1 to V4 and from V2 to the posterior part of the infero-temporal cortex in the monkey brain (TEO; Nakamura et al., 1993). In humans, diffusion tensor imaging (DTI) studies have not reported direct anatomical connectivity between V1 and the FFA in the majority of brain connectivity patterns tested but direct connections between early visual areas V3 and V3a and the FFA (Kim et al., 2006). Second, in addition to the right hemisphere V1-FFA relationships that we identified using Granger causality, there was a dominant influence of the right FFA towards several posterior regions: the right lateral ventral occipital cortex (vLOC), next to the lesion, and several areas in the left hemisphere, including the left OFA (Dricot et al., in preparation). Obviously, the right OFA cannot be included in this network because it is damaged in the patient's brain. However, preliminary analyses using Granger Causality in normal participants tested during face processing tasks also suggest a dominant influence of the right FFA towards the ipsilateral OFA (Dricot et al., in preparation). Considering these observations altogether, the right FFA activation may indeed reflect an early stage of processing, possibly following direct early visual inputs in primary visual area or extrastriate cortex, and influencing in turn several ispilateral and contralateral posterior areas.

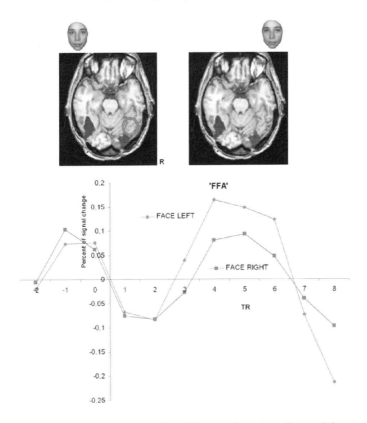

Figure 8.6. The right FFA of the patient PS is activated earlier and larger for contralateral presentation of faces (the right hemisphere is on the right here, for sake of clarity) than ispilateral presentation, against the hypothesis that the right FFA activation originates from transcallosal connections from left posterior visual areas (e.g. left OFA).

To summarize, the neuroimaging investigations carried out mainly on the prosopagnosic patient PS and reinforced by studies of other brain-damaged cases of prosopagnosia strongly suggest that in the normal brain: (1) the posteriorly located right OFA is a necessary component of the face perception system; (2) the anteriorly located FFA, also a necessary component of the face perception system, can be activated through a direct pathway from early visual areas, bypassing the OFA; (3) face preferential response in the OFA may either originate from early visual inputs also, or may depend on inputs from the ipsilateral FFA.

8.3.5 Holistic and fine-grained discrimination of individual faces: a role for an FFA-OFA reentrant loop?

How can a patient like PS be deeply prosopagnosic and yet show a preferential response for faces in the FFA (and in the pSTS) that looks perfectly normal in terms of localization, size and height of the differential fMRI signal between faces and objects?

A

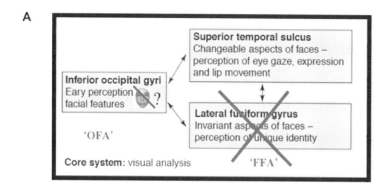

B

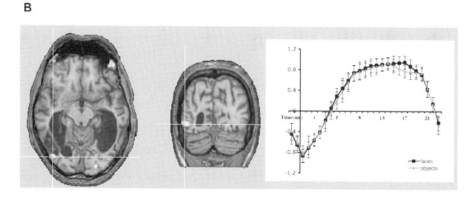

Figure 8.7. The patient NS (Delvenne et al., 2004) is an acquired case of visual agnosia and prosoagnosia, presenting lesions to the right middle fusiform gyrus, as well as the parahippocampal gyrus, bilaterally. (A) In the right hemisphere, his lesion damages the whole territory of the right FFA, but largely sparing the right inferior occipital cortex, as represented schematically here onto Haxby et al. (2000) neuroanatomical model of face perception. However, when performing the exact same face localizer experiment as the patient PS (parameters in Schiltz et al., 2006) there was no evidence for any face-preferential activation three face localizer runs, besides a small spot of activation in the pSTS ($p < 0.05$, uncorrected). This absence of face-preferential activation was not due to a lower signal in visual areas, which were activated for both faces and objects above the fixation cross baseline (here the percent signal change for faces and objects in an area of the right inferior and middle occipital cortex, posterior to the lesioned cortex, activated equally strongly for faces and objects).

To understand this apparent paradox, one should be reminded that the FFA activation emerges by differentiating pictures of faces and non-face object categories (a face lo-calizer), something that the patient PS is perfectly able to do behaviorally (e.g. Schiltz et al., 2006). Like other cases of prosopagnosia, her difficulties are apparent when she has to process individual exemplars of faces: either discriminate different individual faces, or recognize an individual familiar face. Hence, populations of neurons in her

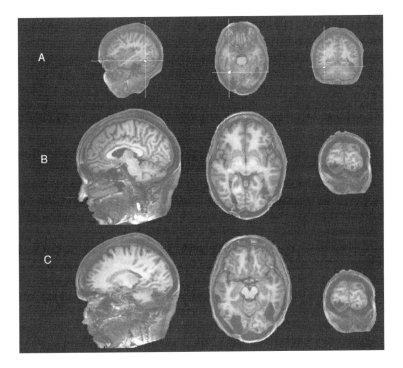

Figure 8.8. Granger causality (Roebroeck et al., 2005) was applied to a face localizer experiment with the patient PS. (A) The right FFA as activated in a face localizer is taken as the source searching across the whole brain for regions influencing and being influenced by the right FFA. (B) The main site of influence to the right FFA during the presentation of faces (but not objects) was located in the ipsilateral primary visual cortex (in green color, 6, -92, -11). (C) In blue, regions receiving direct influences from the right FFA, controlaterally in the left hemisphere (including the left OFA) and in the right vLOC. (From Dricot et al., in preparation). See CD-ROM for color version.

FFA can carry out the categorization of the stimulus as a face, even when it is extremely simplified or degraded (Figure 8.9). However, unlike neurons in the same area of the normal brain, they may just be unable to code for individual faces.

A FFA that does not discriminate individual faces

To test the intriguing hypothesis that cells in PS's FFA may be unable to code for individual faces, PS and control participants were presented with blocks or pairs of identical face stimuli in fMRI as compared with the successive presentation of different face stimuli. Whereas neural activation was lower for repeated facial identities in the right FFA of normal participants consistent with many studies (e.g. Gauthier et al., 2000b; Grill-Spector and Malach, 2001, Eger et al., 2004; Gilaie Dotan and Malach, 2007), there was no significant difference in the level of activation for the patient PS whether different or identical face identities were presented successively (Schiltz et al.,

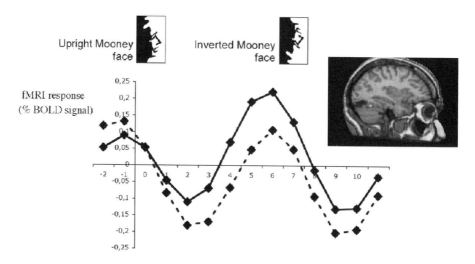

Figure 8.9. The right FFA of the patient PS is activated for pictures of Mooney faces, in line with her preserved behavioral ability to categorize a face as a face (Schiltz et al., 2006), to detect faces in visual scenes presented rapidly and to perceive faces in these two-tone images (scale in TR, one TR = 1250 ms).

2006; see Figure 8.10). That is, despite showing a larger response to faces than objects in the normal range, PS's right FFA showed an absence of face identity adaptation effect. To be more accurate, the level of signal in PS's right FFA was as large as in normal participants when identical faces were presented repeatedly but failed to show a release from adaptation when different faces were presented (Figure 8.10).

Hence, contrary to what our initial observations suggested, PS's right FFA does not work normally: while being involved in the categorization of the stimulus as a face (as opposed to other objects), the signal in this area does not carry sufficient coding information to discriminate individual faces. Originally, these observations were made during an orthogonal task that the patient was able to perform as well as normal participants (color detection task, see Schiltz et al., 2006), both in a block design and an event-related (ER) paradigm. Interestingly, they stand out even during an ER individual face discrimination task in the scanner for which the patient performs well below controls and more slowly but better than at chance (Dricot et al., 2008). Again, these results have been recently replicated with the patient DF, also showing (bilateral) FFA activation without release to face identity adaptation (Steeves et al., 2007).

This observation of a dissociation, in the same brain area, between an intact face categorization and an impaired face individualization has several theoretical consequences. First, the anomalous activation to conditions with different faces in the FFA of the prosopagnosic patient PS, in line with her behavioral impairment, points towards a critical function of this region in individual face perception. Second, and most importantly, these observations suggest that successful individual face perception in the FFA may require the right OFA to be intact: without a contribution of the right OFA, which is also showing face identity adaptation effects in the normal brain (see Schiltz et al.,

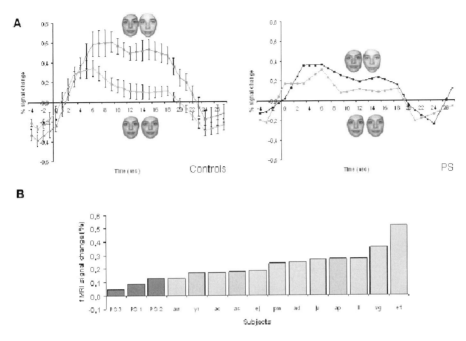

Figure 8.10. Lack of release from identity adaptation effect for the prosopagnosic patient PS in the right FFA (adapted from Schiltz et al., 2006). (A) Left: Activation in normal subjects is larger when pictures of different faces are presented successively during a block (18 seconds, 18 different face stimuli) than when the same facial identity is repeated throughout the block. Right: For the patient PS, the two conditions do not show a significant difference: there is a lack of release from identity adaptation in the right FFA. (B) Adaptation indexes (different – same faces / sum) for the patient PS (replicated two times, 3 × 3 runs) and for each normal participant in the same experiment (in pink color: aged-matched controls). See CD-ROM for color version.

2006), the coding for facial identity is impaired. This is observed in fMRI-adaptation paradigms, as described above, but also in the face localizer experiment where different facial identities are presented: initially, neural activation to faces in the right FFA of PS is as large or even larger than in the normal brain but the BOLD response is not sustained and drops down below normal range (Figure 8.11). Hence, averaging over the entire time window of activation for faces may mask any difference between PS's and normal participants' right FFA during a face localizer (Rossion et al., 2003). However, a closer look at the time course of activation, in particular when long stimulation blocks and recording epochs are used, reveals an abnormally functioning FFA in the patient's brain. We have attributed this nonsustained response of the FFA to the lack of reentrant inputs from the OFA which contribute to individualization of the face representations in the normal brain (see the discussion section in Schiltz et al., 2006). According to this hypothesis, the FFA of the patient PS may show a normal response

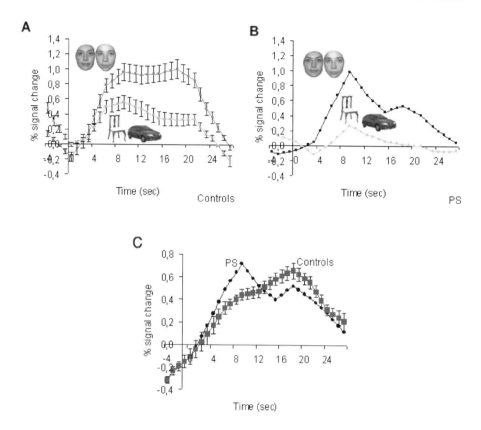

Figure 8.11. Typical BOLD signal in the right FFA observed for a face localizer (TR 3000 ms; blocks of 18 secs, see methods in Rossion et al., 2003; Schiltz et al., 2006) for normal participants (A) and the patient PS (B). Note that relative to controls the BOLD response is not sustained for PS when different faces are presented. However, subtracting the reponse to object stimuli from the response to face stimuli leads to an overall response in the normal range for PS when the whole timecourse is considered (Rossion et al., 2003). The lack of sustained activation, presumably because of identity adaptation in the absence of OFA inputs, would cause a significant decrease of the differential response to faces for PS, only apparent with long stimulation blocks. (Figure adapted from Schiltz et al., 2006.)

profile in simple face detection tasks (e.g. Figure 8.9), but is likely to shown smaller or abnormal responses relative to controls when individual faces have to be discriminated and should benefit from the OFA inputs (a so-called dynamic diaschisis effect, Price et al., 2001).

To summarize, we have shown that the preferential activation for faces in the lateral part of the right middle fusiform gyrus ("rFFA") can arise in the absence of face preferential inputs coming from posterior areas such as the right OFA. However, without any contribution from the right OFA, the activation level in the "rFFA" when different faces are presented drops down to the level of identical faces.

The neural microgenesis of face perception

Based on these observations, we suggest reformulating the neurofunctional organization of face perception in the human brain, to incorporate the following elements (see Figure 8.12; Rossion, 2008). Following early processing in striate and extrastriate visual areas, face stimuli would activate high-level visual areas of the fusiform gyrus (and possibly pSTS) through a direct pathway, leading to the earliest face preferential response at a relatively anterior location in the ventral visual stream (FFA). Neurons in this nonretinotopic visual area have presumably a relatively large receptive field, as in the area TE of the monkey IT (between 30 and 50 degrees, Boussaoud et al., 1991), allowing an initial representation of the whole face stimulus, even when it is perceived out of the foveal view (i.e. a face popping out, somewhere in the visual scene). This initial representation would be rather coarse, sufficient for accurate detection and categorization of the stimulus as a face for instance, but insufficient for the fine-grained analysis required to identify the particular person whose face is presented. This process is preserved for the patient PS who shows normal behavioral and neural face categorization/detection function even for degraded high-contrast stimuli such as Mooney faces (Figure 8.9). However, in the normal brain, following this initial categorization process, the face representation would be progressively refined to allow the extraction of local features and their integration to form a full percept of an individual face supporting identification (a structural encoding code, according to the terminology of Bruce and Young's (1986) functional model of face processing). This is where lower-visual areas such as the OFA may be called upon during this microgenesis of face perception (Sergent, 1986). That is, through reentrant signaling, the higher order face-sensitive populations of neurons in the FFA may lead to or enhance face preferential responses in lower level visual areas – the OFA, where populations of neurons with smaller receptive fields would help refining the face representation. In other words, global and coarse information in higher visual areas would serve as a header to set up the processing of fine information related to facial identity in lower visual areas. Given their smaller receptive fields, neurons in the OFA may be fine-tuned to subserve such fine discrimination, which are critical in real life situations (e.g. recognizing the same identity across age differences, changes in lighting, discriminating siblings or twins, etc.). Reentrant connectivity between the two areas would then support the full extraction of individual face representations (Figure 8.2).

If we consider patients such as PS, the initial categorization of the stimulus as a face in the right FFA, which allows her to categorize faces vs. objects, to detect faces in visual scenes, or even to perceive a whole Mooney face stimulus, cannot be followed by an integration with lower visual areas in the right hemisphere to refine the initial face representation. Consequently, there is an absence of facial identity discrimination in the FFA of PS, and a decrease of the hemodynamic FFA response in the absence of sustained reentrant interactions with the right OFA (Figures 8.10 and 8.11).

This proposal of a neural microgenesis of face perception, starting with a coarse categorization in high visual areas followed by a refinement through reentrant interac-

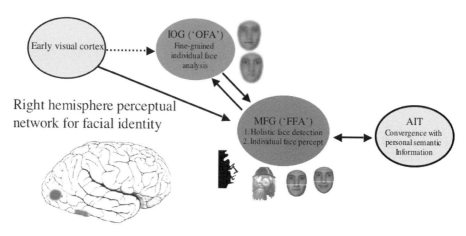

Figure 8.12. Reformulating the neurofunctional organization of face perception in the human brain. Following early visual analysis, visual stimuli are detected as whole faces in high visual cortices (1): in the middle fusiform gyrus (MFG), leading to preferential activation for these stimuli (FFA). The crude representation of the face stimulus is then refined through reentrant interactions with lower visual areas (2), leading to a face preferential activation in the inferior occipital gyrus (IOG, OFA). This refinement allows the extraction of a full percept of an individual face. A lesion of the OFA does not prevent face preferential activation in the FFA but leads to an absence of individual face adaptation effects in this area.

tions with lower visual areas (Rossion et al., 2003), is in agreement with the presence of massive cortical bidirectional connections (Felleman and Van Essen, 1991) and the hypothesis of reentrant phasic signaling between areas of the visual cortex (Edelman, 1978, 1993). It is a proposal that is not particularly challenging or novel, but is inspired from several sources. Starting with Mumford (1992), a number of authors have indeed suggested that through feedback connections, higher level perceptual computations and representations that involve high resolution details, fine geometry and spatial precision may involve lower visual areas (Mumford, 1992; Lee et al., 1998; Bullier et al., 2001; Galuske et al., 2002). These proposals have perhaps been more extensively formulated in the reverse hierarchy theory (RHT) of visual perception proposed by Hochstein and Ahissar (2002). According to RHT, explicit perception begins at high-level visual cortex, representing the gist of the scene or an object at the basic level. This is performed on the basis of a first order approximation of low-level inputs. The details are not represented at this stage, and the representation is then refined by recruiting lower visual areas, with smaller receptive fields neurons, through feedback connections. RHT has been derived from perceptual learning experiments and has been proposed to account for many phenomena of vision and attention such as the initial and fast perception of object categories (including face detection), feature search "popout" effects, and whole superiority effects (see Hochstein and Ahissar, 2002).

The revised cortical model of face perception proposed here is largely in agreement with this RHT framework. In fact, faces are perhaps the best candidates for a coarse-whole to fine-parts scheme: faces are often detected very far away, out of foveal vision and/or with their features too small to resolve. Hence, a whole face stimulus can be detected without and before any detailed analysis and decomposition of the individual features (Sergent, 1986; Loftus and Harley, 2004). In visual scenes, faces can be detected extremely rapidly (Rousselet et al., 2003). More to the point, a whole face is perceived readily even when there are no facial features, or when they are not easily discernable, such as in a painting of the sixteenth century artist Giuseppe Arcimboldo (e.g. "The Vegetable Gardener") or in a two-tone Mooney face (Figure 8.9). Besides being compatible with multiple sources of evidence, an initial, rapid, feedforward categorization of the stimulus as a face followed by reentrant interactions with lower visual areas is thus (eco)logically valid and highly plausible. Moreover, this initial categorization and the reentrant interactions between high and low level visual processes would probably take place predominantly in the right hemisphere for faces, consistent with the evidence that early face categorization and individual discrimination effects are observed most significantly in this hemisphere (Jacques et al., 2007).

With respect to the RHT, the present proposal differs according to at least two aspects. First, in order to obtain a first approximation of the visual stimulus in high-level visual areas it may not be necessary for the feedforward initial processing of visual information to go through the hierarchy of visual areas, as proposed in the RHT framework. That is, direct connections from low-level visual areas such as V1/extrastriate cortex to high-level visual areas such as the FFA can bypass the hierarchy of intermediate visual areas, including the OFA (Figure 8.12). Otherwise, there would not be any activation of the FFA in brain-damaged patients with posterior occipital lesions such as PS and DF. Second, and this is a related point, it may be incorrect to refer to a feedback from the FFA to the OFA, as we initially proposed (Rossion et al., 2003). Rather, the initial input to the OFA could possibly originate from the FFA, or the two areas may exchange information largely in parallel. Consequently, rather than feedback, it would be more appropriate to hypothesize the presence of phasic reentrant connections (Edelman, 1978, 1993) between these areas, as leading to a full individual face percept.

Interestingly, this revised neural model of the microgenesis of face perception is also largely compatible with neurophysiological evidence. For instance, single cell recordings in the monkey brain have shown that the representation of faces in IT which emerges rapidly (70–130 ms, average latency 100 ms in the monkey brain, Kiani et al., 2005) is that of a global face stimulus which cannot be decomposed in parts without altering the cell's response (Desimone et al., 1984; Wang et al., 1996). The very same neurons in these areas appear to carry out both coarse- and fine-grained categorization of faces at different timescales (100–150 ms, Sugase et al., 1999). Event-related potential (ERP) recordings on the human scalp as well as the latency of saccadic reaction times also indicate that objects and faces are detected in visual scenes well before a perceptual decision at 150 ms (Thorpe et al., 1996; Rousselet et al., 2003; Kirchner and Thorpe, 2006). ERPs indicate that segmented faces are reliably discriminated from other object categories at about 130 ms (onset of occipitotemporal N170 peak; see Rossion and Jacques, 2008 for a review), and recent evidence collected in our laboratory indicates that individual representations of faces are discriminated slightly later, at about 160 ms, within the time window of the same component (Jacques and Rossion,

2006; Jacques et al., 2007). Thus, overall, a reasonable amount of evidence supports the possibility of a rapid coarse categorization of the face stimulus in high level visual areas such as the right fusiform gyrus (FFA) followed by a refinement through reentrant interactions with lower visual areas, in particular the ipsilateral OFA.

To be fair and complete it is necessary to mention and discuss the potential evidence against the view advocated here and which would rather support a hierarchical feed-forward two stages model, with an initial face categorization in posterior lower visual areas such as the OFA followed by individual face representations in the FFA. For instance, using fMRI adaptation to facial identity, Rotshtein et al. (2005) showed that the OFA was more sensitive to the physical aspects of the face stimulus than the FFA. Following an earlier work that we performed with morphed individual faces in PET (Rossion et al., 2001) these authors used fMRI to show release from adaptation to two faces that differed physically in the OFA, regardless of whether the subject perceived the two faces as being two photographs of the same person or of different identities. This finding contrasts with the FFA, which showed release from adaptation when the two pictures of faces were perceived as different identities but not when they were perceived as the same identity. This evidence was taken in favor of a hierarchical model of face processing in the ventral stream, with only the FFA but not the OFA being sensitive to individual representations of faces. However, as we indicated previously (Schiltz et al., 2006), the presence of a fine discrimination sensitivity (release from adaptation when two faces slightly differ physically) in the OFA is compatible with our findings and with the view advocated here. Furthermore, while our model calls upon reentrant interactions between these areas (Figure 8.12), it is also in favor of a higher level of abstraction in the FFA than the OFA, following the initial input to the face system in the FFA. As a matter of fact, holistic representations are stronger in the FFA than the OFA, in particular in the right hemisphere (Schiltz and Rossion, 2006). The only finding in the study of Rotshtein et al. (2005) that is difficult to reconcile with our view is that of an absence of release from adaptation when the faces differ only physically in the FFA. This would indeed suggest that this area does not discriminate highly similar faces, even following reentrant inputs from the OFA. In this context, it is interesting to note that a recent fMRI study using morphed faces did not replicate this latter observation of Rotshtein et al.'s (2005) study: the FFA (and the OFA) was sensitive to small physical differences between the faces along a morphed continuum, mirroring the subject's discrimination abilities (Gilaie-Dotan and Malach, 2007).

More recently, Fairhall and Ishai (2007) applied Dynamic Causal Modeling (DCM) to fMRI data during face processing to investigate the connectivity between these areas. These authors reported a predominantly feedforward connectivity between the OFA and FFA which could be interpreted as being in disagreement with the model out-lined on Figure 8.12. However, unlike Granger Causality, DCM is a modeling method that requires specific hypotheses. Thus, the brain regions included in the model, the anatomical connectivity between them and the modulations by experimental conditions have to be specified (Penny et al., 2004). In line with Haxby et al.'s (2000) earlier pro-posal, Fairhall and Ishai (2007) constrained their model by considering the OFA as the entry node of the system, such that the functional connections tested mediated the prop-agation of face-selective responses in the OFA around the face system. The model is thus biased, even though the authors mention that there was no evidence for a potential contribution of backwards connections from the FFA and STS to the OFA to the model. This purely hierarchical feedforward interpretation, without any feedback, is rather surprising, given that there should certainly be important feedback connections between these areas, consistent with the presence of massive reentrant connections in the visual system (Felleman and Van Essen, 1991). Furthermore, the regions of interest defined by Fairhall and Ishai (2007) were obtained after contrasting faces and scrambled faces, and may thus contain a large number of voxels that do not respond preferentially to faces (over objects), but simply to shape information (i.e. LOC), making it difficult to compare with our proposal. While it would be interesting to apply DCM to appropriate fMRI data to test the functional pathways leading to face preferential responses, there are probably better ways to test the model, as described below (see also Rossion, 2008). In particular, the finding of a dominant OFA to FFA functional relationship by Fairhall and Ishai (2007) does not rule out the view advocated here that the initial activation for faces emerges in the FFA through a rapid direct pathway, bypassing the OFA. When the two areas then interact with each other, it may well be that a substantial directional relationship takes place in the posterior-anterior (OFA to FFA) direction. In the absence of precise timing information, as could be collected from MEG studies or neurophysiological recordings in the monkey face-selective patches of activation (see below), this issue is difficult to clarify.

Finally, while the view advocated here is compatible with a number of sources, it disagrees with other purely hierarchical computational models of face processing such as the HMAX architecture proposed by Riesenhuber and colleagues (Riesenhuber and Poggio, 1999; Jiang et al., 2006). While this hierarchical model may perhaps account for some characteristics of face processing obtained from both behavioral and neuroimaging signals (Jiang et al., 2006), it cannot account for the observations of an activation of the FFA without a posterior OFA, as observed in the cases of PS and DF. Being based on a simple combination of features through several stages of increasing complexity, it is also at odds with several phenomena characterizing normal face perception, such as the perception of faces made of nonface features (e.g. Arcimboldo's paintings). In addition, it cannot account for the observation that inversion affects more the perception of spatial relationships between facial features than local information on these features (e.g. Freire et al., 2000; Goffaux and Rossion, 2007), and with the widely acknowledged norm-based coding of individual faces (e.g. Rhodes et al., 1987; Leopold et al., 2001). My view is that this hierarchical computational architecture will need to be substantially revised to incorporate top-down connections and processes, or it will prove increasingly incompatible with numerous neural and functional key aspects of face perception (i.e. the whole before the parts, see Sergent, 1986).

All in all, I believe that there is currently no substantial evidence against the neurofunctional framework proposed here from neuroimaging studies of brain-damaged patients, which is rather in agreement with the nature of face perception.

To conclude this section, I have derived from the neuroimaging studies of brain-damaged patients (mainly PS) the proposal that there is a direct feedfoward activation from V1/extrastriate areas to the right FFA, which bypasses the visual areas located along the hierarchy in the ventral stream. This early face preferential activation is that of a global percept, allowing fast categorization of the stimulus as a face. However, the first face representation is too coarse for perceptual tasks requiring the extraction of a more detailed individual representation. In the normal brain, the face representation is thus progressively (i.e. within tens of milliseconds, between 100–200 ms following stimulus onset) refined, calling upon lower-visual areas through reentrant interactions. This may cause the emergence or increase of face preferential responses in the OFA, in the normal brain. This process cannot take place in the patients PS and DF, who present damage to the inferior occipital cortex, without any evidence of OFA activation. Consequently, these patients are severely impaired at perceiving individual faces.

This proposal is consistent with several sources of evidence, as reviewed above, but is inconsistent with a strict hierarchical view of the face processing pathway as initially suggested (Haxby et al., 2000) and often taken for granted in the literature. Direct tests of this proposal inspired by neuroimaging studies of brain-damaged patients should benefit from independent work using this approach (i.e. combining functional neuroimaging and lesion studies). Further evaluation of the model may also come from two different methods in future investigations. First, transcranial magnetic stimulation (TMS) could be used to interrupt the flow of information coming out of the identified right OFA in individual brains. In many participants of our experiments, the OFA appears to be located close to the external surface of the cortex suggesting that it should be possible to create relatively selective temporary interruption of cortical function in this area. Behaviorally, disrupting the processing of information in the right OFA using TMS should leave intact face detection but rather cause impairments in individual face discrimination and recognition tasks. This has been recently reported by Pitcher et al. (2007) in an rTMS and dual pulse TMS study, even though these authors used an average localization rather than individually defined "OFAs," making it difficult to ensure that they truly affected the OFA area in all of their participants. Furthermore, if repetitive TMS coupled with fMRI (e.g. Bestmann et al., 2004; Sack et al., 2007) is applied to the OFA territory, one should still observe a normal onset of preferential activation for faces in the ipsilateral FFA, which may nevertheless not be as sustained as without TMS, due to the lack of reentrant OFA inputs. This is a direct and strong prediction of the model outlined on Figure 8.2.

Another promising method to test the directionality and the timecourse of the OFA-FFA interaction (or of "face areas" in general) during normal face processing is fMRI recordings in the monkey brain (Logothetis et al., 2001). Using this method, several studies have identified similar areas of face preferential response in the monkey occipito-temporal cortex (Tsao et al., 2003; Pinsk et al., 2005). Electrophysiological recordings have shown a high face-selectivity of the neurons responses (Tsao et al., 2006) in three patches located in the STS, emerging at a latency of about 100 ms, as in traditional IT recordings. However, there was no information reported in these studies about possible differential time courses of neural activation in different face patches, and the relationship between these areas and the human FFA and OFA remains unclear. Nevertheless, the discovery of these face-selective small regions in fMRI recordings in the monkey brain may offer the exciting opportunity to create animal models of prosopagnosia, by lesioning these regions selectively and temporarily (e.g. through cooling methods, see Hupé et al., 2001) to investigate their functional connectivity. Insofar as the nonhuman primate face perception system is highly homologous to humans, I would again predict that anterior areas can show a preferential response to faces independently of such responses in lower visual areas.

8.4 Conclusions and future directions

Of the most important observations made principally but not exclusively on the brain-damaged prosopagnosic patient PS, I can summarize the following:

(1) The preferential response to faces in the inferior occipital cortex, termed the OFA, is not an epiphenomenon. It is usually neglected in the neuroimaging face literature, which concentrates most often exclusively on the FFA (e.g. Kleinschmidt and Cohen, 2006). Yet the OFA appears to play a critical role in face perception. A lesion of the right OFA is instrumental in causing cause prosopagnosia.

(2) A lesion of the right FFA may also cause prosopagnosia, as suggested by others (Barton et al., 2002), and there is also evidence that prosopagnosia can follow more anterior temporal structures sparing both the FFA and OFA structurally (e.g. Gainotti et al., 2003; Bukach et al., 2006). However, a conventional structural imaging approach is not sufficient to derive conclusions about the critical sites causing prosopagnosia because there is a large amount of interindividual variability in the localization functional areas. Most importantly, functional imaging may reveal abnormal face processing in areas left intact by the lesions, because they are deprived of inputs from other areas.

(3) A lesion of the right OFA will usually concern the ventral part of the lateral occipital complex (vLOC) as well, causing impairments for both face and object perception. In rare cases such as PS, the damage has spared the vLOC, leading to prosopagnosia without object agnosia.

(4) Even without any contribution of the right OFA, the right FFA may yet show intact categorization of the visual stimulus as a face suggesting direct striate/extrastriate inputs, bypassing the hierarchy of visual areas. This initial representation can be that of a whole face. This contradicts a view according to which the OFA would be the necessary "front end" of the face perception system, extracting facial features first (Haxby et al., 2000).

(5) Without reentrant inputs from the right OFA, the FFA is unable to derive a full perceptual representation of an individual face. Discriminating individual unfamiliar faces can be achieved to a certain extent by acquired prosopagnosic patients but the FFA plays little or no role in this function if deprived of OFA inputs.

Collectively, these studies show that there is a network of visual areas with a right hemispheric dominance that is involved in deriving full perceptual representations of individual faces, a function that is fundamental for our social interactions. A subset of these areas show a preferential response to faces, such as the right FFA and the OFA and appear to be critical for this function. Obviously, a large number of questions remain open, both about the neurofunctional organization of the patient PS and other acquired prosopagnosic patients, as well as about the functional neuroanatomy of face perception in the normal brain. Why is the FFA not recruited at all for individual face perception without the OFA, even though the patient can perform individual face discrimination above chance level? Is the vLOC or other areas coding for residual individual face discrimination in prosopagnosia by means of low-level analysis of single face features such as the mouth (see Dricot et al., 2008)? Why is there no sign of functional reorganization in PS's brain? Where is the initial FFA activation coming from, both in the normal brain and in patients such as PS and DF? What is the role of the left hemisphere, in particular the left FFA and OFA, in normal face perception? Besides the right OFA, whose lesion is instrumental in causing prosopagnosia, which are the other regions – such as the right FFA and anterior temporal areas – that are also necessary to subtend normal face perception?

Answering these questions will be fundamental to establish the neural dynamics of face perception at the system level in the human brain. While there are certainly multiple methods of cognitive neuroscience that will contribute to reach this goal, I hope to have provided a convincing illustration that a fruitful and inspiring approach in this field is the combination of functional imaging with the study of brain-damaged cases of prosopagnosia. Because acquired prosopagnosic patients with well-preserved low-level visual processes are extremely rare, present a large degree of variability in terms of their functional and neural impairments, and need to be characterized in depth for these studies, I advocate a single-case approach as described here rather than studies which treat variable patients as a group. In line with a cognitive neuropsychology approach at the functional level (Caramazza, 1986; Shallice, 1988), this single-case methodology can constrain and inspire neurofunctional models of normal face processing. This methodology is important not only to characterize the function(s) of brain areas and to clarify the necessity of certain areas for a given function but also to understand the functional connectivity between brain areas. Using this approach for a number of years, my colleagues and I have derived here a number of predictions about the functional neuroanatomy of face perception. Even if these predictions and the simple scheme proposed here are proved wrong by future investigations, the approach itself should not be abandoned, as it is undoubtedly a powerful source of inspiration for deriving hypotheses about how the human brain perceives faces.

Acknowledgments

I am supported by the Belgian National Foundation for Scientific Research (FNRS). I would like to thank the colleagues who contributed significantly to the empirical studies of the patient PS described in this chapter, Christine Schiltz, Bettina Sorger, Laurence Dricot, Rainer Goebel, Eugène Mayer, Roberto Caldara, Meike Ramon, Thomas Busigny, Mohamed Seghier, Philippe Lefèvre, Jean-Jacques Orban de Xivry. In addition, Christine Schiltz, Laurence Dricot, Jennifer Steeves, Thomas Busigny and Adélaïde de Heering provided useful comments on a previous version of this chapter. Finally and most importantly, I am greatly indebted to PS for her willingness to participate in our studies, her patience, and enthusiasm. Over the years she has been an invaluable source of inspiration not only for the studies summarized here but also for my understanding of prosopagnosia and how our face perception system works in general.

References

Avidan, G., Hasson, U., Hendler, T., Zohary, E. and Malach, R. (2002). Analysis of the neuronal selectivity underlying low fMRI signals. *Curr. Biol.*, 12: 964–972.

Barton, J. J., Press, D. Z., Keenan, J. P. and O'Connor, M. (2002). Lesions of the fusiform face area impair perception of facial configuration in prosopagnosia. *Neurol.*, 58: 71–78.

Benton, A. L. and Van Allen, M. W. (1968). Impairment in facial recognition in patients with cerebral disease. *Cortex*, 4: 344–358.

Bestmann, S., Baudewig, J., Siebner, H. R., Rothwell, J. C. and Frahm, J. (2004). Functional MRI of the immediate impact of transcranial magnetic stimulation on cortical and subcortical motor circuits. *Eur. J. Neurosci.*, 19: 1950–1962.

Bodamer, J. (1947). Die-Prosop-agnosie. Arch. Psychiatr. Nervenkrankh. 179: 6–54. English translation by Ellis, H. D. and Florence, M. (1990). *Cog. Neuropsychol.*, 7: 81–105.

Boussaoud, D., Desimone, R. and Ungerleider, L. G. (1991). Visual topography of area TEO in the macaque. *J. Comp. Neurol.*, 306: 554–575.

Bouvier, S. E and Engel, S. A. (2006). Behavioral deficits and cortical damage loci in cerebral achromatopsia. *Cereb. Cortex.*, 16: 183–191.

Bruce, V. and Young, A. W. (1986). Understanding face recognition. *Brit. J. Psychol.*, 77: 305–327.

Bukach, C. M., Bub, D. N., Gauthier, I. and Tarr, M. J. (2006). Perceptual expertise effects are not all or none: spatially limited perceptual expertise for faces in a case of prosopagnosia. *J. Cogn. Neurosci.*, 18: 48–63.

Bullier, J., Hupé, J. M., James, A. C. and Girard, P. (2001). The role of feedback connections in shaping the responses of visual cortical neurons. *Prog. Brain Res.*, 134: 193–204.

Busigny, T. and Rossion, B. (in preparation). Normal face detection in a case of acquired prosopagnosia.

Caldara, R., Schyns, P., Mayer, E., Smith, M., Gosselin, F. and Rossion, B. (2005). Does prosopagnosia take the eyes out from faces? Evidence for a defect in the use of diagnostic facial information in a brain-damaged patient. *J. Cogn. Neurosci.*, 17: 1652–1666.

Caramazza, A. (1986). On drawing inferences about the structure of normal cognitive systems from the analysis of patterns of impaired performance: the case for single-patient studies. *Brain Cogn.*, 5: 41–46.

Chen, C. C., Kao, K. L. and Tyler, C. W. (2007). Face configuration processing in the human brain: the role of symmetry. *Cereb. Cortex*, 17: 1423–1432.

Clarke, S., Lindemann, A., Maeder, P., Borruat, F. X. and Assal, G. (1997). Face recognition and postero-inferior hemispheric lesions. *Neuropsychologia*, 35: 1555–1563.

Damasio, H. and Damasio, A. R. (1989). *Lesion Analysis in Neuropsychology*. New York: Oxford University Press.

Damasio, A. R., Damasio, H. and Van Hoesen, G. W. (1982). Prosopagnosia: anatomic basis and behavioral mechanisms. *Neurology*, 32: 331–341.

Davidoff, J. and Landis, T. (1990). Recognition of unfamiliar faces in prosopagnosia. *Neuropsychologia*, 28: 1143–1161.

De Haan, E. H., Heywood, C. A., Young, A. W., Edelstyn, N. and Newcombe, F. (1995). Ettlinger revisited: the relation between agnosia and sensory impairment. *J. Neurol. Neurosurg. Psychiat.*, 58: 350–356.

De Renzi E. (1986). Prospagnosia in two patients with CT scan evidence of damage confied to the right hemisphere. *Neuropsychologia*, 24: 385–389.

De Renzi, E. and Pellegrino, G. (1998). Prosopagnosia and alexia without object agnosia. *Cortex*, 45: 403–415.

Delvenne, J.-F., Seron, X., Coyette, F. and Rossion, B. (2004). Evidence for perceptual deficits in associative visual (prosop)agnosia: a single-case study. *Neuropsychologia*, 42: 597–612.

Desimone, R., Albright, T. D., Gorss, C. G. and Bruce, C. (1984). Stimulus-selective properties of interior temporal neurons in the macaque. *J. Neurosci.*, 4: 2051–2062.

Dricot, L., Sorger, B., Schiltz, C., Goebel, R., Rossion, B. (2008). The roles of 'face' and 'non-face' areas during individual face discrimination: evidence by fMRI adaptation in a brain-damaged prosopagnosic patient. *NeuroImage*, 40: 318–332.

Edelman, G. M. (1978). Group selection and phasic reentrant signaling: a theory of higher brain function. In F. O. Schmitt (ed.) *The Mindful Brain*. Cambridge, MA: MIT Press.

Edelman, G. M. (1993). Neural Darwinism: selection and reentrant signaling in higher brain function. *Neuron*, 10: 115–125.

Eger, E., Henson, R. N., Driver, J. and Dolan, R. J. (2004). Bold repetition decreases in object-responsive ventral visual areas depend on spatial attention. *J. Neurophysiol.*, 92: 1241–1247.

Ellis, H. D. and Florence, M. (1990). Bodamer's (1947) paper on prosopagnosia. *Cog. Neuropsy.*, 81–105.

Ellis, H. D. and Young, A. W. (1989). Are faces special? In A. W. Young and H. D. Ellis (eds.) *Handbook of Research on Face Processing*. Amsterdam: Elsevier Science Publishers, pp. 1–26.

Ettlinger, G. (1956). Sensory deficits in visual agnosia. *J. Neurol., Neurosur Psy.*, 19: 297–301.

Fairhall, S. L. and Ishai, A. (2007). Effective connectivity within the distributed cortical network for face perception. *Cereb. Cortex*, 17: 2400–2406.

Fang, F., Murray, S. O. and He, S. (2007). Duration-dependent FMRI adaptation and distributed viewer-centered face representation in human visual cortex. *Cereb. Cortex*, 17: 1402–1411.

Farah, M. J. (1990). *Visual Agnosia: Disorders of Object Recognition and What They Tell Us About Normal Vision*. Cambridge, MA: MIT Press.

Felleman, D. J. and Van Essen, D. C. (1991). Distributed hierarchical processing in the primate cerebral cortex. *Cereb. Cortex*, 1: 1–47.

Freire, A., Lee, K. and Symons, L. A. (2000). The face-inversion effect as a deficit in the encoding of configural information: direct evidence. *Perception*, 29: 159–170.

Gainotti, G., Barbier, A. and Marra, C. (2003). Slowly progressive defect in the recognition of familiar people in a patient with right anterior temporal atrophy. *Brain*, 126: 792–803.

Galuske, R. A., Schmidt, K. E., Goebel, R., Lomber, S. G. and Payne, B. R. (2002). The role of feedback in shaping neural representations in cat visual cortex. *Proc. Nat. Acad. Sci USA*, 99: 17083–17088.

Gauthier, I., Behrmann, M. and Tarr, M. J. (1999). Is prosopagnosia a general deficit in subordinate-level categorization? *J. Cogn. Neurosci.*, 11: 349–370.

Gauthier, I., Skudlarski, P., Gore, J. C. and Anderson, A. W. (2000a). Expertise for cars and birds recruits brain areas involved in face recognition. *Nat. Neurosci.*, 3: 191–197.

Gauthier, I., Tarr, M. J., Moylan, J., Skudlarski, P., Gore, J. C. and Anderson, A. W. (2000b). The fusiform "face area" is part of a network that processes faces at the individual level. *J. Cogn. Neurosci.*, 12: 495–504.

Gilaie-Dotan, S. and Malach, R. (2007). Sub-exemplar shape tuning in human face-related areas. *Cereb. Cortex*, 17: 325–338.

Goffaux, V. and Rossion, B. (2007). Face inversion disproportionately impairs the perception of vertical but not horizontal relations between features. *J. Exp. Psychol.: Hum. Percept. Perf.*, 33: 995–1002.

Goldsmith, Z. G. and Liu, G. T. (2001). Facial recognition and prosopagnosia: past and present concepts. *Neuro-ophthalmol.*, 25: 177–192.

Gosselin, F. and Schyns, P. G. (2001). Bubbles: a technique to reveal the use of information in recognition tasks. *Vision Res.*, 41: 2261–2271.

Grill-Spector, K. and Malach, R. (2001). fMR-adaptation: a tool for studying the functional properties of human cortical neurons. *Acta Psychol.*, 107: 293–321.

Grill-Spector, K., Kushnir, T., Edelman, S., Avidan, G., Itzchak, Y. and Malach, R. (1999). Differential processing of objects under various viewing conditions in the human lateral occipital complex. *Neuron*, 24: 187–203.

Grill-Spector, K., Henson, R. and Martin, A. (2006). Repetition and the brain: neural models of stimulus-specific effects. *Trends Cogn. Sci.*, 10: 14–23.

Grill-Spector, K., Sayres, R. and Ress, D. (2006a). High-resolution imaging reveals highly selective nonface clusters in the fusiform face area. *Nat. Neurosci.*, 9: 1177–1185.

Haig, N. D. (1985). How faces differ – a new comparative technique. *Perception*, 14: 601–615.

Halgren, E., Dale, A. M., Sereno, M. I., Tootell, R. B. H., Marinkovic, K. and Rosen, B. (1999). Location of human face-selective cortex with respect to retinotopic areas. *Hum. Brain Mapp.*, 7: 29–37.

Haxby, J. V., Hoffman, E. A. and Gobbini, M. I. (2000). The distributed human neural system for face perception. *Trends Cogn. Sci.*, 4: 223–233.

Haxby, J. V., Gobbini, M. I., Furey, M. L., Ishai, A., Schouten, J. L. and Pietrini, P. (2001). Distributed and overlapping representations of faces and objects in ventral temporal cortex. *Science*, 293: 2425–2430.

Hécean, H. and Angelergues, R. (1962). Agnosia for faces (prosopagnosia). *Arch. Neurol.*, 7: 92–100.

Henke, K., Schweinberger, S. R., Grigo, A., Klos, T. and Sommer, W. (1998). Specificity of face recognition: recognition of exemplars of non-face objects in prosopagnosia. *Cortex*, 34: 289–296.

Hochstein, S. and Ahissar, M. (2002). View from the top: hierarchies and reverse hierarchies in the visual system. *Neuron*, 36: 791–804.

Hupé, J. M., James, A. C., Girard, P., Lomber, S. G., Payne, B. R. and Bullier, J. (2001). Feedback connections act on the early part of the responses in monkey visual cortex. *J. Neurophysiol.*, 85: 134–145.

Jacques, C. and Rossion, B. (2006). The speed of individual face categorization. *Psych. Sci.*, 17: 485–492.

Jacques, C., d'Arripe, O. and Rossion, B. (2007). The time course of the face inversion effect during individual face discrimination. *J. Vision*, 7: 1–9.

James, T. W., Culham, J., Humphrey, G. K., Milner, A. D. and Goodale, M. A. (2003). Ventral occipital lesions impair object recognition but not object-directed grasping: an fMRI study. *Brain*, 126: 2463–2475.

James, T. W., Humphrey, G. K., Gati, J. S., Menon, R. S. and Goodale, M. A. (2000). The effects of visual object priming on brain activation before and after recognition. *Curr. Biol.*, 10: 1017–1024.

Jiang, X., Rosen, E., Zeffiro, T., Vanmeter, J., Blanz, V. and Riesenhuber, M. (2006). Evaluation of a shape-based model of human face discrimination using FMRI and behavioral techniques. *Neuron*, 50: 159–172.

Joubert, S., Felician, O., Barbeau, E., Sontheimer, A., Barton, J. J., Ceccaldi, M. and Poncet, M. (2003). Impaired configurational processing in a case of progressive prosopagnosia associated with predominant right temporal lobe atrophy. *Brain*, 126: 2537–2550.

Kanwisher, N., McDermott, J. and Chun, M. M. (1997). The fusiform face area: a module in human extrastriate cortex specialized for face perception. *J. Neurosci.*, 17: 4302–4311.

Kleinschmidt, A. and Cohen, L. (2006). The neural bases of prosopagnosia and pure alexia: recent insights from functional neuroimaging. *Curr. Opin. Neurol.*, 19: 386–391.

Kiani, R., Esteky, H. and Tanaka, K. (2005). Differences in onset latency of macaque inferotemporal neural responses to primate and non-primate faces. *J. Neurophysiol.*, 94: 1587–1596.

Kim, M., Ducros, M., Carlson, T., Ronen, I., He, S., Ugurbil, K. and Kim, D. S. (2006). Anatomical correlates of the functional organization in the human occipitotemporal cortex. *Magn. Reson. Imaging*, 24: 583–590.

Kirchner, H. and Thorpe, S. J. (2006). Ultra-rapid object detection with saccadic eye movements: visual processing speed revisited. *Vision Res.*, 46: 1762–1776.

Landis, T., Regard, M., Bliestle, A. and Kleihues, P. (1988). Prosopagnosia and agnosia from noncanonical views: an autopsied case. *Brain*, 11: 1287–1297.

Lee, T. S., Mumford, D., Romero, R. and Lamme, V. A. (1998). The role of the primary visual cortex in higher level vision. *Vision Res.*, 38: 2429–2454.

Leopold, D. A., O'Toole, A. J., Vetter, T. and Blanz, V. (2001). Prototype-referenced shape encoding revealed by high-level aftereffects. *Nat. Neurosci.*, 4: 89–94.

Levine, D. N. and Calvanio, R. (1989). Prosopagnosia: a defect in visual configural processing. *Brain Cog.*, 10: 149–170.

Levy, J., Trevarthen, C. and Sperry, R. W. (1972). Perception of bilateral chimeric figures following hemispheric disconnection. *Brain*, 95: 61–78.

Loffler, G., Yourganov, G., Wilkinson, F. and Wilson, H. R. (2005). fMRI evidence for the neural representation of faces. *Nat. Neurosci.*, 8: 1386–1390.

Loftus, G. R. and Harley, E. M. (2004). Why is it easier to identify someone close than far away? *Psychon. Bull. Rev.*, 12: 43–65.

Logothetis, N. K., Pauls, J., Augath, M., Trinath, T. and Oeltermann, A. (2001). Neurophysiological investigation of the basis of the fMRI signal. *Nature*, 412: 150–157.

Malach, R., Reppas, J. B., Benson, R. R., Kwong, K. K., Jiang, H., Kennedy, W. A., Ledden, P. J., Brady, T. J., Rosen, B. R. and Tootell, R. B. (1995). Object-related activity revealed by functional magnetic resonance imaging in human occipital cortex. *Proc. Natl. Acad. Sci. USA*, 92: 8135–8139.

Mazard, A., Schiltz, C. and Rossion, B. (2006). Recovery from adaptation to facial identity is larger for upright than inverted faces in the human occipito-temporal cortex. *Neuropsychologia*, 44: 912–922.

McCarthy, G., Puce, A., Gore, J. C. and Allison, T. (1997). Face-specific processing in the human fusiform gyrus. *J. Cogn. Neurosci.*, 9: 605–610.

Meadows, J. C. (1974). The anatomical basis of prosopagnosia. *J. Neurol. Neurosurg. Psych.*, 37: 489–501.

Milner, A. D., Perrett, D. I., Johnston, R. S., Benson, P. J., Jordan, T. R., Heeley, D. W., Bettucci, D., Mortara, F., Mutani, R. and Terazzi, E. (1991). Perception and action in 'visual form agnosia'. *Brain*, 114: 405–428.

Mumford, D. (1992). On the computational architecture of the neocortex. II. The role of cortico-cortical loops. *Biol. Cybern.*, 66: 241–251.

Nakamura, H., Gattass, R., Desimone, R. and Ungerleider, L. G. (1993). The modular organization of projections from areas V1 and V2 to areas V4 and TEO in macaques. *J. Neurosci.*, 13: 3681–3691.

Orban de Xivry, J. J., Ramon, M., Lefèvre, P. and Rossion, B. (submitted) Reduced fixation on the eyes area of personally familiar faces following acquired prosopagnosia.

Penny, W. D., Stephan, K. E., Mechelli, A. and Friston, K. J. (2004). Modelling functional integration: a comparison of structural equation and dynamic causal models. *NeuroImage*, 23: suppl. 1: S264–274.

Pinsk, M. A., DeSimone, K., Moore, T., Gross, C. G. and Kastner, S. (2005). Representations of faces and body parts in macaque temporal cortex: a functional MRI study. *Proc. Nat. Acad. Sci. USA*, 102: 6996–7001.

Price, C. J. and Friston, K. (2002a). Functional imaging studies of neuropsychological patients: applications and limitations. *NeuroCase*, 8: 345–354.

Price, C. J. and Friston, K (2002b). Degeneracy and cognitive anatomy. *Trends Cog. Sci.*, 6: 416–421.

Price, C. J., Mummery, C. J., Moore, C. J., Frackowiak, R. S. and Friston, K. J. (1999). Delineating necessary and sufficient neural systems with functional imaging studies of neuropsychological patients. *J. Cogn. Neurosci.*, 11: 371–382.

Price, C. J., Warburton, E. A., Moore, C. J., Frackowiak, R. S. and Friston, K. J. (2001). Dynamic diaschisis: anatomically remote and context-sensitive human brain lesions. *J. Cogn. Neurosci.*, 13: 419–429.

Puce, A., Allison, T., Bentin, S., Gore, J. C. and McCarthy, G. (1998). Temporal cortex activation in humans viewing eye and mouth movements. *J. Neurosci.*, 18: 2188–2199.

Puce, A., Allison, T., Gore, J. C. and McCarthy, G. (1995). Face-sensitive regions in human extrastriate cortex studied by functional MRI. *J. Neurophysiol.*, 74: 1192–1199.

Quaglino, A. and Borelli, G. (1867). Emiplegia sinistra con amaurosi – guarigione – perdita totale della percezione dei colori e della memoria della configurazione degli oggetti. *Giornale d'Oftalmologia Italiano*, 10: 106–117. English translation by S. Deall Salla and A. W. Young (2003) Quaglino's 1867 case of prosopagnosia. *Cortex*, 39: 533–540.

Ramon, M. and Rossion, B. (2007). What's lost in prosopagnosia? An investigation of familiar face processing in a single-case of pure prosopagnosia working in a kindergarten. *J. Vision*, 7: 122.

Rhodes, G., Brennan, S. and Carey, S, (1987). Identification and ratings of caricatures: implications for mental representations of faces. *Cog. Psychol.*, 19: 473–497.

Riesenhuber, M., Jarudi, I., Gilad, S. and Sinha, P. (2004). Face processing in humans is compatible with a simple shape-based model of vision. *Proc. Biol. Sci.*, 271: S448–450.

Riesenhuber, M. and Poggio, T. (1999). Hierarchical models of object recognition in cortex. *Nat. Neurosci.*, 2: 1019–1025.

Roebroeck, A., Formisano, E. and Goebel, R. (2005). Mapping directed influence over the brain using Granger causality and fMRI. *NeuroImage*, 25: 230–242.

Rossion, B. (2008). Constraining the cortical face network by neuroimaging studies of acquired prosopagnosia. *NeuroImage*, 40: 423–426.

Rossion, B. and Jacques, C. (2008). Does physical interstimulus variance account for early electrophysiological face sensitive responses in the human brain? Ten lessons on the N170. *NeuroImage*, 39: 1959–1979.

Rossion, B. and Pourtois, G. (2004). Revisiting Snodgrass and Vanderwart's object databank: the role of surface detail in basic level object recognition. *Percept.*, 33: 217–236.

Rossion, B., Dricot, L., Devolder, A., Bodart, J. M., Crommelinck, M., de Gelder, B. and Zoontjes, R. (2000a). Hemispheric asymmetries for whole-based and part-based face processing in the human fusiform gyrus. *J. Cogn. Neurosci.*, 12: 793–802.

Rossion, B., Gauthier, I., Tarr, M. J.,Despland, P., Bruyer, R., Linotte, S. and Crommelinck, M. (2000b). The N170 occipito-temporal component is delayed and enhanced to inverted faces but not to inverted objects: an electrophysiological account of face-specific processes in the human brain. *NeuroReport*, 11: 69–74.

Rossion, B., Schiltz, C., Robaye, R., Pirenne, D. and Crommelinck, M. (2001). How does the brain discriminate familiar and unfamiliar faces: a PET study of face categorical perception. *J. Cogn. Neurosci.*, 13: 1019-1034.

Rossion, B., Caldara, R., Seghier, M., Schuller, A. M., Lazeyras, F. and Mayer, E. (2003). A network of occipito-temporal face-sensitive areas besides the right middle fusiform gyrus is necessary for normal face processing. *Brain*, 126: 2381–2395.

Rotshtein, P., Henson, R. N., Treves, A., Driver, J. and Dolan, R. J. (2005). Morphing Marilyn into Maggie dissociates physical and identity face representations in the brain. *Nat. Neurosci.*, 8: 107–113.

Rousselet, G. A., Mace, M. J. and Fabre-Thorpe, M. (2003). Is it an animal? Is it a human face? Fast processing in upright and inverted natural scenes. *J. Vision*, 5: 440–455.

Sack, A. T., Kohler, A., Bestmann, S., Linden, D. E., Dechent, P. and Goebel, R. (2007). Imaging the brain activity changes underlying impaired visuospatial judgments: simultaneous fMRI, TMS, and behavioral studies. *Cereb. Cortex*, 17: 2841–2852.

Sayres, R. and Grill-Spector, K. (2006). Object-selective cortex exhibits performance-independent repetition suppression. *J. Neurophysiol.*, 95: 995–1007.

Schiltz, C. and Rossion, B. (2006). Faces are represented holistically in the human occipito-temporal cortex. *NeuroImage*, 32: 1385–1394.

Schiltz, C., Sorger, B., Caldara, R., Ahmed, F., Mayer, E., Goebel, R. and Rossion, B. (2006). Impaired face discrimination in acquired prosopagnosia is associated with abnormal response to individual faces in the right middle fusiform gyrus. *Cereb. Cortex*, 4: 574–586.

Schweich, M. and Bruyer, R. (1993). Heterogeneity in the cognitive manifestations of prosopagnosia : the study of a group of single cases. *Cog. Neuropsychol.*, 10: 529–547.

Sergent, J. (1984). Configural processing of faces in the left and the right cerebral hemispheres. *J. Exp. Psychol. Hum. Percept. Perform.*, 10: 554–572.

Sergent, J. (1986). Microgenesis of face perception. In H. D. Ellis, M. A. Jeeves, F. Newcombe and A. M. Young (eds.) *Aspects of Face Processing*. Dordrecht: Martinus Nijhoff, pp. 17–33.

Sergent, J. (1988). Face perception and the right hemisphere. In L. Weiskrantz (ed.) *Thought Without Language*. Oxford, UK: Clarendon Press, pp. 108–131.

Sergent, J. and Signoret, J.-L. (1992). Varieties of functional deficits in prosopagnosia. *Cereb. Cortex*, 2: 375–388.

Sergent, J., Ohta, S. and MacDonald, B. (1992). Functional neuroanatomy of face and object processing: a positron emission tomography study. *Brain*, 115: 15–36.

Shallice, T. (1988). *From Neuropsychology to Mental Structure*. Cambridge, UK: Cambridge University Press.

Sorger, B., Goebel, R., Schiltz, C. and Rossion, B. (2007). Understanding the functional neuroanatomy of prosopagnosia. *NeuroImage*, 35: 852–856.

Steeves, J., Culham, J. C., Duchaine, B. C., Pratesi, C. C., Valyear, K. F., Schindler, I., Humphrey, G. K., Milner, A. D. and Goodale, M. A. (2006). The fusiform face area is not sufficient for face recognition: evidence from a patient with dense prosopagnosia and no occipital face area. *Neuropsychologia*, 44: 594–609.

Steeves, J., Goltz, H., Dricot, L., Sorger, B., Peters, J., Goebel, R., Milner, A. D., Goodale, M. A. and Rossion, B. (2007). Face-selective activation in the middle fusiform gyrus in a patient with acquired prosopagnosia: abnormal modulation for face identity. *J. Vision*, 7: 627.

Sugase, Y., Yamane, S., Ueno, S. and Kawano, K. (1999). Global and fine information coded by single neurons in the temporal visual cortex. *Nature*, 400: 869–873.

Thorpe, S., Fize, D. and Marlot, C. (1996). Speed of processing in the human visual system. *Nature*, 381: 520–522.

Tononi, G., Sporns, O. and Edelman, G. M. (1999). Measures of degeneracy and redundancy in biological networks. *Proc. Natl. Acad. Sci. USA*, 1696: 3257–3262.

Tovée, M. J. (1998). Face processing: getting by with a little help from its friends. *Curr. Biol.*, 8: R17–R320.

Tsao, D. Y., Freiwald, W. A., Knutsen, T. A., Mandeville, J. B. and Tootell, R. B. (2003). Faces and objects in macaque cerebral cortex. *Nat. Neurosci.*, 6: 989–695.

Tsao, D. Y., Freiwald, W. A., Tootell, R. B. and Livingstone, M. S. (2006). A cortical region consisting entirely of face-selective cells. *Science*, 311: 670–674.

Valentine, T. (1991). A unified account of the effects of distinctiveness, inversion, and race in face recognition. *Quart. J. Exp. Psychol.*, 43A: 161–204.

Wang, G., Tanaka, K. and Tanifuji, M. (1996). Optical imaging of functional organization in the monkey inferotemporal cortex. *Science*, 272: 1665–1668.

Wigan, A. L. (1844). *A New View of Insanity: The Duality of the Mind.* London: Longman.

Winston, J. S., Henson, R. N., Fine-Goulden, M. R. and Dolan, R. J. (2004). fMRI-adaptation reveals dissociable neural representations of identity and expression in face perception. *J. Neurophysiol.*, 92: 1830–1839.

Yin, R. K. (1969). Looking at upside-down faces. *J. Exp. Psychol.*, 81: 41–145.

Young, A. W., Hellawell, D. and Hay, D. C. (1987). Configurational information in face perception. *Perception*, 16: 747–759.

Yovel, G. and Kanwisher, N. (2005). The neural basis of the face inversion effect. *Curr. Biol.*, 15: 2256–2262.

9 An integrative approach towards understanding the psychological and neural basis of congenital prosopagnosia

G. Avidan, C. Thomas and M. Behrmann

9.1 Background

Faces have distinctive evolutionary and social significance and, therefore, it is not surprising that face perception is probably the most developed visual perceptual skill in humans. At an input level, faces are perceptually similar homogeneous exemplars drawn from a single class and are all composed of essentially the same local elements (e.g. two eyes, a nose, cheeks and a mouth) in the same spatial layout (e.g. eyes above the nose). Despite this fundamental visual similarity, individual faces convey a large amount of critical information upon which we, as human observers, rely heavily for social interaction and communication. A quick look at a person's face reveals valuable information such as age, gender, emotional state, gaze direction, and useful speech cues. We can also identify individuals accurately and rapidly across radically different viewing conditions (e.g. lighting, vantage points) and structural changes of the face as the person ages or conveys different expressions. Moreover, notwithstanding some individual differences (Rotshtein et al., 2007), we can represent the unique identity of an almost unlimited number of faces and, when presented with a familiar face, can easily come up with the name of the person as well as other relevant biographical information that pertains to the individual.

Cortical Mechanisms of Vision, ed. M. Jenkin and L. R. Harris. Published by Cambridge University Press.
© Cambridge University Press 2009.

Faces are also interesting at the neural level. It has been shown that there are specific cells in monkey inferior temporal cortex which are selectively activated by faces (see Gross, 2005 for a recent review) and, recently, face selective patches have also been uncovered in nonhuman primates using functional magnetic resonance imaging (fMRI) (Tsao et al., 2003, 2006). As will be discussed in more detail below, mostly as a result of neuropsychological studies, we have long known that regions in human occipitotemporal cortex are critically involved in face recognition. However, the advent of noninvasive imaging techniques, particularly fMRI, has enabled researchers to investigate these regions in healthy human subjects directly. One key area which is located on the ventral surface of the temporal lobe in the fusiform gyrus consistently shows the strongest preferential response to faces in comparison with other occipitotemporal regions (Sergent et al., 1992; Puce et al., 1995; Kanwisher et al., 1997; McCarthy et al., 1997). In recognition of its central role in face processing, this region has been labeled the fusiform face area, or FFA, and is considered to serve as a critical face processing module in the human brain (Kanwisher et al., 1997). However, a number of other regions in human occipitotemporal cortex, such as the lateral occipital region and the superior temporal sulcus (STS), despite evincing a somewhat less consistent activation, have also been shown to play a major role in face processing (Puce et al., 1998; Ishai et al., 1999; Gauthier et al., 2000; Haxby et al., 2000, 2001; Hoffman and Haxby, 2000; Rossion et al., 2003; Gobbini and Haxby, 2007). Moreover, in addition to these "core regions" of face processing (in the terminology of Haxby et al. (2000)), there are a number of other regions outside the occipitotemporal cortex that belong to an extended face recognition system and play a critical role in other aspects of face perception such as emotional and semantic processing (Fairhall and Ishai, 2007; Gobbini and Haxby, 2007; Ishai, 2007). For example, the amygdalae serve as part of the extended network and are involved in extracting information regarding facial expressions, particularly that of fear (Adolphs et al., 1995; Whalen et al., 1998). Thus, although the FFA may play a pre-eminent role in face perception, there is growing consensus that different aspects of face processing require the coordinated activity of many brain regions and that it may be the case that face perception is accomplished by the net activity of a well-connected face processing network (Fairhall and Ishai, 2007; Summerfield et al., 2006) with some nodes within this network, such as the FFA, being particularly necessary and critical for the process (Ishai, 2007).

9.1.1   Congenital prosopagnosia

Interestingly, although face recognition is quick, efficient, and effortless for most people, it is extremely difficult, if not impossible, for individuals who suffer from a specific disorder termed prosopagnosia. Acquired prosopagnosia (AP), the term referring to the loss of face recognition abilities, occurs in individuals who were premorbidly normal but who sustained brain damage to the ventral visual cortex in adulthood. The existence and profile of AP has been recognized for several decades (Bodamer, 1947) and has provided a unique window into the psychological and neural substrate of face processing. In recent years, however, attention has been drawn to an analogous impairment, congenital prosopagnosia (CP), which refers to the impairment in face processing that is apparent from birth in the absence of any noticeable brain damage or an obvious cortical alteration, and that occurs in the presence of intact sensory and intellectual functions (Bentin et al., 1999; Duchaine et al., 2004; Behrmann and Avidan, 2005; Behrmann et al., 2005; Le Grand et al., 2006; Dobel et al., 2007). This condition is to be differentiated from developmental prosopagnosia (DP) which, although evident from early life too as in the case of CP, is associated with brain injury as a result of, for example, respiratory arrest or a major fall early in the course of development (for example, see Barton et al., 2003).

Oftentimes, the introspection of an individual with CP describes the problem well, as in the quote below.

> "I'm glad I was able to spend some time with you. It's nice that now when I write to you, I can picture you in my mind. Well, "picture you" may not be quite the right words. I just realized my mental picture is medium height, slender build, longish black wavy hair." Face? Well, it's there: two eyes, a nose, and a mouth."[1]

Individuals with CP can certainly detect a face among other visual stimuli (Behrmann et al., 2007), and as reflected in this quote, notice the different features comprising the face (eyes, nose, mouth), and so, their face recognition problem cannot be attributed to early level of processing (this observation was also confirmed by more formal testing; for example see Behrmann et al., 2005; Le Grand et al., 2006). However, for reasons that we still do not completely understand, the features comprising the face are not "glued" together to form a unique, recognizable identity. The description cited above is similar to the numerous personal anecdotes provided by other CP individuals and typically include not only the failure to recognize faces, even those of close family members, but also the compensatory strategies adopted to assist their recognition (such as increased reliance on hair style, body build, voice or gait). Interestingly, such comments are remarkably like those reported by AP patients. Critically however, unlike AP in which the face impairment is dramatically apparent after the onset of the brain insult, CP may go undetected as the individual has no means of comparison with normal face processing skills. The consequences of this is that some CP individuals may experience lasting frustration and socially debilitating consequences (see Duchaine and Nakayama, 2005; but also Dobel et al., 2007 for recent findings suggesting that individuals with CP are socially well adapted and integrated, which are somewhat contradictory to this common view).

All forms of prosopagnosia present researchers with the unique opportunity to delve into the systems that support normal face processing. But CP is somewhat of a special case as it enables researchers to conduct careful functional imaging studies in the absence of cortical damage (such as in cases of AP and DP). Thus, the unfortunate, but singular circumstances of CP, in which a relatively circumscribed behavioral impairment in the domain of face processing exists with an apparently normal brain, provide us with the prospect of pinpointing the brain mechanisms underlying normal face representation and perception. Furthermore, CP allows us to explore the necessary and sufficient brain activations that are required to ensure intact face recognition.

---

[1] Taken from an email sent to one of the authors by CP subject IT after spending an extensive three days of testing in our lab with the author.

In addition, given that CP individuals never develop normal face recognition despite seemingly normal exposure to faces throughout their life, CP raises a host of theoretical questions regarding the psychological and neural conditions required for the initial acquisition of normal face processing and possible limitations on the time period during which this acquisition can occur. Intriguingly, CP also serves as a model to explore whether, and to what extent face processing is amenable to targeted intervention programs and, if so, what underlying neural changes might serve as the correlate accompanying the behavioral improvement.

Finally, a unique aspect of CP, which is reminiscent of other neurodevelopment disorders such as specific language impairments (Lai et al., 2001; Fisher et al., 2003) and congenital amusia (Peretz and Hyde, 2003) is that it apparently runs in families and there have been many reports now documenting the familial component of the disorder (De Haan, 1999; Behrmann and Avidan, 2005; Dobel et al., 2007; Duchaine et al., 2007; Kennerknecht et al., 2008). The presence of this familial component indicates that CP may have a genetic underpinning and indeed, one recent report suggests that CP is compatible with an autosomal-dominant mode of transmission with a point mutation as the basis of the disorder (monogenic disorder) (Grueter et al., 2007). This possible genetic linkage opens up the exciting avenue of understanding not only the genetic predisposition to the disorder but also the link between a specific genetic makeup and high-level cognitive functions, such as face processing (and see Andersson et al., 2008 for another demonstration of such a link).

The main goal of the present chapter is to explore the possible underlying neural bases of CP, at both the functional and structural levels. We start by briefly reviewing the behavioral profile characterizing these individuals and then discuss the neural profile of CP, highlighting findings from a number of methodological avenues which examine the neural mechanisms potentially giving rise to CP.

9.2   Behavioral profile of congenital prosopagnosia

Normal face perception is a multifaceted process and, hence, defining what constitutes a face processing deficit is not a trivial task. For example, face processing requires the detection of a face among other types of visual stimuli, the discrimination between different faces even if they are unfamiliar, and finally, the recognition, in which the exact identification of a specific individual face is derived. Although CP has attracted much scientific attention recently, many aspects of its behavioral profile and underlying neural mechanism are still unclear. Thus, while most researchers would agree that the hallmark of the disorder is the inability to recognize familiar faces, the extent of the impairment in other tasks related to face and nonface processing is not yet fully agreed upon (Duchaine and Nakayama, 2004; Behrmann et al., 2005; Le Grand et al., 2006; Bentin et al., 2007; Duchaine et al., 2007). Since the focus of the present chapter is primarily on the neural profile of CP, the reader is directed to recent publications, which extensively review the behavioral profile of this impairment (Dobel et al., 2007; Behrmann et al., in press). Here, we only briefly describe data from two behavioral tasks which are robust in uncovering the impairment in face processing in CP across a number of investigations.

9.2.1 Famous faces

The first task examined the ability of individuals with CP to identify well-known faces. To this end, we presented photographs of famous individuals (embedded within the same number of photographs of unknown people), one at a time, to the CP participants as well as to matched control subjects. None of the photographs contained any obvious diagnostic cues (see Figure 9.1a) such as hats or beards and subjects were given unlimited duration to make their response. Possible responses included the name of the individual, some contextual information (e.g. actor), which we coded as "correct", "don't know" or an incorrect name.

Figure 9.1A depicts the mean of the control group for each response type as well as the mean of the CP group and the individual performance level for each CP individual tested on this measure. Scores more than two standard deviations below the control mean of all subjects (i.e. below 55.1%) were considered atypical. As evident from this figure, all CP individuals performed well below the mean of the control group ($p < 0.0001$ for correct responses), although there is some variability, with better subjects scoring around 60% accuracy and others only achieving around 30% accuracy. However, even subject MT, whose score was just within the normal range of the control group (62.5%), scored well below his own age and gender-matched controls who scored 89.28% on average. As is clear, there are significantly more ($p < 0.0001$) "don't know" responses for the CP than control subjects and finally, the trend towards the increased "incorrect name" responses in CP ($p < 0.05$) suggests that these participants are familiar with popular culture and celebrities and know the names but cannot assign them to the correct face. These findings serve as a clear marker of the face recognition impairment in all CP individuals.

9.2.2 Face discrimination

Although the behavioral performance of the CP individuals on famous faces recognition is obviously poor, the source of the impairment remains to be elucidated. One possibility is that these individuals do actually recognize the faces but have lost the memory of the names of these individuals, a disorder referred to as prosopamnesia (Tippett et al., 2000; Williams et al., 2007). Alternatively, the problem might arise in the perceptual rather than in the memorial system per se. To adjudicate between these two possibilities, we had the CP individuals make same/different discriminations between a pair of novel faces. If performance is still poor under these conditions, the interpretation favors a perceptual disorder. If, however, performance is within normal bounds, then we might be more inclined to think of a mnemonic basis for the impaired recognition performance.

To address this issue, we had the CP individuals and their controls make a face matching judgment between a target face presented at the top of the screen and two choices presented below, to the left and right. Participants simply indicated their responses using one of two response keys to report that the match was on the left or the right. The mean RT for the control group and the CP subjects is shown in Figure 9.1b. As is evident, the controls' RT is considerably faster than that of the CP individuals ($p < 0.0001$), each of whom performs far more slowly than the control subjects (except for

a. Recognition of famous faces   **b. Unfamiliar face discrimination**

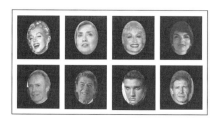   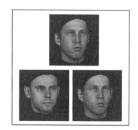

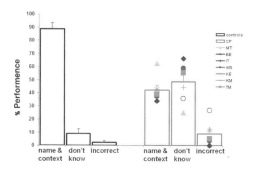   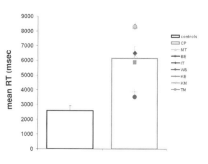

Figure 9.1. (A) Example stimuli and performance level of controls and seven CP individuals on a famous faces questionnaire. The mean of the controls is indicated by the black bars, the mean performance of the CP subjects is indicated by the gray bars and the performance of each CP is denoted by a specific symbol. Providing either the correct name or correct contextual information was considered as a correct response (leftmost bar for each group). Other possible responses were "don't know" or "incorrect" in which the wrong name was provided. CP individuals recognized far fewer famous faces compared with their matched control counterparts. In all figures, error bars indicate standard error of the mean across subjects in each group. (B) Example stimuli and performance level of seven CP individuals relative to controls. The faces in this experiment were presented for unlimited exposure duration and so the dependent measure of interest is reaction time. As can be seen, the CP individuals were significantly slower at face discrimination than the controls, even for unfamiliar faces. (Adapted from Avidan and Behmann, 2008.)

subject WS whose performance is just at the edge of the normal range). These findings reflect the impairment in novel face matching for the CP individuals and suggest that their difficulty in recognition is not simply one of remembering the face. A perceptual component to the disorder is clearly implicated by these results.

9.3 Neural profile of congenital prosopagnosia

As outlined above, CP offers a unique scenario in which a clear deficit in face processing exists in the absence of any other known behavioral deficits (although it is sometimes accompanied by some difficulty in object processing; see Behrmann et al., 2005; Duchaine et al., 2007; Righart and de Gelder, 2007) and with an apparently intact brain. Thus, in addition to its inherent interest as a neurodevelopmental disorder, CP can also be used as a model for understanding the neural substrates underlying normal face processing. Much of our own work has been focused on elucidating the neural substrate supporting face processing and we have adopted an integrative approach using a variety of noninvasive functional and structural imaging techniques. Specifically, at the outset, we first investigated whether CP could be accounted for by a functional alteration in cortical face-related regions. To this end, we have used fMRI to examine the nature of face representation in CP both in the pre-eminent face processing cortical region, the FFA, but also in other face-related regions in occipitotemporal cortex. We then addressed the issue of whether CP could be explained by a localized anatomical alteration within occipitotemporal cortex by systematically analyzing high resolution structural MR images of CP individuals. Finally, given that face processing is probably mediated by a network of brain regions (Haxby et al., 2000; Fairhall and Ishai, 2008; Gobbini and Haxby, 2007; Ishai, 2008) and, hence, depends on the connectivity between these regions we have also used a relatively new technique, Diffusion Tensor Imaging (DTI) and tractography, to examine the structural integrity of the white matter tracts that link the "core" face processing regions in ventral occipital cortex, to the "extended" regions in anterior temporal and frontal cortices (see Section 9.1). Here, we review the main findings of these investigations and consider them in relation to the existing literature.

9.3.1 Functional profile of congenital prosopagnosia: Can CP be accounted for by a functional alteration in face processing regions in occipitotemporal cortex?

Many years of research in AP reveal that, despite the large variability in lesion size and extent across patients, the common underlying site of injury leading to this impairment is in the occipitotemporal cortex, and, more specifically, that the critical site of injury is in the vicinity of the right fusiform gyrus (Damasio et al., 1982, 1990; Sergent and Signoret, 1992; De Renzi, 1997; Wada and Yamamoto, 2001; Bouvier and Engel, 2006). These neuropsychological findings imply that this region is likely necessary in order to ensure intact face processing. In addition, as reviewed in Section 9.1, many imaging studies in healthy individuals have demonstrated the involvement of the FFA in face processing (Sergent et al., 1992; Puce et al., 1995; Kanwisher et al., 1997; McCarthy et al., 1997; Halgren et al., 1999; Ishai et al., 1999; Haxby et al., 2000). However, given the essence of the technique, findings from fMRI studies are correlational in nature: the BOLD signal bears a relationship to some behavior but is not necessarily causally related to it. As such, fMRI studies only allow one to deduce that the FFA is involved in face processing but do not permit us to conclude whether the FFA is actually necessary and sufficient for these behavioral processes to be completed. Critically, CP, in which a clear impairment in face processing exists offers the unique opportunity to examine whether the FFA is not only necessary for face processing as implied from AP, or more generally involved in face perception as suggested by fMRI studies with normal individuals, but is actually sufficient in order to allow intact face processing. Thus, reduced or absent FFA activation in CP should strongly predict that in the absence of this activation, face processing is abnormal. The flip side is that normal FFA activation should predict that face processing is intact.

To date, a number of studies have investigated the functional properties of the occipitotemporal region in relation to face processing in CP using fMRI, ERP and MEG. Despite these numerous attempts, the existing results are far from clear cut, with some studies showing normal activation in FFA in CP individuals while others show an abnormal pattern of response. We start this section with only a brief description of the extant electrophysiological findings which we have recently reviewed elsewhere (Behrmann et al., 2008) and then discuss the fMRI findings in length.

In normal subjects, there is a typical face selective waveform peaking at about 130 to 200 msec after stimulus onset that can be detected in both ERP (N170) and MEG (M170). Both methods have been used to examine the physiological patterns in CP but, as yet, the findings are equivocal. On the one hand, several studies have revealed reduced face selectivity in individuals with CP (Bentin et al., 1999, 2007; Kress and Daum, 2003) but, in another ERP study, the authors found that three participants with DP (they are referred to as DP in this paper but given that they do not have any evidence for brain injury we would call them CP) exhibited normal N170 while only one subject exhibited reduced face selectivity in the N170 response (Minnebusch et al., 2007). Such heterogeneity is also apparent in a MEG study (Harris et al., 2005) in which two out five CP individuals exhibited a normal response but the remaining three individuals did not exhibit a face-selective response in their MEG pattern. Whether the large variability obtained in electrophysiological studies with CP reflects a true heterogeneity within the CP population and whether this heterogeneity is associated with a specific behavioral profile, given that there is also substantial behavioral variability across studies, remains to be resolved (Duchaine and Nakayama, 2004; Behrmann et al., 2005; Le Grand et al., 2006; Bentin et al., 2007; Dobel et al., 2007; Duchaine et al., 2007). The hope is that as more individuals are tested and the procedures become increasingly standardized and widespread in usage, the emerging pattern will become clearer and some consistency might emerge.

Using fMRI, several studies have now revealed normal face-selective activation in the FFA (Hasson et al., 2003; Avidan et al., 2005) as well as in other face-related foci in CP. This finding was initially somewhat surprising and counterintuitive given the vast literature implicating this region as a critical face processing module in the human brain. As such, the expectation was that in CP, the FFA should evince abnormal function when face processing is impaired. In a study which included four individuals with CP (Avidan et al., 2005), we documented normal bilateral FFA activation in CP in terms of the overall signal strength, selectivity to faces, and spatial extent of the BOLD signal. These findings were obtained by employing a conventional face localizer experiment in which static images (line drawings) from several visual categories (faces, houses, objects, and patterns) were presented in a block design fashion. Importantly, in this same experiment, normal patterns of activation were also obtained in other face-related foci in occipitotemporal cortex such as the lateral occipital region. Interestingly, these normal activations (even in FFA) were obtained while CP subjects performed a discrimination task (one-back task) on which they exhibited poorer performance relative to controls, thus exhibiting a clear dissociation between apparently normal brain activation, as reflected in the BOLD signal, and impaired behavioral performance. Since the publication of these data, we have replicated a similar pattern of results in three more CP subjects (one of these subjects has completed the one-back task described here and all three evinced normal response on another face mapping task – see below for further details). Using this approach, similar findings were also obtained in a different subject, YT, described in Hasson et al. (2003). A further CP subject, SO, investigated by a different group of researchers, also exhibited face-selective activation in the right FFA that was similar to that of controls (von Kriegstein et al., 2005).

Although the BOLD signal uncovered in the CP individuals in FFA was robust, one concern that we had regarding the conventional localizer paradigm was that, because of the nature of the paradigm, the FFA activation might have been elevated artifactually. During this fMRI scan, the CP subjects completed a one-back task (discriminating between consecutive images) – this task engaged working memory and was highly demanding for the CP participants, as reflected in their relatively poor performance particularly for faces. Both the involvement of working memory and the task difficulty could potentially have elevated the activity in the FFA, as has been previously shown in healthy individuals (Druzgal and D'Esposito, 2003). Moreover, the stimuli were simple line drawings and the subjects were required to maintain constant fixation throughout – two factors that make the experiment very different from natural situations in which faces are normally viewed.

To circumvent some of the limitations of this initial study, we conducted a second mapping experiment but, this time, the stimuli were presented as short video clips containing real images of people, landscapes, buildings, and moving or manipulated objects, rather than static images. In addition, subjects were instructed to watch these clips naturally without performing any task and were also allowed to move their eyes freely. Interestingly, it was also the case that when using this more naturalistic paradigm, normal face-selective activation was obtained in all face-related foci bilaterally (FFA, lateral occipital cortex, superior temporal sulcus – STS) in the same CP individuals who participated in the initial conventional mapping experiment. We have recently replicated this result in three additional individuals with CP and the pattern of normal face-selective activation in all these seven subjects and in seven typical controls subjects is presented in Figure 9.2. As is evident from the figure, the pattern of activation obtained in CP is very similar to that of controls, further suggesting that their FFA functionality is normal.

In contrast to these robust findings, abnormal face-related BOLD activation in the FFA in a single CP subject has been recently reported (Bentin et al., 2007). The source of the discrepancy between this latter study and the results presented above are not obvious, but, as mentioned in relation to the electrophysiological findings, it may be related to the substantial heterogeneity among CP individuals. In addition, another study failed to show face-selective activation in three prosopagnosic individuals (Had-

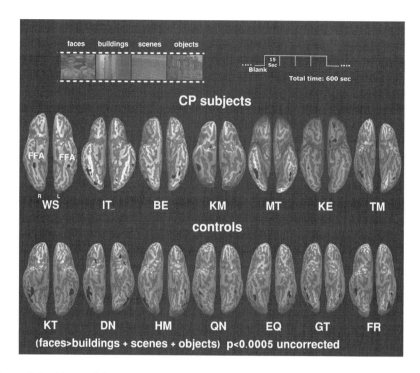

Figure 9.2. Maps of face-related activation in the fusiform face area (FFA) of seven CP subjects and seven controls. For each subject, the data are presented on an inflated brain representation shown from a ventral view. As is evident, the CP individuals exhibit similar activation patterns to those of controls, thus indicating normal face-related activation in the fusiform gyrus. The maps were obtained from the motion picture experiment in which short video clips were presented to the subjects (top of figure) and face activation was obtained by contrasting the BOLD signal generated during the perception of faces with that of all other stimuli (buildings, scenes, objects) at $p < 0.0005$ for each subject (uncorrected).

jikhani and de Gelder, 2002); however two out of the three participants tested in this study suffered a brain injury at childhood and so do not qualify as pure cases of CP and this may clearly account for their lack of face selectivity. The third case described in this study does fit our definition of CP but still, for reasons that are not clear, failed to show any face-selective activation in occipitotemporal cortex.

The fMRI findings, reviewed so far, reveal that many (although not all) CP individuals exhibit an apparently normal activation pattern in the fusiform gyrus as well as in other face-related foci in occipitotemporal cortex in studies using functional fMRI measurements. However, due to the nature of the BOLD signal which averages the activation across a large number of neurons (Levy et al., 2004), a face-selective signal could result from a number of different underlying mechanisms (Avidan et al., 2002). As such, the presence of a face-selective signal does not per se indicate that the computations taking place in the FFA are indeed normal. For example, it could be that neurons in the FFA are activated by the presence of a face but in CP, unlike in normal subjects, they are not sensitive to the identity of the face. If this were the case, we might obtain an average response which is face-selective despite the fact that the neurons are not sensitive to the critical information about the face.

One technique that can be used in order to overcome this problem is that of fMR adaptation (fMR-A). This technique takes advantage of the fact that repeated presentation of visual stimuli such as faces results in reduced neuronal activation and reduction of the BOLD response in the FFA as well as in other high order visual areas (Li et al., 1993; Grill-Spector et al., 1999; Avidan et al., 2002; Pourtois et al., 2005; Rotshtein et al., 2005; Gilaie-Dotan and Malach, 2007). As such, fMR-A has been used to study the sensitivity of the neuronal properties of higher order visual areas at a subvoxel resolution. More specifically, it has been used to examine the sensitivity of such regions and particularly the FFA to various parameters such as the viewing angle (Grill-Spector et al., 1999; Pourtois et al., 2005) or the identity of the face (Rotshtein et al., 2005). We have also adopted this technique with the express purpose of examining the sensitivity of the FFA in CP individuals to face repetition. We and others have shown that at the behavioral level, CP individuals are impaired at deciding whether two faces are the same or different and this is true even for unfamiliar faces (see Figure 9.1b, and Behrmann et al., 2005; Bentin et al., 2007; Duchaine et al., 2007). The fMR-A technique can allow us to assess whether this behavioral difficulty is reflected in the fMRI signal. In our previous work (Avidan et al., 2005), we scanned 10 healthy control subjects and four individuals with CP in a block design paradigm (Figure 9.3a) (see Behrmann et al., 2005 for the behavioral profile of the CP subjects who participated in the experiment). Subjects viewed blocks of stimuli containing 12 different face images or 12 repetitions of an identical face (the original experiment also included stimuli from other categories such as vehicles but the results of these other categories are beyond the scope of this chapter and the reader is referred to (Avidan et al., 2005) for more details on this issue). We have previously shown that, in control subjects, the repeated presentation of the identical image leads to a substantial signal reduction (Avidan et al., 2002) and this effect is depicted on the left graph on Figure 9.3b (compare the dark gray bar to the light gray bar). This is entirely consistent with the plethora of studies showing visual adaptation and the magnitude of the adaptation is within the expected range (Grill-Spector et al., 1999; Pourtois et al., 2005). Most interesting and, as can be seen in the right panel of Figure 9.3b, the four CP individuals actually exhibited the same response pattern as the controls; this was true both at the level of the overall signal but, more critically, at the level of the repetition suppression; that is, the signal reduction following repeated presentation of the same stimulus. Thus, these findings indicate that the FFA response of CP individuals is indeed sensitive to face repetition and provides us with another apparent dissociation between the behavioral performance in these individuals and their BOLD signal.

The use of a block design paradigm in general, and particularly in the context of a repetition suppression experiment, has been frequently criticized (e.g. Kourtzi and Kanwisher, 2000). The main argument against this kind of a design is that during the course of an experimental block, subjects may lose interest and become less attentive to the stimuli and this is especially true if a block contains many repetitions of the same stimulus such as in the design depicted on Figure 9.3a. Thus, the claim is that, in

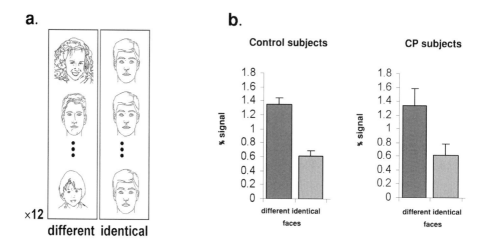

Figure 9.3. (a) Experimental design of the block design repetition suppression experiment. Line drawings of faces were presented in blocks containing 12 different images or 12 repeated presentations of the same face. (b) Results of the block design repetition suppression experiment. Left graph: control subjects, right graph: CP subjects. As evident, both groups exhibited substantial signal reduction during the repeated vs. different conditions (compare dark with light gray bars), indicating neural adaptation. (Adapted from Avidan et al., 2005.)

such cases, the signal attenuation might not be attributable to the repetition suppression effect but might also be related to reduced attention which has been shown to lead to signal reduction in higher order visual areas (O'Craven et al., 1999; Kastner and Ungerleider, 2000; Avidan et al., 2003).

To circumvent such possible alternative explanations for the apparently normal signal attenuation in CP, we recently conducted another repetition suppression study in which we employed a rapid event-related design rather than a block design. Unlike in the previous design, here, two consecutive faces appeared briefly on the screen. In each pair, the two face images could be two images of two different individuals (for example, a picture of Bill Clinton and a picture of Clint Eastwood) or a repetition of the exact same image of the same individual (see Figure 9.4). The experiment also included a third condition in which the two images within a pair were two different pictures of the same person (e.g. two different photographs of Bill Clinton), but the discussion of this condition is beyond the scope of this chapter (but see Avidan and Behrmann, 2008 for more details on this condition). During the entire experiment, the subjects' task was to decide whether the two consecutive images within a pair were of the same individual or two different individuals.

In order to examine the effects of face familiarity on the activation pattern in FFA, as well as other cortical regions, half of the faces presented in this experiment were of famous people whereas the other half of the images were of unknown individuals. The issue of familiarity effects remains controversial despite much research, and is only mentioned here briefly in relation to the repetition effect. The reader is referred to our papers, as well as many other papers, for a more comprehensive discussion of this topic (Gorno-Tempini et al., 1998; George et al., 1999; Henson et al., 2000, 2003; Leveroni et al., 2000; Nakamura et al., 2000; Gorno-Tempini and Price, 2001; Eger et al, 2005; Avidan and Behrmann, 2008).

Twelve healthy controls and six CP individuals participated in the experiment (all CP subjects whose behavioral data is presented in Figure 9.1 except for subject TM). For each subject, the left and right FFA were independently localized using an external face localizer experiment (motion picture experiment, see Avidan et al., 2005).

The specific experimental design employed here allowed us to examine the effect of face repetition and its interaction with face familiarity. In line with previously reported results (Kourtzi and Kanwisher, 2001; Pourtois et al., 2005; Rotshtein et al., 2005), the control subjects exhibited a clear repetition effect (that is, signal reduction for repeated presentation of the same face). As expected, given the rapid event-related presentation adopted in this experiment, the effect of the repeated versus nonrepeated images was weaker compared with the block design experiment, but, nevertheless, it was still significant. Interestingly, a significant interaction was found between face familiarity and face repetition. But again, even more surprising, the very same results were observed for the CP subjects. That the group of six CP individuals exhibited a similar pattern of activity indicates that their FFA response is indeed sensitive to face repetition even when very stringent experimental conditions are employed.

Thus, the emerging view from the cumulative evidence reviewed here is that many individuals with CP exhibit activity in their occipitotemporal cortex and particularly in the FFA and that this activity mirrors that of normal subjects in all examined parameters: signal amplitude, face selectivity and spatial extent of the activity. Moreover, and as evident from the more taxing experimental designs, the BOLD signals obtained from the CP individuals also exhibit sensitivity to face repetition. All these findings, and particularly the latter ones, suggest that the FFA functions normally in CP and that the computations related to face processing and representation in this region are intact and probably normal. These results challenge existing accounts of face processing and suggest that the FFA may be necessary for face recognition (as evident from AP studies) but is certainly not sufficient for these processes, as implied from modular views of face processing (Fodor, 1983; Kanwisher et al., 1997; Kanwisher, 2000; McKone et al., 2007). Finally, these results point to alternative neural mechanisms, beyond a specific functional alteration in the FFA, as being involved in the impairment in CP, and these other possibilities are explored in the next sections.

As a concluding remark for this section, it is important to note that it is still possible that the BOLD signal in the CP individuals is not fully normal but that limited spatial and temporal resolution of the fMRI method (several millimeters in space and 1 sec in time in the case of rapid event-related designs) prevent us from observing the abnormality of the activation or computational properties in the FFA. Our conclusions, therefore, have to be considered with caution and are still provisional given the limitations of the present technology.

Familiar   Unknown

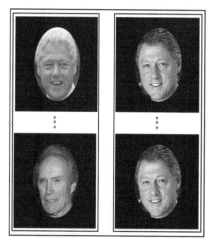 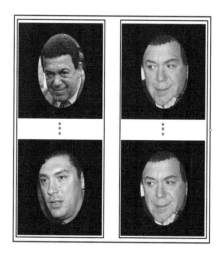

different   identical   different   identical

Figure 9.4. Experimental design of the rapid event-related repetition suppression experiment. Each trial was composed of two briefly presented consecutive face images that could be either different or identical. In order to examine the effect of face familiarity on FFA activation, half of the faces presented in the experiment were of famous faces and half were of unknown individuals. (Adapted from Avidan and Behrmann, 2008.)

9.4   Structural profile of cognitive prosopagnosia

In the previous section, we have seen that several fMRI studies imply that CP individuals exhibit normal BOLD signal in the fusiform face area (FFA), the pre-eminent region involved in face processing. These findings are consistent across studies, and replicable even under challenging experimental conditions. These results imply that the quality of the representation or computation in occipitotemporal cortex and particularly in the FFA is not different in individuals with CP compared with controls and that these regions, as far as we can tell, function normally. As such, these neural systems cannot simply account for the impairment in face recognition in these CP people. What then might be the underlying neural basis of this deficit? Many studies have revealed that face processing is not completed at the level of the FFA, but rather that a network of cortical nodes (as well as subcortical regions which are beyond the scope of this chapter) is involved in face perception and recognition (Haxby et al., 2001; Fairhall and Ishai, 2007; Gobbini and Haxby, 2007; Ishai, 2008). Thus, it could be that the propagation of output from the occipitotemporal cortex to more anterior regions involved in face processing is disrupted in CP and this disruption gives rise to this impairment.

In the next section, we address this possibility by examining the integrity of the face processing network, first by carefully investigating whether any localized structural alterations exist anywhere along the network of face processing that may account for the disorder in CP. We then employ a detailed analysis of the underlying white matter connectivity linking the various loci which are apparently involved in face processing by employing the diffusion tensor imaging (DTI) technique.

9.4.1 Structural volumetric/morphometric analyses: Can CP be accounted for by localized structural alterations?

Interestingly, conventional inspection, even by expert neuroradiologists, of the structural brain scans of individuals with CP that have been reported so far in the literature, has not revealed any obvious alterations or structural abnormalities in these individuals (e.g. Jones and Tranel, 2001). One exception to this rule is a single case study of subject YT, who appeared to have a smaller right temporal lobe compared with controls (Bentin et al., 1999). Structural abnormalities or lesions may sometimes go undetected even in cases of known neurological injury (e.g. Barton et al., 2001). Moreover, there are several neurodevelopmental disorders such as developmental dyslexia (e.g. Brown et al., 2001; Casanova et al., 2005), amusia (Hyde et al., 2006) and developmental dyscalculia (difficulties in numerical representation) (Molko et al., 2003) in which only the application of more sophisticated analysis tools allows investigators to reveal structural alterations. We therefore set out to explore the possibility of a subtle structural alteration in CP by adopting a comprehensive analysis of the inferior occipitotemporal cortex in a group of six CP individuals for whom we found normal fMRI activation profile in FFA and 12 matched control participants (Behrmann et al., 2007). Behavioral performance for five out of these six subjects (KM, TM, MT, BE, IT) is presented in Figure 9.1.

Examination of the structural brain images was carried out using two complementary techniques: first, we conducted sulcal tracing and sulcal depth and deviation analyses in occipitotemporal cortex to detect any morphometric abnormality in these regions in individuals with CP compared with controls. We then parcellated the occipitotemporal region into several anatomical substructures and obtained volumetric measures for each of these structures in order to test whether any of these regions would exhibit abnormal volume (enlarged or reduced volume) that may hint at a structural alteration. The specific procedures used for these analyses were adopted from several studies of other neurodevelopmental populations in whom no obvious cortical lesion is evident and the reader is referred to Behrmann et al. (2007) for more technical details.

The analysis of sulcal deviation and sulcal depth was carried out for each CP and control but, to permit direct comparisons between subjects, all brains were spatially normalized to a standard T1-MRI template. Specifically, the occipitotemporal and collateral sulci were manually traced on the inferior surface of the brain (see Figure 9.5a). Importantly, all tracings were conducted by an expert neuroradiologist who was blind to the identity and performance profile of the individual participants so that any experimenter bias would be eliminated. To quantify and compare the sulcal morphometry across the CP and control groups, we measured both the distance of the collateral (C) and occipitaltemporal (OT) sulci from the midline as well as the depth of the sulci in several locations (see Figure 9.5a). These two sulci border the fusiform gyrus, which is primarily involved in face processing, medially and laterally, and thus tracing them also allowed us to label this gyrus. The fusiform gyrus was further bisected into an anterior and a posterior portion (anterior fusiform – aF, posterior fusiform – pF). The depth of the C and OT sulci was measured by a straight line between the deepest point and the surface opening of the sulcus.

The results of the sulcal tracing for the CP and control individuals are shown in Figure 9.5b and, as is evident by observation, there are no obvious group differences in the organization or length of the collateral or occipitotemporal sulci even when the tracings from the two groups are overlayed (Figure 9.5b, rightmost brain illustration). The quantification of the distance of the sulci from the midline permitted a systematic comparison of any sulcal deviations between the groups beyond visual inspection. Importantly, statistical analyses revealed that the sulcal path and extent of deviation from the midline was equivalent in the two groups. Similar findings were also obtained in the analysis of the depth of the two sulci. These findings clearly indicate that there are no differences in sulcal morphometry and patterning for the CP compared with the control group, and therefore, rule out any gross changes in the shape of the brains of the two groups.

In order to compare further the structural characteristics of the brain of CP and controls beyond the sulcal morphometry procedure described above, for each participant we also quantified the volume of nine different subregions within the occipitotemporal lobe. These regions included the fusiform gyrus (subdivided into anterior and posterior, see Figure 9.5a), hippocampus, parahippocampus, superior temporal gyrus and middle and inferior temporal gyrus (subdivided into anterior and posterior portions). These structures were manually traced on alternate slices for each CP subject and each control separately for the left and right hemispheres and their volumes were head-size corrected. For more details regarding the tracing and volume calculation procedure, the reader is referred to Behrmann et al. (2007).

We conducted a statistical analysis comparing the volumes of all subregions across CPs and controls and this is presented in Figure 9.5c. Interestingly, we have found that, overall, the CP group had a larger volume than the controls in the anterior and the posterior portion of the middle temporal gyrus (averaged across both hemispheres). Of greater interest perhaps is that the CP individuals had reduced volume (albeit in a slightly larger temporal lobe) of the anterior fusiform compared with controls (Figure 9.5c). Importantly, this region in the anterior fusiform gyrus was located anteriorly to the functionally defined FFA as delineated in the fMRI studies and does not overlap it (see Figure 9.2 and Avidan et al., 2005). Furthermore, the FFA region overlapped with the anatomically defined posterior fusiform and critically, in this region, no structural alterations were observed. Of much importance, we found that these volumetric alterations in the anterior fusiform gyrus were correlated with the behavioral profile in CP, suggesting that these changes have functional significance. Specifically, we found a correlation between the volume of the anterior fusiform and the level of performance on the famous face recognition questionnaire (Figure 9.1a) such that reduced performance was accompanied by a smaller volume. Finally, as is also evident in Figure 9.5c, CP also exhibited enlarged volume in both the anterior and posterior portions of the

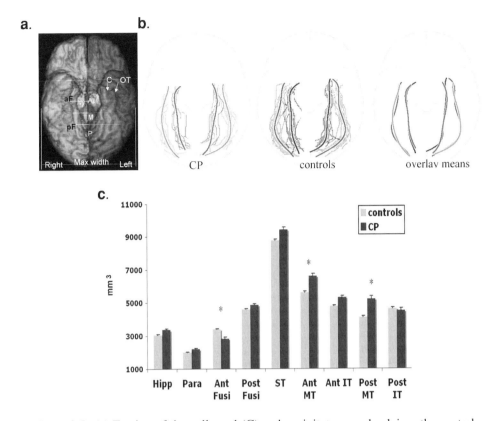

Figure 9.5. (a) Tracing of the collateral (C) and occipitotemporal sulci on the ventral aspect of the brain. In addition, the anterior (aF) and posterior fusiform (pF) are also indicated. Note also the schematic depiction of the method for assessing the maximal width of the brain. (b) Tracing of the C and OT sulci in CP, controls and the overlay of the average tracing of the two groups. (c) Volume of nine subregions in occipitotemporal cortex for CP and controls. CP subjects exhibited reduced volume in the anterior fusiform and enlarged volume in the anterior and posterior middle temporal (MT) sulcus. Abbreviations: Hipp, hippocampus; Para, parahippocampal gyrus; Ant Fusi, anterior fusiform; Post Fusi, posterior fusiform; ST, superior temporal sulcus; Ant MT, anterior middle temporal sulcus; Ant IT, anterior inferior temporal sulcus; post MT, posterior middle temporal sulcus; post IT, posterior inferior temporal sulcus. (Reprinted with permission from Behrmann et al., 2007.)

middle temporal gyrus. However, unlike the correlation found between behavioral performance and reduced anterior fusiform volume, the enlarged middle temporal volume was not related to any behavioral measure. One possible explanation for this might be that this enlarged volume is a result of a compensatory response for the reduced volume in the anterior fusiform and therefore is not directly related to the behavioral profile in CP.

Taken together, systematic evaluation of high resolution structural MR images revealed very specific alterations in the brains of individuals with CP. The main alteration and the only change that was correlated with reduced behavioral performance in face identification was observed in the anterior portion of the fusiform gyrus. Importantly, this region did not overlap with the functionally defined FFA which seems to function normally in CP and no structural alterations were observed in the more posterior fusiform which overlaps the FFA. Thus, these findings are consistent with our hypothesis that in CP the FFA functions normally and it is the propagation of information to (or from) more anterior regions such as the anterior fusiform which is disrupted. These findings are also consistent with converging evidence obtained from several different techniques such as fMRI and neuropsychological investigations (Bright et al., 2005), ERP (Puce et al., 1999); and single unit recordings and computational accounts (Bussey et al., 2005) showing that the anterior temporal cortex is involved in fine-grained discrimination and recognition – processes which are impaired in CP. Unfortunately, fMRI activity in these more anterior regions is not always visible as a result of susceptibility artifacts and this could be one of the reasons why we did not observe and compare this more anterior activation in our fMRI studies. However, there are now reports suggesting that more advanced techniques and higher field strength would enable better detection of the activation in these foci (Kriegeskorte et al., 2007) and we hope to successfully image them and examine their activity in our future studies.

It is important to note that the reduced volume observed in this study cannot be attributed particularly to gray or white matter and so we cannot be sure whether this volume reduction in anterior fusiform is attributed to neuronal tissue, white matter, or both. Such details would help us in refining our understanding of the underlying mechanism leading to CP and would also further constrain models of face processing in the normal brain. In the following section, we specifically examine the integrity of the white matter connectivity in CP using innovative structural imaging methods.

9.4.2   Structural analyses of white matter connectivity: Can CP be accounted for by a disruption of white matter connectivity in the face processing network?

In the previous section, we addressed the issue of whether localized structural alterations could account for CP. However, it is now widely recognized that face processing is accomplished by the concerted activity of a network of regions rather than of a single location. The advent of new structural imaging techniques such as diffusion tensor imaging (DTI) and tractography (Mori and Zhang, 2006) which permits imaging of white matter fibers in the human brain in vivo, has allowed us to specifically examine the integrity of the underlying white matter connectivity relating the various nodes of the face processing network. Given the apparent role of the FFA as a necessary node in this network, we focused our analysis on the main fiber tracts connecting this region with the anterior portion of the temporal lobe (the same region which revealed structural alterations in the previous section) and with the frontal lobe. These include two long-range fiber tracts that pass through the fusiform gyrus: (i) the inferior longitudinal fasciculus (ILF), which passes through the fusiform and lingual gyri and the cuneus and traverses the superior, inferior and middle temporal gyri as well as the hippocampus and parahippocampus and (ii) the inferior frontooccipital fasciculus (IFOF), which projects between the lingual, fusiform and inferior temporal gyri and the inferolateral and dorsolateral frontal cortex (Catani et al., 2003). Both the temporal and frontal lobes have been shown to be important for completion of face identification and for fine detailed discrimination (Puce et al., 1999; Bar et al., 2006; Summerfield et al., 2006) and so the rationale behind this analysis was that any alterations in these tracts will have adverse consequences for face recognition and therefore may account for the behavioral profile in CP. We have recently used a similar approach in another study examining face processing abilities and aging and so the reader is referred to this paper for the more technical aspects of this work and for the establishment of the various dependent measures used in this study (Thomas et al., 2008). Briefly, the dependent measurers that we have used included the number of fibers, number of voxels through which the fibers pass (index of volume) and the average fractional anisotropy (FA) of the fibers in the tracts of interest. Given that variations in the number of fibers and voxels across the entire brain are expected as a function of individual whole brain volume, the dependent measures pertaining to specific fiber tracts were normalized by dividing them by the whole brain measures and expressing them as percentages (%fibers, %voxels). For each subject, all these measurements were obtained separately from each hemisphere. It is currently accepted that the number of fibers and number of voxels reflect gross measurements of a tract, while the FA reflects the microstructural properties of the axons within a voxel. However, the exact dependent measures one should use remains controversial and so, in this initial DTI investigation, we chose to examine all measures, keeping in mind that a reduction in all three measures would further attest to the reliability of the findings. Six individuals with CP (all subjects whose performance is presented in Figure 9.1 except for TM) and 17 age and gender matched controls participated in this study.

The main question we aimed to address was whether CP subjects would differ from controls in any of the dependent measures that reflect the structural integrity of the ILF and IFOF. Interestingly, we found that CP individuals exhibited reduced structural integrity in all dependent measures (%voxels, %fibers, mean FA) in both left and right ILF and IFOF compared with controls, thus exhibiting evidence for reduction in both macro- and microstructural integrity of these specific tracts. It is important to note that the CP group did not differ from controls with regard to the overall white matter connectivity at the whole brain level thus stressing that it is not the case that CP subjects just have overall reduced connectivity – rather they exhibit reduced white matter integrity only in specific locations.

This study has allowed us to uncover specific white matter alterations in the cortical fiber tracts specifically connecting the fusiform gyrus with anterior temporal and frontal regions (ILOF and ILF). These results were very specific and no evidence for reduced connectivity was found in the overall brain connectivity or in another control tract that we examined, involving information transfer in the frontal cortex (i.e. forceps minor). It is important to note that DTI can only tell us that there is reduced structural connectivity but does not provide any information regarding the directionality of the information flow. It is well known that information flows in a bidirectional fashion such that regions like the FFA propagate information to more anterior temporal and frontal cortex, but they also receive reciprocal connections from the very same regions. The exact role of this top-down information is not fully determined but several hypotheses have been raised (Hochstein and Ahissar, 2002; Bar et al., 2006; Kveraga et al., 2007). In any case, it is of course a viable possibility that connectivity in both directions is disrupted in the face processing network in CP and critical feedback information does not propagate back to earlier visual areas.

9.5   Concluding remarks

Using an integrative approach in which both functional and structural imaging techniques were combined, we have been able to elucidate some of the neural mechanisms that might give rise to the behavioral profile observed in CP. Specifically, we have argued that CP might be accounted for by a failure of information propagation along both the core and extended face-related systems. Thus, activity patterns obtained using fMRI revealed normal face-related processing in occipitotemporal cortex, implying that these regions and particularly the FFA are functioning normally in CP. In addition, detailed analyses of structural MR images of the same CP individuals revealed an anatomical alteration in the anterior temporal fusiform gyrus, in a region located anteriorly to the functionally defined FFA. This finding further supports the hypothesis that information from the intact FFA is not being properly propagated to more anterior temporal cortex or propagated back from these regions to the FFA. Finally, analysis of the white matter connectivity in major fiber tracts connecting the FFA to anterior temporal and frontal cortex revealed reduced connectivity in CP compared with controls which was strictly confined to the face processing system. We would like to propose that this converging evidence indicates that face processing requires the net activity along the entire face network with no specific region being sufficient to complete this process on its own. We would further like to stress that our studies do not undermine the criticality or necessity of regions such as the FFA for face processing, a claim which is strongly supported by numerous lesions studies. Rather, our work points out that these regions, while necessary, may not be sufficient for successful recognition to occur. Moreover, we do not make the claim that other regions such as frontal cortex or anterior temporal cortex are neither necessary nor sufficient but rather we point out that they are intimately involved in intact face processing. The findings from CP stand in contrast with AP in which the lesion is to a more localized region (possibly a particular node in the face network) such as the FFA although, of course, damage to a node can affect propagation of information through the face circuit.

While substantial advancements have been made in understanding the neural mechanism underlying CP, this research is far from being complete and there are still many open questions. One major caveat has to do with technological limitations that pertain to both functional and structural research. Thus, the noninvasive techniques currently used are limited in either the temporal, spatial resolution or both and so do not allow us to study directly the activity of single neurons or specific small neuronal networks. Although we have used techniques such as the fMR adaptation to circumvent such limitations, it could still be the case that the fMRI signal masks the abnormality of the function of occipitotemporal cortex in CP, and future and more advanced techniques may be able to uncover this if it exists. In addition, in relation to the structural investigations, the DTI technique is still in its early days and future studies may be able to reveal much more fine-grained alteration in white matter connectivity compared with the present results. For example, at the moment, the exact underlying mechanisms which accompany reductions in white matter integrity such as those observed from the DTI explorations are still not clear, and the hope is that future studies will provide some answers to these questions. Moreover, we plan to combine the fMRI data with the DTI in order to investigate both structural and functional aspects of connectivity in the same individuals. Finally, as was alluded to in the introduction, a common finding in CP is its familial aspect and so an exciting research avenue which is already being pursued (Grueter et al., 2007; Kennerknecht et al., 2007) is to decipher the exact genetic makeup that underlies CP. Thus, it will be of major interest to find out how these specific genetic findings are related to the structural alterations reported here and to the specific behavioral profile of CP individuals. Such investigations will provide an unprecedented opportunity to bridge genetics, brain structure and function, and unique aspects of human behavior such as face processing. Moreover, such investigations could lay the foundation to formulate a deeper understanding of other neurodevelopmental disorders.

References

Adolphs, R., Tranel, D., Damasio, H. and Damasio, A. R. (1995). Fear and the human amygdala. *J. Neurosci.*, 15: 5879–5891.

Andersson, F., Glaser, B., Spiridon, M., Debbane, M., Vuilleumier, P. and Eliez, S. (2007). Impaired activation of face processing networks revealed by functional magnetic resonance imaging in 22q11.2 deletion syndrome. *Biol. Psychiatry*, 63: 49–57.

Avidan, G. and Behrmann, M. (2008). Implicit familiarity processing in congenital prosopagnosia. *J. Neuropsychol.*. 2: 141–164.

Avidan, G., Hasson, U., Hendler, T., Zohary, E. and Malach, R. (2002). Analysis of the neuronal selectivity underlying low fMRI signals. *Curr. Biol.*, 12: 964–972.

Avidan, G., Hasson, U., Malach, R. and Behrmann, M. (2005). Detailed exploration of face-related processing in congenital prosopagnosia: 2. Functional neuroimaging findings. *J. Cogn. Neurosci.*, 17: 1150–1167.

Avidan, G., Levy, I., Hendler, T., Zohary, E. and Malach, R. (2003) Spatial vs. object specific attention in high-order visual areas. *NeuroImage*, 19: 308–318.

Bar, M., Kassam, K. S., Ghuman, A. S., Boshyan, J., Schmid, A. M., Dale, A. M., Hamalainen, M. S., Marinkovic, K., Schacter, D. L., Rosen, B. R. and Halgren, E. (2006). Top-down facilitation of visual recognition. *Proc. Natl. Acad. Sci. USA*, 103: 449–454.

Barton, J. J., Cherkasova, M., O'Connor, M. (2001). Covert recognition in acquired and developmental prosopagnosia. *Neurologia*, 57: 1161–1168.

Barton, J. J., Cherkasova, M. V., Press, D. Z., Intriligator, J. M., O'Connor, M. (2003). Developmental prosopagnosia: a study of three patients. *Brain Cogn.*, 51: 12–30.

Behrmann, M. and Avidan, G. (2005). Congenital prosopagnosia: face-blind from birth. *Trends Cogn. Sci.*, 9: 180–187.

Behrmann, M., Avidan, G., Gao, F. and Black, S. (2007). Structural imaging reveals anatomical alterations in inferotemporal cortex in congenital prosopagnosia. *Cereb. Cortex*, 17: 2354–2363.

Behrmann, M., Avidan, G. and Humphreys, K. (in press). Congenital and acquired prosopagnosia. In D. Bub, D. I. Gauthier and M. Tarr (eds.) *Perceptual Expertise: Bridging Brain and Behavior*, Oxford, UK: Oxford University Press.

Behrmann, M., Avidan, G., Marotta, J. J. and Kimchi, R. (2005). Detailed exploration of face-related processing in congenital prosopagnosia: 1. Behavioral findings. *J. Cogn. Neurosci.*, 17: 1130–1149.

Bentin, S., Degutis, J. M., D'Esposito, M. and Robertson, L. C. (2007). Too many trees to see the forest: performance, event-related potential, and functional magnetic resonance imaging manifestations of integrative congenital prosopagnosia. *J. Cogn. Neurosci.*, 19: 132–146.

Bentin, S., Deouell, L. Y. and Soroker, N. (1999). Selective visual streaming in face recognition: evidence from developmental prosopagnosia. *NeuroReport*, 10: 823–827.

Bodamer, J. (1947). Die prosop-Agnosie. *Archiv für Psychiatrie und Nervenkrankheiten*, 179: 6–53.

Bouvier, S. E. and Engel, S. A. (2006). Behavioral deficits and cortical damage loci in cerebral achromatopsia. *Cereb. Cortex*, 16: 183–191.

Bright, P., Moss, H. E., Stamatakis, E. A. and Tyler, L. K. (2005). The anatomy of object processing: the role of anteromedial temporal cortex. *Quart. J. Exp. Psychol. B*, 58: 361–377.

Brown, W. E., Eliez, S., Menon, V., Rumsey, J. M., White, C. D. and Reiss, A. L. (2001). Preliminary evidence of widespread morphological variations of the brain in dyslexia. *Neurology*, 56: 781–783.

Bussey, T. J., Saksida, L. M. and Murray, E. A. (2005). The perceptual-mnemonic/feature conjunction model of perirhinal cortex function. *Quart. J. Exp. Psychol. B*, 58: 269–282.

Casanova, M. F., Christensen, J. D., Giedd, J., Rumsey, J. M., Garver, D. L. and Postel, G. C. (2005). Magnetic resonance imaging study of brain asymmetries in dyslexic patients. *J. Child Neurol.*, 20: 842–847.

Catani, M., Jones, D. K., Donato, R. and Ffytche, D. H. (2003). Occipito-temporal connections in the human brain. *Brain*, 126: 2093–2107.

Damasio, A. R., Damasio, H. and Van Hoesen, G. W. (1982). Prosopagnosia: anatomic basis and behavioral mechanisms. *Neurology*, 32: 331–341.

Damasio, A. R., Tranel, D. and Damasio, H. (1990) Face agnosia and the neural substrates of memory. *Ann. Rev. Neurosci.*, 13: 89–109.

De Haan, E. H. (1999). A familial factor in the development of face recognition deficits. *J. Clin. Exp. Neuropsychol.*, 21: 312–315.

De Renzi, E. (1997). Prosopagnosia. In T. E. Feinberg and M. Farah (eds.) *Behavioral Neurology and Neuropsychology*. New York: McGraw-Hill, pp. 245–256.

Dobel, C., Bolte, J., Aicher, M. and Schweinberger, S. R. (2007). Prosopagnosia without apparent cause: overview and diagnosis of six cases. *Cortex*, 43: 718–733.

Druzgal, T. J. and D'Esposito, M. (2003). Dissecting contributions of prefrontal cortex and fusiform face area to face working memory. *J. Cogn. Neurosci.*, 15: 771–784.

Duchaine, B. and Nakayama, K. (2005). Dissociations of face and object recognition in developmental prosopagnosia. *J. Cogn. Neurosci.*, 17: 249–261.

Duchaine, B., Germine, L. and Nakayama, K. (2007). Family resemblance: ten family members with prosopagnosia and within-class object agnosia. *Cogni. Neuropsychol.*, 24: 419–430.

Duchaine, B. C. and Nakayama, K. (2004). Developmental prosopagnosia and the Benton Facial Recognition Test. *Neurologia*, 62: 1219–1220.

Duchaine, B. C., Dingle, K., Butterworth, E. and Nakayama, K. (2004). Normal greeble learning in a severe case of developmental prosopagnosia. *Neuron*, 43: 469–473.

Eger, E., Schweinberger, S. R., Dolan, R. J. and Henson, R. N. (2005). Familiarity enhances invariance of face representations in human ventral visual cortex: fMRI evidence. *NeuroImage*, 26: 1128–1139.

Fairhall, S. L. and Ishai, A. (2007). Effective connectivity within the distributed cortical network for face perception. *Cereb. Cortex*, 17: 2400–2406.

Fisher, S. E., Lai, C. S. and Monaco, A. P. (2003). Deciphering the genetic basis of speech and language disorders. *Ann. Rev. Neurosci.*, 26: 57–80.

Fodor, J. A. (1983). *The Modularity of Mind: An Essay on Faculty Psychology*. Cambridge, MA: MIT Press.

Gauthier, I., Tarr, M. J., Moylan, J., Skudlarski, P., Gore, J. C. and Anderson, A. W. (2000). The fusiform "face area" is part of a network that processes faces at the individual level. *J. Cogn. Neurosci.*, 12: 495–504.

George, N., Dolan, R. J., Fink, G. R., Baylis, G. C., Russell, C. and Driver, J. (1999). Contrast polarity and face recognition in the human fusiform gyrus. *Nat. Neurosci.*, 2: 574–580.

Gilaie-Dotan, S. and Malach, R. (2007). Sub-exemplar shape tuning in human face-related areas. *Cereb. Cortex*, 17: 325–338.

Gobbini, M. I. and Haxby, J. V (2007). Neural systems for recognition of familiar faces. *Neuropsychologia*, 45: 32–41.

Gorno-Tempini, M. L. and Price, C. J. (2001). Identification of famous faces and buildings: a functional neuroimaging study of semantically unique items. *Brain*, 124: 2087–2097.

Gorno-Tempini, M. L., Price, C. J., Josephs, O., Vandenberghe, R., Cappa, S. F., Kapur, N., Frackowiak, R. S. and Tempini, M. L. (1998). The neural systems sustaining face and proper-name processing. *Brain*, 121: 2103–2118.

Grill-Spector, K., Kushnir, T., Edelman, S., Avidan, G., Itzchak, Y. and Malach, R. (1999). Differential processing of objects under various viewing conditions in the human lateral occipital complex. *Neuron*, 24: 187–203.

Gross, C. G. (2005). Processing the facial image: a brief history. *Am. Psychol.*, 60: 755–763.

Grueter, M., Grueter, T., Bell, V., Horst, J., Laskowski, W., Sperling, K., Halligan, P. W., Ellis, H. D. and Kennerknecht, I. (2007). Hereditary prosopagnosia: the first case series. *Cortex*, 43: 734–749.

Hadjikhani, N. and de Gelder, B. (2002). Neural basis of prosopagnosia: an fMRI study. *Hum. Brain Mapp.*, 16: 176–182.

Halgren, E., Dale, A. M., Sereno, M. I., Tootell, R. B. H., Marinkovic, K. and Rosen, B. R. (1999) Location of human face-selective cortex with respect to retinotopic areas. *Hum. Brain Mapp.*, 7: 29–37.

Harris, A. M., Duchaine, B. C. and Nakayama, K. (2005). Normal and abnormal face selectivity of the M170 response in developmental prosopagnosics. *Neuropsychologia*, 43: 2125–2136.

Hasson, U., Avidan, G., Deouell, L. Y., Bentin, S. and Malach, R. (2003). Face-selective activation in a congenital prosopagnosic subject. *J. Cogn. Neurosci.*, 15: 419–431.

Haxby, J. V., Gobbini, M. I., Furey, M. L., Ishai, A., Schouten, J. L. and Pietrini, P. (2001). Distributed and overlapping representations of faces and objects in ventral temporal cortex. *Science*, 293: 2425–2430.

Haxby, J. V., Hoffman, E. A. and Gobbini, M. I. (2000). The distributed human neural system for face perception. *Trends Cogn. Sci.*, 4: 223–233.

Henson, R., Shallice, T. and Dolan, R. (2000). Neuroimaging evidence for dissociable forms of repetition priming. *Science*, 287: 1269–1272.

Henson, R. N., Goshen-Gottstein, Y., Ganel, T., Otten, L. J., Quayle, A. and Rugg, M. D. (2003). Electrophysiological and haemodynamic correlates of face perception, recognition and priming. *Cereb. Cortex*, 13: 793–805.

Hochstein, S. and Ahissar, M. (2002). View from the top: hierarchies and reverse hierarchies in the visual system. *Neuron*, 36: 791–804.

Hoffman, E. A. and Haxby, J. V. (2000). Distinct representations of eye gaze and identity in the distributed human neural system for face perception. *Nature Neurosci.*, 3: 80–84.

Hyde, K. L., Zatorre, R. J., Griffiths, T. O., Lerch, J. P. and Peretz, I. (2006). Morphometry of the amusic brain: a two site study. *Brain*, 129: 2562–2570.

Ishai, A. (2008). Let's face it. It's a cortical network. *NeuroImage*, 40: 415–419.

Ishai, A., Ungerleider, L. G., Martin, A., Schouten, H. L. and Haxby, J. V. (1999). Distributed representation of objects in the human ventral visual pathway. *Proc. Nat. Acad. Sci. USA*, 96: 9379–9384.

Jones, R. D. and Tranel, D. (2001). Severe developmental prosopagnosia in a child with superior intellect. *J. Clin. Exp. Neuropsychol.*, 23: 265–273.

Kanwisher, N. (2000). Domain specificity in face perception. *Nat. Neurosci.*, 3: 759–763.

Kanwisher, N,. McDermott, J. and Chun, M. M. (1997). The fusiform face area: a module in human extrastriate cortex specialized for face perception. *J. Neurosci.*, 17: 4302–4311.

Kastner, S. and Ungerleider, L. G. (2000). Mechanisms of visual attention in the human cortex. *Ann. Rev. Neurosci.*, 23: 315–341.

Kennerknecht, I., Pluempe, N. and Welling, B. (2008). Congenital prosopagnosia – a common hereditary cognitive dysfunction in humans. *Front. Biosci.*, 13: 3150–3158.

Kourtzi, Z. and Kanwisher, N. (2000). Cortical regions involved in perceiving object shape. *J. Neurosci.*, 20: 3310–3318.

Kourtzi, Z. and Kanwisher, N. (2001). Representation of perceived object shape by the human lateral occipital complex. *Science*, 293: 1506–1509.

Kress, T. and Daum, I. (2003). Event-related potentials reflect impaired face recognition in patients with congenital prosopagnosia. *Neurosci. Let.*, 352: 133–136.

Kriegeskorte, N., Formisano, E., Sorger, B. and Goebet, P. (2007). Individual faces elicit distinct fMRI response patterns in human anterior temporal cortex. *Proc. Nat. Acad. Sci. USA*, 104: 20600–20605.

Kveraga, K., Ghuman, A. S. and Bar, M. (2007). Top-down predictions in the cognitive brain. *Brain Cogn.*, 65: 145–168.

Lai, C. S., Fisher, S. E., Hurst, J. A., Vargha-Khadem, F. and Monaco, A. P. (2001). A forkhead-domain gene is mutated in a severe speech and language disorder. *Nature*, 413: 519–523.

Le Grand, R., Cooper, P. A., Mondloch, C. J., Lewis, T. L., Sagiv, N., de Gelder, B. and Maurer, D. (2006). What aspects of face processing are impaired in developmental prosopagnosia? *Brain Cogn.*, 61: 139–158.

Leveroni, C. L., Seidenberg, M., Mayer, A. R., Mead, L. A., Binder, J. R. and Rao, S. M. (2000). Neural systems underlying the recognition of familiar and newly learned faces. *J. Neurosci.*, 20: 878–886.

Levy, I., Hasson, U. and Malach, R. (2004). One picture is worth at least a million neurons. *Curr. Biol.*, 14: 996–1001.

Li, L., Miller, E. K. and Desimone, R. (1993). The representation of stimulus familiarity in anterior inferior temporal cortex. *J. Neurophysiol.*, 69: 1918–1929.

McCarthy, G., Puce, A., Gore, J. C. and Allison, T. (1997). Face specific processing in the human fusiform gyrus. *J. Cog. Neurosci.*, 9: 605–610.

McKone, E., Kanwisher, N. and Duchaine, B. C. (2007). Can generic expertise explain special processing for faces? *Trends Cogn. Sci.*, 11: 8–15.

Minnebusch, D. A., Suchan, B., Ramon, M. and Daum, I. (2007). Event-related potentials reflect heterogeneity of developmental prosopagnosia. *Eur. J. Neurosci.*, 25: 2234–2247.

Molko, N., Cachia, A., Riviere, D., Mangin, J. F., Bruandet, M., Le Bihan, D., Cohen, L. and Dehaene, S. (2003). Functional and structural alterations of the intraparietal sulcus in a developmental dyscalculia of genetic origin. *Neuron*, 40: 847–858.

Mori, S. and Zhang, J. (2006). Principles of diffusion tensor imaging and its applications to basic neuroscience research. *Neuron*, 51: 527–539.

Nakamura, K., Kawashima, R., Sato, N., Nakamura, A., Sugiura, M., Kato, T., Hatano, K., Ito, K., Fukuda, H., Schormann, T. and Zilles, K. (2000). Functional delineation of the human occipito-temporal areas related to face and scene processing. A PET study. *Brain*, 123: 1903–1912.

O'Craven, K. M., Downing, P. E., Kanwisher, N. (1999). fMRI evidence for objects as the units of attentional selection. *Nature*, 401: 584–587.

Peretz, I. and Hyde, K. L. (2003). What is specific to music processing? Insights from congenital amusia. *Trends Cogn. Sci.*, 7: 362–367.

Pourtois, G., Schwartz, S., Seghier, M. L., Lazeyras, F. and Vuilleumier, P. (2005). View-independent coding of face identity in frontal and temporal cortices is modulated by familiarity: an event-related fMRI study. *NeuroImage*, 24: 1214–1224.

Puce, A., Allison, T., Bentin, S., Gore, J. C. and McCarthy, G. (1998). Temporal cortex activation in humans viewing eye and mouth movements. *J. Neurosci.*, 18: 2188–2199.

Puce, A., Allison, T., Gore, J. C. and McCarthy, G. (1995). Face-sensitive regions in human extrastriate cortex studied by functional MRI. *J. Neurophysiol.*, 74: 1192–1199.

Puce, A., Allison, T. and McCarthy, G. (1999). Electrophysiological studies of human face perception. III: Effects of top-down processing on face-specific potentials. *Cereb. Cortex*, 9: 445–458.

Righart, R. and de Gelder, B. (2007). Impaired face and body percetion in developmental prosopagnosia. *Proc. Natl. Acad. Sci. USA*, 104: 17234–17238.

Rossion, B., Caldara, R., Seghier, M., Schuller, A. M., Lazeyras, F. and Mayer, E. (2003). A network of occipito-temporal face-sensitive areas besides the right middle fusiform gyrus is necessary for normal face processing. *Brain*, 126: 2381–2395.

Rotshtein, P., Geng, J. J., Driver, J. and Dolan, R. J. (2007). Role of features and second-order spatial relations in face discrimination, face recognition, and individual face skills: behavioral and functional magnetic resonance imaging data. *J. Cogn. Neurosci.*, 19: 1435–1452.

Rotshtein, P., Henson, R. N., Treves, A., Driver, J. and Dolan, R. J. (2005). Morphing Marilyn into Maggie dissociates physical and identity face representations in the brain. *Nat. Neurosci.*, 8: 107–113.

Sergent, J. and Signoret, J.-L. (1992). Functional and anatomical decomposition of face processing: evidence from prosopagnosia and PET study of normal subjects. *Phil. Trans. Roy. Soc. (Lond) B*, 335: 55–61; discussion 61–52.

Sergent, J., Ohta, S. and MacDonald, B. (1992). Functional neuroanatomy of face and object processing. A positron emission tomography study. *Brain*, 115: 15–36.

Summerfield, C., Egner, T., Greene, M., Koechlin, E., Mangels, J. and Hirsch, J. (2006). Predictive codes for forthcoming perception in the frontal cortex. *Science*, 314: 1311–1314.

Thomas, C., Moya, L., Avidan, G., Humphreys, K., Jung, K. J., Peterson, M. A. and Behrmann, M. (2008). Reduction in white matter connectivity, revealed by DTI, may account for age-related changes in face perception. *J. Cogn. Neurosci.*, 20: 268–284.

Tippett, L. J., Miller, L. A. and Farah, M. J. (2000). Prosopamnesia: a selective impairment in face learning. *Cogn. Neuropsychol,*, 17: 241–255.

Tsao, D. Y., Freiwald, W. A., Knutsen, T. A., Mandeville, J. B. and Tootell, R. B. (2003). Faces and objects in macaque cerebral cortex. *Nat. Neurosci.*, 6: 989–995.

Tsao, D. Y., Freiwald, W. A., Tootell, R. B. and Livingstone, M. S. (2006). A cortical region consisting entirely of face-selective cells. *Science*, 311: 670–674.

von Kriegstein, K., Kleinschmidt, A., Sterzer, P. and Giraud, A.-L. (2005). Interaction of face and voice areas during speaker recognition. *J. Cogn. Neurosci.*, 17: 367–376.

Wada, Y. and Yamamoto, T. (2001). Selective impairment of facial recognition due to a haematoma restricted to the right fusiform and lateral occipital region. *J. Neurol. Neurosur. Psy.*, 71: 254–257.

Whalen, P. J., Rauch, S. L., Etcoff, N. L., McInerney, S. C., Lee, M. B. and Jenike, M. A. (1998). Masked presentations of emotional facial expressions modulate amygdala activity without explicit knowledge. *J. Neurosci.*, 18: 411–418.

Williams, M. A., Berberovic, N. and Mattingley, J. B. (2007). Abnormal FMRI adaptation to unfamiliar faces in a case of developmental prosopamnesia. *Curr. Biol.*, 17: 1259–1264.

10 Object ontology in temporal lobe ensembles

R. Baez-Mendoza and K. L. Hoffman

10.1 About ontologies

Imagine you are hungry and facing a fruit bowl bursting with ripe goodies. You would like to eat one of the objects in that fruit bowl, but do not know which one to take first. You could start with the red round one or the elongated yellow arc or the tiny red balloons hanging from a branch; there are also big orange spheres and smaller ones. Whatever your decision is, the first step will be to discriminate from among the objects found in the fruit bowl: in the general class "fruits" and in the class "fruits that I can eat from the fruit bowl" each individual fruit has a series of attributes like shape, size, color and tastiness. Some of these attributes can be shared: persimmons and oranges are both orange; plums and nectarines have a similar size and shape. To purposely act upon our hunger we group the fruits in the fruit bowl based on their attributes, their relations, and their classes or categories; we have an ontology for these objects.

In computer science, ontology is defined as an explicit specification of a conceptualization (Gruber, 1993). For AI systems, what "exists" is that which can be represented. The systematic description includes specification of the concepts – like apple, banana and orange – and relationships that can exist among these concepts – in our example, based on attributes such as color, shape or seasonal availability. Thus, ontology can be viewed as a way of modeling knowledge about individuals, their attributes and their relationships to other individuals.

The word ontology was borrowed from philosophy where it is defined as the study of being or existence and, as such, tries to answer the question "what exists?" often with special attention to the relations between particulars and universals, between intrinsic and extrinsic properties, and between essence and existence. What ontology has in common in both computer science and philosophy is the representation of entities, ideas and events along with their properties and relations according to a system of categories. One of the cornerstones of the cognitive revolution was the computer as a

Cortical Mechanisms of Vision, ed. M. Jenkin and L. R. Harris. Published by Cambridge University Press.

metaphor of the mind. Whereas this analogy is deficient in many respects, ontologies remain useful in the sense that our brains may form them and use them to structure and, in fact, exploit the underlying patterning of the myriad objects we encounter on a daily basis. What is the nature of this organization and where in the brain might it be specified?

10.2   The temporal lobe in primates

Imagine that you could not tell an apple from an orange by looking at them, even if you noticed that they had a slightly different form and color, even though hearing, speaking or reading the words "apple" or "orange" conjured into mind two different fruits. This condition is called visual agnosia and in humans is caused by lesions in the temporal lobe (Humphreys and Riddoch, 1987; Farah, 1990).

Temporal lobe lesions in monkeys also produce visual agnosia. While studying the neural basis of the mescaline experience, Heinrich Klüver and Paul Bucy (1939) removed the temporal lobe of several monkeys. They observed that although mescaline still seemed to produce its psychotropic effects, lobotomized monkeys showed visual agnosia, as part of a set of maladaptive behaviors (Klüver and Bucy, 1939). Further work by Mortimer Mishkin and colleagues in the 1950s showed that visual agnosia in monkeys was caused by lesions restricted to the inferior convexity of the temporal cortex or inferior temporal (IT) cortex (Mishkin, 1954; Mishkin and Pribram, 1954).

Lesion data suggest that the temporal lobe contains neurons that are important for perceiving and discriminating objects. Yet, anatomically the temporal lobe is many synapses removed from sensory inputs about those objects.

Visual sensory information reaches the temporal and parietal lobes by a number of corticocortical stages beginning in the primary visual cortex. One pathway passes dorsally through extrastriate cortex to end in the posterior parietal lobule and the frontal lobe; the other passes ventrally through extrastriate cortex to reach the IT cortex within the temporal lobe (Ungerleider and Mishkin, 1982).

IT is a large region of cortex that extends anteriorly from the inferior occipital sulcus to the sphenoid bone and from the fundus of the superior temporal sulcus (STS) to the fundus of the occipitotemporal sulcus. Based on different criteria researchers have further parcelated this area. One of the most common subdivisions is based on the laminar organization of projections and divides IT in anterior, central and posterior IT (Felleman and Van Essen, 1991). An earlier classification is based on topography and cytoarchitectonics, and parcelates IT into areas TEa and TEm in the fundus of the superior temporal sulcus, TE1, TE2 and TE3 anteriorly and TEO posteriorly (Von Bonin and Bailey, 1947; Iwai and Mishkin, 1969).

According to Logothetis and Sheinberg (1996; for further anatomical descriptions see Felleman and Van Essen, 1991; Seltzer and Pandya, 1994), area TEO receives feedforward cortical inputs from areas V2, V3, and V4 and has interhemispheric connections mediated mainly via the corpus callosum. Sparser inputs arise from areas V3A, V4t, and MT. Each of these areas receives feedback connections from TEO. TEO feeds forward to TE, which sends feedback projections to TEO. Cortical projections of area

TE include those to TH, TF, STP, frontal eye fields (FEF), and area 46. Area TE has both direct and indirect connections to limbic structures.

Regional variations in the pyramidal cell phenotype may determine the complexity of cortical circuitry and, in turn, influence neural activity and how information is conveyed by neural activity. Pyramidal cells in TEO and in TE are fundamentally different. Those cells located in layer V in TEO have smaller bifurcations and have fewer spines than those in TE (Elston, 2002) or those in layer III TEO (Elston, 2003). In macaque visual cortex, the differences in arbor size result in a more than hundred-fold difference in the region of the visual map sampled by individual pyramidal cells in the primary visual area (V1) and cytoarchitectonic area TEO (Elston, 1998). Therefore, the difference in the total number of putative excitatory inputs along the dendrite and differences in their density may influence local summation of postsynaptic potentials or cooperation between inputs. Such summation is more likely to occur in highly spinous than in less spinous dendrites (Elston, 2002). In addition, whereas dendritic properties are conserved across species in early visual areas, in TE there is a dramatic expansion in size and arborization from marmosets to macaques to humans.

Unfortunately, too little is known about the exact connectivity among cells in the temporal lobe. But what is known suggests that IT may have a far greater integrative capacity than "earlier" visual areas (Elston, 2002), while still maintaining a topographic map in which neighboring neurons tend to receive similar inputs relative to distant neurons. Why the mass expansion of dendrites compared with early visual areas and across species? How might this affect cortical function in IT?

10.3   Object ontologies in the temporal lobe

10.3.1   Hierarchical visual processing in temporal lobe

Visual processing in the cortex is classically modeled as a hierarchy of increasingly sophisticated representations which accounts for the progressive increase in the complexity of physiological receptive fields, and the pyramidal cells' "appetite" for more complex stimuli as we move anteriorly in the occipitotemporal visual processing stream.

This account is based on the pioneering work of Hubel and Wiesel (1962, 1968) who discovered simple and complex cells in the cat striate cortex. Simple cells increase their firing rate to bars that have certain orientation and phase in their receptive field; that is in the area of the visual field where a stimulus can elicit a response. Complex cells also have limited receptive fields and their firing rate or response also depends on the bar orientation but is phase independent. These findings led Hubel and Wiesel to propose that an array of simple cells with different phase-dependent responses "feed" complex cells with information about their "visual" input, and then complex cells integrate this information and fire accordingly (Hubel and Wiesel, 1962, 1968).

A typical example of a hierarchical computational model extended to the level of object recognition is the MAX model of Riesenhueber and Poggio (1999). In this model, striate and extrastriate cortex are view-based modules which analyze the retinal image and then feed forward information about their specific response field to anterior IT and prefrontal cortex. View-invariant response units arise from a nonlinear MAX operation using the appropriate input from the previous modules. The information coded by these units is then fed forward and pooled together by object-tuned units whose information about the objects in the environment can then be used to accomplish goal-directed behavior (Riesenhueber and Poggio, 1999, 2002; Freedman et al., 2001).

Another influential theory of how IT cells accomplish object representation was put forward by Tanaka et al. (2000, 2003) who proposed that TE is parceled in columns that respond to similar object features, forming a continuous map of complex feature space and that object representation is achieved by binding the activity of these feature columns.

10.3.2   Functional visual processing in the temporal lobe?

Gibson (1979) proposed that perception should be understood by analyzing the structure of the organism's environment, its ecology. By shifting the focus of analysis from the organism to the environment that the organism acts upon to survive, Gibson emphasized the informational basis of perception rather than its mechanistic basis in the brain. This theoretical shift led into a reappreciation of what the function of perception is, and for that matter the function of the visual system: to reflect what we need to know about the environment to effectively act upon it. Indeed, Gibson's ecological optics theory emphasizes perceiving as an active exploration of the environment and the informational consequences of this fact.

Though it is a major contribution to our understanding of perception, ecological optics has difficulties in explaining how we are able to represent objects, for example the reconstruction of a three-dimensional face in the real world from the two-dimensional image in the retina.

As an alternative to a hierarchical theory of object ontology in IT, it is suggested that IT, instead of being organized around similar object features, is organized around an object's functional significance. Indeed, cells in IT and perirhinal cortex can hold a representation of pairs of arbitrary visual stimuli (Miyashita, 1988; Sakai and Miyashita, 1991; Erickson and Desimone, 1999; Messinger et al., 2001) that, in turn, are functionally important since monkeys are rewarded for selecting the correct pairing of the stimuli. In a similar delayed match-to-sample task, supposedly "unimodal" IT neurons show delay activity that is selective for the auditory stimulus that was paired to a visual stimulus, and not to other auditory stimuli (Colombo and Gross, 1994; Gibson and Maunsell, 1997). Therefore, the visual representation of an object in IT cortex can be associated to any other visual or even auditory stimulus representations *provided those pairings are functionally important for the subject*.

These two ontologies could be mutually exclusive or they can coexist. Therefore, using the ontology of objects in the temporal lobe pokes at the literal interpretation of existence while also suggesting we need to determine the organization of activity in the temporal lobe; that is, the vocabulary and grammar. The functional and featural accounts are but two such ontologies.

10.4   An instantiation of an object ontology: individuals

In an attempt to reveal a class of extremely selective cells (the so-called "grandmother cells") in the human temporal lobe, a remarkable degree of featural invariance was brought to light (Quiroga et al., 2005). According to the visual hierarchy account of temporal lobe organization, similarities in stimulus space lead to similar responses in the temporal lobe. But there can be no greater dissimilarity in the sensory inputs than stimuli transmitted through different modalities. How can a sound be "similar" to a sight? By analogy, our written language provides an arbitrary relationship between a visually presented object and that object's "name"; they share no systematic visual features. Yet cells in the human temporal lobe have been found that are selective for a large range of images of a particular celebrity's face but not to other faces, and even to the written name of that celebrity but not to other celebrities' names. Regardless of the specificity of these cells within a modality, the correspondence that ignores featural similarities across all those faces while favoring the arbitrary but functional mapping between an image and the written referent of the object in that image, makes an interesting case for the functional organization of objects in the temporal lobe. Were these images a fluke? If this is an ontology in the temporal lobe in general, it should be seen in human and monkey temporal lobes alike. But how to "name" objects for monkeys? How to find the relevant or "functional" attributes for monkeys?

Human and nonhuman primates live in cooperative and, at the same time, competitive societies; therefore the ability to recognize and remember the group members and their relationships to one another is vital for resource exploration and exploitation. Indeed, nonhuman primates spend much of their time watching conspecifics to acquire information about them. Evidence that these behaviors involve individuation stems from experiments measuring the discrimination of the bodies, faces, and vocalizations of individuals.

Macaques given the opportunity to watch the "private behavior" of another monkey do so at a constant level but, when given the opportunity to watch another monkey, they later increase their viewing time to the original monkey. It is inferred from this that they benefited more from comparing monkeys' behavior (Humphrey and Keeble, 1976). Since rhesus monkeys value acquiring information from conspecifics, watching other monkeys' faces is rewarding enough to ensure that presenting monkey face pictures acts as a reinforcer (Anderson, 1998). Furthermore, macaques are able to individuate conspecifics (Humphrey, 1974) even when looking only at their faces (Dahl et al., 2007). In an elegant study, Dahl and colleagues exposed rhesus monkeys to unfamiliar conspecific monkey faces and various nonconspecific animal pictures in a habituation-dishabituation paradigm and observed that, even without explicit training, monkeys showed a selective ability to differentiate conspecific faces but not non-conspecific pictures; that is, they recognized individual macaques and not just the basic category "macaque." Although faces are the only visual stimulus known to be individuated by macaques, they also value observing other body parts: female perinea can be used as a powerful reward (Deaner et al., 2005). Other sensory modalities are also used for individuation; in particular, rhesus are able to recognize kin based on their vocalizations (Rendall et al., 1996). This evidence suggests that macaques have an understanding of the individual, though our comprehension of the neural correlates of their understanding is incomplete.

10.5   An empirical test of featural versus functional representation of individuals in the temporal lobe

We addressed the following questions: first, are neural signals from the temporal lobe modulated by modality (visual and auditory)? Second, are these signals also modulated by the familiarity that the subject holds with the monkeys used as stimuli or are they exclusively stimulus or modality dependent? Finally, can a population of neural signals from the temporal lobe amodally represent individuals? To test these questions we presented a set of familiar and unfamiliar monkey stimuli consisting of video clips of faces and perinea, as well as vocalizations, while recording neural activity from the right temporal lobe (Baez-Mendoza, 2007).

To generate the stimulus set we filmed a subject monkey's cagemates, as well as three age- and weight-matched unfamiliar monkeys. From the films we extracted two neutral face clips, two hindquarter clips and two exemplars of the monkeys' coos. One 6-year-old adult male rhesus monkey weighing 10.25 kg participated in the experiments. For any given trial in the passive viewing task, six stimuli from the same feature category (face, perineum or vocalization) were presented after which the monkey received a juice reward. The trial started when the monkey maintained gaze in a 2° by 2° window around a 0.5° fixation spot for 500 ms. One example from each individual was presented in random order. The subject needed to maintain gaze within a visual stimulus, 18° by 14° of visual angle and to maintain fixation during the 100 ms inter-stimulus interval when no visual stimulus was presented. Failure to do so aborted the current stimulus and initiated a 2500 ms delay, after which the monkey was required to redirect his gaze to the fixation spot and the aborted stimulus was presented again followed by the remaining stimuli from the same trial. To signal the boundaries of where the eye gaze could go during a trial, a yellow rectangle of the same dimensions as the stimulus was shown on the monitor for the duration of the block of stimuli. In this way, the subject had to maintain his gaze in the same area during both audio and visual trials. The task had at least ten repetitions of each stimulus (20 for each of the attributes of a given monkey) and the category blocks were presented pseudorandomly without replacement.

For electrophysiological recordings we used a chronically implanted tetrode-drive (Neuralynx Inc., Tucson, AZ, USA). This prototype drive consisted of a Y-shaped titanium body that fits into the recording chamber attached to the skull. A 42-electrode series of shuttles allows the independent movement of each tetrode. The inner diameter of the vertically oriented recording chamber was 23 mm, directly above the right temporal lobe and implanted under sterile surgical conditions. We recorded neural activity in parallel from the upper bank STS, lower bank STS, ventral IT cortex (AMTS) and the hippocampus. Positions were confirmed through an MR scan following recordings. The data presented here came from five recording sessions in which 12–20 tetrodes were recorded simultaneously, for a total sample of 81 recording sites. Peristimulus time histograms (PSTHs) containing 100 ms before stimulus onset and 1000 ms during stimulus presentation were constructed for each recording site and stimulus. Local field potential (LFP) power was estimated for each trial and recording site with a Discrete

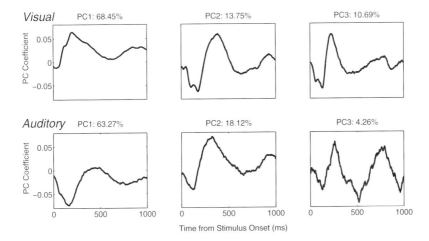

Figure 10.1. Principal components of temporal lobe LFP waveforms to visual and auditory stimuli. The percentage of explained variance above each subplot. The PCA inputs were the trial-averaged LFP waveforms from each site, evoked in response to visual or auditory stimuli.

Fourier Transform (DFT) with 256 points and bandwidth of 0–500 Hz. For all null hypothesis statistical tests, the alpha level was set to 0.05 and corrected for multiple comparisons by dividing by the sample size.

10.5.1 Modality selectivity

To characterize the LFP waveform in response to either a visual or auditory stimulus we used principal components analysis (PCA). The input was the averaged full LFP responses after stimulus onset from each site to visual or auditory stimuli averaged across trials. The first principal component for visual stimuli had a positive slow rise peaking at 204 ms and went back to zero about 650 ms later. In contrast, the first principal component of the auditory responses had a sharper negative rise that peaked at about 164 ms and went back to zero at about 400 ms. The second principal component for both modalities was very similar: a biphasic waveform. In both cases, the first two principal components explained over 80% of the variance; see Figure 10.1.

We were further interested in testing the dependence of responses on stimulus modality. To do so we used the LFP waveform timecourse as well as LFP responses in the frequency domain since LFP activity has been demonstrated to be sensitive to stimulus parameters independent of the local unit activity (Kruse and Eckhorn, 1996; Mehring et al., 2003; Siegel and Konig, 2003; Rickert et al., 2005; Kreiman et al., 2006; Liu and Newsome, 2006; Wilke et al., 2006). First, we tested whether the averaged LFP visual or auditory response during a 50 ms window around the time of maximum absolute amplitude after stimulus onset was significantly greater than zero (i.e. baseline). This definition we call MAXDIFF. Based on MAXDIFF, 55% of recorded sites responded to auditory stimuli, 69% responded to visual stimuli, and 35% responded

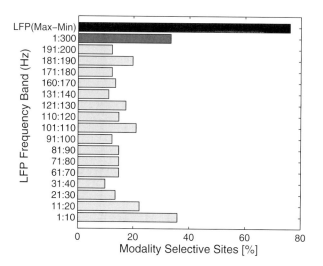

Figure 10.2. Proportion of modality selective sites as a function of LFP frequency band. The black bar shows the percentage of modality selective sites when the LFP response is defined as the average amplitude at the point of maximum difference between auditory and visual responses (MAXDIFF). The numbers next to each gray bar correspond to the frequency band from which the total power was calculated.

to both modalities. Several of the responses to auditory stimuli arose from areas in IT cortex traditionally thought to be unimodal visual (e.g. Baylis et al., 1987; Riesenhuber and Poggio, 1999, 2000).

The second LFP measure was obtained by converting the 1000 ms responses into the frequency domain, and calculating the power found in 10 Hz increments from 1 to 200 Hz (excluding those around 50 and 150 Hz, which could contain line noise). Power obtained from visual and auditory trials was then compared using a paired samples t-test. The third LFP measure was the sum of the power in the range 1–300 Hz, compared across modality. The results are summarized in Figure 10.2. As far as we are aware analysis of the frequency domain of the temporal lobe LFPs has been limited. We chose an analysis replicating a previous one used for analyzing IT cortex LFP responses to visual stimuli (Kreiman et al., 2006), and we extended this to analyze both visual and auditory modalities. In the case of modality selectivity, the LFP response definition by Kreiman and colleagues provided a very similar proportion of selective sites to the selectivity we observed in the bins at lower frequencies. The selectivity seen in Figure 10.2 suggests that the low-frequency components of the LFP are the most informative about stimulus modality.

10.5.2   Category and familiarity

The next step was to analyze the LFP response to stimuli from familiar or unfamiliar monkeys (a variable we call "familiarity") depending on the feature category. We compared familiarity effects only for a given category of stimulus (face, call, perineum), since the auditory responses were commonly quite different as a class from the visual stimuli (see Figures 10.1 and 10.2). For the statistical analysis, we performed a two-way ANOVA on the LFP response with two levels for the familiarity factor: familiar and unfamiliar, and three levels for the category factor: faces, perinea and calls. Figure 10.3 shows some examples of normalized LFP waveforms in response to the three stimulus categories and Figure 10.4 shows familiarity effects evoked by stimuli of a given category.

Since most sites had a modality effect, we expected and confirmed that most sites had a different response between visual categories, faces and perinea, and calls. However, we were surprised to find that only one site had a differential LFP response between faces and perinea. The present electrode sites may simply not be the ones whose signals differentiate faces and perinea: only a mere fraction of the temporal lobe was sampled. Face and hand selectivity has been demonstrated since the discovery of face cells (see Gross, 2005, for review). More recently, evidence of category-selective organization in the macaque was provided by Pinsk and workers who measured the BOLD of monkeys passively fixating faces and body parts with fMRI and found bilaterally face-selective areas in the STS and adjacent to them body-selective areas (Pinsk et al., 2005). Yet, to our knowledge, no studies have compared face activity with that of the perineum. Both potentially convey information about the status of the individual and both contain similar low-level visual features (symmetric high-spatial-frequency features surrounded by a furry external contour). It remains a possibility that some of the reports of "face" cells could, in fact, be described as "coin" cells, as in heads or tails.

We found that about 20% of sites responded differentially to familiar and unfamiliar individuals irrespective of category. About 10% of recording sites had an interaction of familiarity and category. Some sites differentiated between perinea or calls, given the features were extracted from a familiar stimulus monkey, but none differentiated familiar versus unfamiliar faces. These results are in partial accordance with a previous human fMRI study, which found higher BOLD activation for familiar than for unfamiliar faces or voices in the anterior temporal lobe (von Kriegstein and Giraud, 2006) and with lesion case studies of semantic dementia for specific individuals which localize the lesion in the anterior temporal lobe bilaterally (Gainotti et al., 2003).

We cannot exclude the participation of other areas in the representation of familiar individuals. The finding of selectivity for individuals in the human hippocampus, amygdala, parahippocampal gyrus and entorhinal cortex (Quiroga et al., 2005) suggest that these areas are candidates for the representation of familiar individuals. Another area is the posterior cingulate cortex, though at odds with the aforementioned study by von Kriegstein (2006). Shah et al. (2001) showed that the cingulate has a higher activation when humans see faces of familiars or hear their voices than to the same gestures by unfamiliars. One reason for this discrepancy may be the use of familiar and unfamiliar individuals in the latter study compared with recently learned voice-face-name associations in the former. Though our findings cannot disentangle these contradictory results, they do support a role for the temporal lobe in the representation of individuals sharing complete social contact, irrespective of the stimulus modality.

We also assessed different definitions of LFP response based on the frequency domain and then submitted these data to a two-way ANOVA. Whereas category selectivity was maximal for low frequencies (1–10 Hz), familiarity effects were minimal

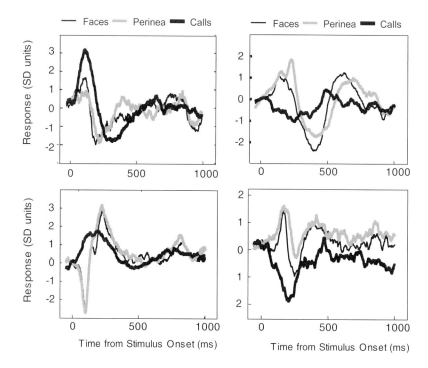

Figure 10.3. Example mean LFP waveforms in response to stimuli from each category. Responses have been normalized to the response during the baseline period for that electrode site.

in the low frequencies, showing the greatest proportion of discrimination in the high gamma-band (e.g. 71–100 Hz, see Figure 10.5). There were, however, fewer familiarity selective sites based on the frequency domain compared with the MAXDIFF definition. In visual areas, attended stimuli induce enhanced responses and an improved synchronization of rhythmic neuronal activity in this frequency range, and it is proposed that this synchronization underlies the binding of attended stimulus features (Gray, 1994; Engel et al., 2001). Though there is accumulating evidence against the binding-by-synchrony hypothesis (Roelfsema et al., 2004), our definition of familiarity is independent of modality, therefore an interesting question is whether neuronal and LFP activity at this frequency range reflect the "binding" of amodal features from an individual. Analysis of our neuronal data examining the LFP coherence and spike-LFP coherence (Engel et al., 2001; Fries et al., 2001; Pesaran et al., 2002; Womelsdorf et al., 2006), and/or cross-correlation between recording sites (Gochin et al., 1991, 1994) could further explore this question.

10.5.3   Coding of individuals

Since we observed that LFPs in the temporal cortex could be sensitive to the presentation modality, the category, and to familiarity, we assessed the selectivity of the LFP for

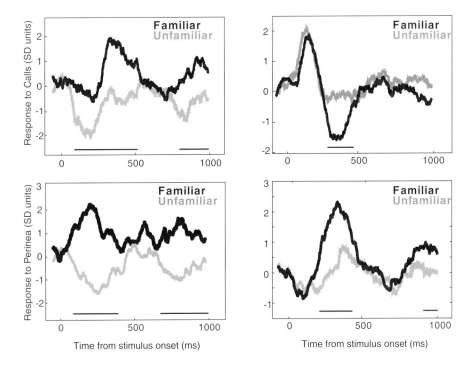

Figure 10.4. Example mean LFP waveforms in response to familiar versus unfamiliar stimuli from a given category. Responses in the top row are to perinea, and in the bottom row, to calls. Each response has been normalized to that of the baseline period for that electrode site. Black horizontal bars at the bottom of each image show time points when the responses to familiar and unfamiliar stimuli were significantly different. Electrode locations included ventral IT and both banks of the STS.

a familiar individual depending on the feature category. As an exploratory analysis of the neural coding for individuals, we reduced the dimensionality of the LFP responses to all the stimuli with PCA, and then ran an NHST on the Euclidean distance of the first ten coefficients for each stimulus between and within familiar or unfamiliar individuals on each category in 50 ms bins across the stimulus presentation period. We found that at the time bin centered at 525 ms after stimulus onset, the distances were greater for the face/call/perineum across individuals than those corresponding to the same familiar individual, and these distances were less than to the attributes of the unfamiliar individuals. In other words, at this time point the LFP from the temporal lobe could be used to differentiate known individuals independently of modality. Interestingly, this time point does not correspond to the point of largest difference for any of the conjunctions we tested before: modality, category and familiarity, and individuals.

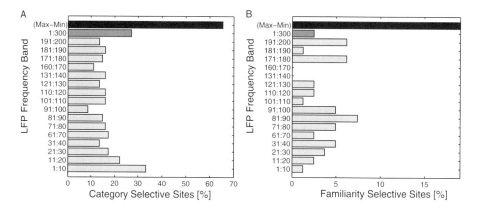

Figure 10.5. Category and familiarity selectivity depending on LFP frequency band. For both plots, the black bar shows the percentage of selective sites when the LFP response is defined as the average amplitude at the point of maximum difference between auditory and visual responses. The numbers next to each gray bar correspond to the frequency band where the total power was summed. Selectivity was determined through a two-way ANOVA of category x familiarity. (A) Percentage of category selective sites. (B) Percentage of familiarity selective sites. Note the change in the scaling of the abscissa between (A) and (B).

10.6   Conclusions

The LFP responses from the temporal lobe are dependent on the sensory modality stimulated and that the population of LFP waveforms in the temporal lobe may contain information about individual identity depending on the stimulus modality. We are, however, cautious about these conclusions for two reasons. First, the recorded LFP possessed a high variability during and across recording sessions. Second, there is no behavioral evidence, yet, indicating that rhesus macaques are capable of amodally individuating.

Nevertheless, this study opens the ground to future studies of neural coding of individuals. One important first step would be to confirm that macaque monkeys are behaviorally capable of amodally individuating. The next steps could go into several directions; one project could involve fMRI in awake monkeys. Since the LFP is highly correlated to BOLD activation (Logothetis et al., 2001; Logothetis, 2002), these preliminary results suggest that an fMRI experiment in awake behaving monkeys could shed light on where the brain might process information about individuals. Another project could focus on analyzing the single unit activity and multiple unit activity of the temporal lobe to our stimulus set; focusing, for example, in the frequency and category effects we found in the temporal and frequency domains. These studies would shed light on how the neural coding of individuals is achieved.

With what we have analyzed, the main effects appear to support a feature-based object ontology. This could be a consequence of the features chosen; perhaps within the visual domain, much greater invariance is possible – as with faces and perinea. Indeed, there is evidence to suggest that functional pairing of stimuli leads to a shared response space across nearby neurons (Erickson et al., 2000). It could also be that many IT areas show feature-based representations, with only the temporal pole or perirhinal cortex getting enough diverse connections to support amodal-functional representations. Or there may be sufficient information about the individual based on a distributed code: the brain doesn't require the "amodal neuron" if it can represent the individual over many neurons that cover the feature space. This would be analogous to how view-invariant representations might arise out of several view-tuned cells. As long as view tuning covers a sufficient amount of "view space," invariance to view can be achieved. Here, pooling feature (i.e. category) selective responses according to the individual they represent could similarly lead to an amodal representation of the individual. Thus, the representational capacity of cells in the temporal lobe is substantial and can arise from multiple mechanisms. This could be topographic, as in maps of feature space, or from other domains of convergence, such as functionally relevant representations of the individual. We are only beginning to understand the full capacity of – and mechanics underlying – temporal lobe activity.

Cross-modal responses in 'unimodal' temporal lobe areas as described here and elsewhere (Colombo and Gross, 1994; Gibson and Maunsell, 1997; Schroeder and Foxe, 2002; Fu et al., 2003; Ghazanfar et al., 2005; Hoffman et al., 2008), serve as an illustration of how adaptive temporal lobe responses may be. To better understand the organization and classification of regions in the temporal lobe (i.e. the ontology) we should consider the unique anatomy and connectivity of this broad area and the "output" of the system: the goal is not to veridically represent what is out there, but to reflect what we need to know to effectively learn about and act upon the environment.

Acknowledgments

We are grateful for the generous support and guidance of Nikos K. Logothetis, in whose lab the experiments were conducted. We would also like to thank the Max Planck Society for their financial support.

References

Anderson, J. R. (1998). Social stimuli and social rewards in primate learning and cognition. *Behav. Processes*, 42: 159–175.

Baez-Mendoza, R. (2007). Neural coding of individuals in the temporal cortex of the macaque. Thesis, Graduate School of Neural and Behavioural Sciences. International Max Planck Research School. Tübingen, Germany.

Baylis, G., Rollis, E. and Leonard, C. (1987). Functional subdivisions of the temporal lobe neocortex. *J. Neurosci.*, 7: 330–342.

Colombo, M. and Gross, C. G. (1994). Responses of inferior temporal cortex and hippocampal neurons during delayed matching to sample in monkeys (*Macaca fascicularis*). *Behav. Neurosci.*, 108: 443–455.

Dahl, C. D., Logothetis, N. K. and Hoffman, K. L. (2007). Individual and holistic processing of faces in rhesus monkeys. *Proc. Roy. Soc. Lond. B*, 274: 2069–2076.

Deaner, R. O., Khera, A. V. and Platt, M. L. (2005). Monkeys pay per view: adaptive valuation of social images by rhesus monkeys. *Curr. Biol.*, 15: 543–568.

Elston, G. N. (1998). Morphological variation of layer III pyramidal neurones in the occipitotemporal pathway of the macaque monkey visual cortex. *Cereb. Cortex*, 8: 278–294.

Elston, G. N. (2002). Cortical heterogeneity: implications for visual processing and polysensory integration. *J. Neurocyt.*, 31: 317–35.

Elston, G. N. (2003). Cortex, cognition and the cell: new insights into the pyramidal neuron and prefrontal function. *Cereb. Cortex*, 13: 1124–1138.

Engel, A. K., Fries, P. and Singer, W. (2001). Dynamic predictions: oscillations and synchrony in top-down processing. *Nat. Rev. Neurosci.*, 2: 704–716.

Erickson, C. A. and Desimone, R. (1999). Responses of macaque perirhinal neurons during and after visual stimulus association learning. *J. Neurosci.*, 19: 10404–10416.

Erickson, C. A., Jagadeesh, B. and Desione, R. (2000). Clustering of perirhinal neurons with similar properties following visual experience in adult monkeys. *Nat. Neurosci.*, 3: 1143–1148.

Farah, M. J. (1990). *Visual Agnosia*. Cambridge, MA: MIT Press.

Felleman, D. J. and Van Essen, D C. (1991). Distributed hierarchical processing in the primate cerebral cortex. *Cereb. Cortex*, 1: 1–47.

Freedman, D. J., Riesenhuber, M., Poggio, T. and Miller, E. K. (2001). Categorical representation of visual stimuli in the primate prefrontal cortex. *Science*, 291: 312–316.

Fries, P., Reynolds, J. H., Rorie, A. E. and Desimone, R. (2001). Modulation of oscillatory neuronal synchronization by selective visual attention. *Science*, 291: 1560–1563.

Fu, K.-M. G., Johnston, T. A., Shar, A. S., Arnold, L., Smiley, J., Hackett, T. A., Garraghty, P. E., and Schroeder, C. E. (2003). Auditory cortical neurons respond to somatosensory stimulation. *J. Neurosci.*, 23: 7510–7515.

Gainotti, G., Barbier, A. and Marra, C. (2003). Slowly progressive defect in recognition of familiar people in a patient with right anterior temporal atrophy. *Brain*, 126: 792–803.

Ghazanfar, A. A., Maier, J. X., Hoffman, K. L. and Logothetis, N. K. (2005). Multisensory integration of dynamic faces and voices in rhesus monkey auditory cortex. *J. Neurosci.*, 25: 5004–5012.

Gibson, J. R. (1979). *The Ecological Approach to Visual Perception*. Boston, MA: Houghton Mifflin.

Gibson, J. R. and Maunsell, J. H. (1997). Sensory modality specificity of neural activity related to memory in visual cortex. *J. Neurophysiol.*, 78: 1263–1275.

Gochin, P. M., Colombo, M., Dorfman, G. A., Gerstein, G. L. and Gross, C. G. (1994). Neural ensemble coding in inferior temporal cortex. *J. Neurophysiol.*, 71: 2325–2337.

Gochin, P. M., Miller, E. K., Gross, C. G. and Gerstein, G. L. (1991). Functional interactions among neurons in inferior temporal cortex of the awake macaque. *Exp. Brain Res.*, 84: 505–516.

Gray, C. M. (1994). Synchronous oscillations in neural systems: mechanisms and functions. *J. Comput. Neurosci.*, 1: 11–38.

Gross, C. (2005). Processing the facial image: a brief history. *Am. Psychologist*, 60: 755-763.

Gruber, T. R. (1993). A translational approach to portable ontology specifications. *Knowl. Acquisit.*, 5: 199–220.

Hoffman, K. L., Ghazanfar, A. A., Gauthier, I. and Logothetis, N. K. (2008). Category-selective responses to faces and objects in primate auditory cortex. *Front. Syst. Neurosci.*, 1, Article 2.

Hubel, D. H. and Wiesel, T. N. (1962). Receptive fields, binocular interaction and function architecture in the cat's visual cortex. *J. Physiol. (Lond.)*, 160: 106–154.

Hubel, D. H. and Wiesel, T. N. (1968). Receptive fields and functional architecture of monkey striate cortex. *J. Physiol. (Lond.)*, 195: 215–243.

Humphrey, N. K. (1974). Species and individuals in the perceptual world of monkeys. *Perception*, 3: 105–114.

Humphrey, N. K. and Keeble, G. R. (1976). How monkeys acquire a new way of seeing. *Perception*, 5: 51–56.

Humphreys, G. W. and Riddoch, M. J. (1987). The fractionation of visual agnosia. In G. W. Humpreys and M. J. Riddoch (eds.) *Visual Object Processing: A Cognitive Neuropsychological Approach*. London: Lawrence Erlbaum.

Iwai, E. and Mishkin, M. (1969). Further evidence on the locus of the visual area in the temporal lobe of the monkey. *Exp. Neurol.*, 25: 585–594.

Klüver, H. and Bucy, P. C. (1939). Preliminary analysis of functions of the temporal lobes in monkeys. *Arch. Neurol. Psychiatry*, 42: 979-1000.

Kreiman, G., Hung, C. P., Kraskov, A., Quiroga, R. Q., Poggio, T. and DiCarlo, J. J. (2006). Object selectivity of local field potentials and spikes in the macaque inferior temporal cortex. *Neuron*, 49: 433–445.

Kruse, W. and Eckhorn, R. (1996). Inhibition of sustained gamma oscillations (35-80 Hz) by fast transient responses in cat visual cortex. *Proc. Nat. Acad. Sci.*, 93: 6112–6117.

Liu, J. and Newsome, W. T. (2006). Local field potential in cortical area MT: stimulus tuning and behavioral correlations. *J. Neurosci.*, 26: 7779–7790.

Logothetis, N. K. (2002). The neural basis of the blood-oxygen-level-dependent functional magnetic resonance imaging signal. *Phil. Trans. Roy. Soc. Lond. B*, 357: 1003–1037.

Logothetis, N. K. and Sheinberg, D. L. (1969). Visual object recognition. *Ann. Rev. Neurosci.*, 19: 577–621.

Logothetis, N. K., Pauls, J., Augath, M., Trinath, T. and Oeltermann, A. (2001). Neurophysiological investigation of the basis of the fMRI signal. *Nature*, 412: 150–157.

Mehring, C., Rickert, J., Vaadia, E., de Oliveira, S. C., Aertsen, A. and Rotter, S. (2003). Inference of hand movements from local field potentials in monkey motor cortex. *Nat. Neurosci.*, 6: 1253–1254.

Messinger, A., Squire, L. R., Zola, S. M. and Albright, T. D. (2001). Neuronal representations of stimulus associations develop in the temporal lobe during learning. *Proc. Nat. Acad. Sci. USA*, 98: 12239–12244.

Mishkin, M. (1954). Visual discrimination performance following partial ablations of the temporal lobe. II. Ventral lobe vs. hippocampus. *J. Comp. Physiol. Psychol.*, 47: 187–193.

Mishkin, M. and Pribram, K. H. (1954). Visual discrimination performance following partial ablations of the temporal lobe. I. Ventral vs. lateral. *J. Comp. Physiol. Psychol.*, 47: 14–20.

Miyashita, Y. (1988). Neuronal correlate of visual associative long-term memory in the primate temporal cortex. *Nature*, 335: 817–820.

Pesaran, B., Pezaris, J. S., Sahani, M., Mitra, P. P. and Andersen, R. A. (2002). Temporal structure in neuronal activity during working memory in macaque parietal cortex. *Nat. Neurosci.*, 5: 805–811.

Pinsk, M. A, Desimone, K., Moore, T., Gross, C. G. and Kastner, S. (2005). Representations of faces and body parts in macaque temporal cortex: a functional MRI study. *Proc. Nat. Acad. Sci. USA*, 102: 6996.

Quiroga, R. Q., Reddy, L., Kreiman, G., Koch, C. and Fried, I. (2005). Invariant visual representation by single neurons in the human brain. *Nature*, 435: 1102–1107.

Rendall, D., Rodman, P. S. and Emond, R. E. (1996). Vocal recognition of individuals and kin in free-ranging rhesus monkeys. *Anim. Behav.*, 51: 1007–1015.

Rickert, J., de Oliveira, S. C., Vaadia, E., Aertsen, A., Rotter, S. and Mehring, C. (2005). Encoding of movement direction in different frequency ranges of motor cortical local field potentials. *J. Neurosci.*, 25: 8815–8824.

Riesenhuber, M. and Poggio, T. (1999). Hierarchical models of object recognition in cortex. *Nat. Neurosci.*, 2: 1019.

Riesenhuber, M. and Poggio, T. (2000), Models of object recognition. *Nat. Neurosci.*, 3: 1199–1204.

Riesenhuber, M. and Poggio, T. (2002). Neural mechanisms of object recognition. *Curr. Opin. Neurobiol.*, 12: 162–168.

Roelfsema, P. R., Lamme, V. A. and Spekreijse, H. (2004). Synchrony and covariation of firing rates in the primary visual cortex during contour grouping. *Nat. Neurosci.*, 7: 982–991.

Sakai, K. and Miyashita, Y. (1991). Neural organization for the long-term memory of paired associates. *Nature*, 354: 152–155.

Schroeder, C. E. and Foxe, J. J. (2002). The timing and laminar profile of converging inputs to multisensory areas of the macaque neocortex. *Cogn. Brain Res.*, 14: 187–198.

Seltzer, B. and Pandya, D. N. (1994). Parietal, temporal, and occipital projections of the superior temporal sulcus in the rhesus monkey: a retrograde tracer study. *J. Comp. Neurol.*, 343: 445–463.

Shah, N. J., Marshall, J. C., Zafiris, O., Schwab, A., Zilles, K., Markowitsch, H. J. and Fink, G. R. (2001). The neural correlates of person familiarity. A functional magnetic resonance imaging study with clinical implications. *Brain*, 124: 804–815.

Siegel, M. and Konig, P. (2003). A functional gamma-band defined by stimulus-dependent synchronization in area 18 of awake behaving cats. *J. Neurosci.*, 23: 4251–4260.

Tanaka, K. (2000). Mechanisms of visual object recognition studied in monkeys. *Spatial Vis.*, 13: 147–163.

Tanaka, K. (2003). Columns for complex visual object features in the inferotemporal cortex: clustering of cells with similar but slightly different stimulus selectivities. *Cereb. Cortex*, 13: 90–99.

Ungerleider, L. G. and Mishkin, M. (1982). Two cortical visual systems. In D. J. Ingle, M. A. Goodale and R. J. W. Mansfield (eds.) *Analysis of Visual Behavior*. Cambridge, MA: MIT Press.

von Bonin, G. and Bailey, P. (1947). *The Neurocortex of Macaca Mulatta*. Urbana, IL: Univ. of Illinois Press.

von Kriegstein, K. and Giraud, A.-L. (2006). Implicit multisensory associations influence voice recognition. *PLoS Biol.*, 4: e326.

Wilke, M., Logothetis, N. K. and Leopold, D. A. (2006). Local field potential reflects perceptual suppression in monkey visual cortex. *Proc. Nat. Acad. Sci. USA*, 103: 17507–17512.

Womelsdorf, T., Fries, P., Mitra, P. P. and Desimone, R. (2006). Gamma-band synchronization in visual cortex predicts speed of change detection. *Nature*, 439: 733–736.

Part III

Frontal cortex

11 How the prefrontal cortex is thought to be involved in response suppression

S. Ovaysikia, A. E. N. Hoover, K. Tahir, A. Tharani and J. F. X. DeSouza

11.1 Functions of the prefrontal cortex

Most of us are able to suppress the urge to respond emotionally when confronted with a frustrating situation. However, patients with prefrontal cortex (PFC) damage act out based on their impulsive urges. Faulty emotional regulation, which can ultimately lead to impulsive violence if not regulated, results from PFC damage. The question is why? It is because the PFC is responsible for inhibition and has a crucial role in the flexible control of behavior.

The PFC can be subdivided into three major regions: orbital, medial, and lateral. It receives input from both the ventral visual stream, which has been implicated in feature and object-related processing, as well as the dorsal visual stream, which is involved in spatial visual processing (Chelazzi et al., 1998). The orbital and medial regions are mostly involved in emotional behavior. The lateral subdivision is maximally developed in humans and provides the cognitive support to the temporal organization of behavior, speech, and reasoning (Fuster, 2001). Such higher cognitive functions are amongst those that develop relatively later in human beings and developmental studies have provided the anatomical evidence for this. It has been shown through neuroimaging studies that the prefrontal areas do not reach full maturity until adolescence in humans (Sowell et al., 1999).

Cortical Mechanisms of Vision, ed. M. Jenkin and L. R. Harris. Published by Cambridge University Press.
© Cambridge University Press 2009.

The PFC has been implicated in execution of many higher cognitive functions including long-term planning, response suppression and response selection. It has also been shown that the prefrontal areas have a particularly critical, executive role in detecting deviations from familiar patterns and inhibiting automatic responses (Nobre et al., 1999). This was demonstrated by Nobre et al. (1999) as they found activation of the PFC when the learned and expected stimulus associations that guide behavior were violated and thus required inhibition of the prepared response and redirection of the focus of attention. When the environment is ambiguous or presents competing demands that are contrary to habit and it makes performance prone to errors, an executive system then needs to exert control to suppress the errors (Schall et al., 2002). Different actions are required depending on the situation; the PFC has a crucial role in this flexible control of behavior.

Working memory in PFC has also been tested using delayed match to sample tasks (Goldman-Rakic, 1992). Another piece of evidence comes from humans with prefrontal cortex lesions (Guitton et al., 1985). These patients perform better on simple memory tasks, such as recalling information after a delay period, than do patients with medial temporal lesions. However, they show marked deficits in more complex memory tasks (Miller et al., 1996).

In this chapter, we will focus on the role of the prefrontal cortex in response suppression and evaluate its consequences for clinical populations and clinical applications. After reviewing the results, implications for future research in neuroprosthetics will be briefly discussed.

11.1.1   Measuring neural responses

Much of the research on neural correlates of behavior has been found using the recent technology of functional magnetic resonance imaging (fMRI). These studies attempt to reveal different patterns of brain activity, which are associated with a specific task of interest compared with a controlled baseline task. The strengths of fMRI include being noninvasive, having high spatial and adequate temporal resolution, and adapting to many types of experimental paradigms. The underlying technique of fMRI is to measure the difference in blood-oxygen-level-dependency, or the BOLD contrast effect. Because fMRI is noninvasive and does not involve exposure to radiation, it has the advantage of repeatability in a single subject. This allows researchers and clinicians to follow changes in brain function in individual subjects over the course of a progressive study or disease, during recovery from injury or stroke, or in response to treatment (Le Bihan et al., 1995).

11.2   Examining response suppression using the anti-saccade task

In pro-saccade trials, individuals must make a reflexive glance towards a presented stimulus. Conversely, in an anti-saccade task (Hallett, 1978), individuals must suppress their reflexive urge to make an eye movement to the stimulus and instead make a saccade in the opposite direction (i.e. to the mirror location) of that stimulus (for more detailed description of methods, see DeSouza et al., 2003, and see DESOUZA slide presentation slides #20 to e #25).[1] Thus, the anti-saccade task has three parts: preparation of which task is required, inhibition of the prepotent response to look at the stimulus (making a pro-saccade) and the inversion of the saccade target vector.

Patients with frontal lobe damage (Guitton et al., 1985; Fukushima et al., 1994; Walker et al., 1998) and schizophrenia (Fukushima et al., 1990; Clementz et al., 1994) have impaired performances on anti-saccade tasks, fueling the popularity of such tasks as a test of frontal cortex function. An increased error rate in anti-saccade trials involving patients with frontal cortex damage suggests a failure of response suppression (Guitton et al., 1985). Much evidence has accumulated to support the claim that the prefrontal cortex is responsible for response suppression in the Stroop (Barkley et al., 1992) and anti-saccade tasks (Guitton et al., 1985; Fukushima et al., 1994; Walker et al., 1998).

11.2.1   The Stroop task

The role of PFC in attentional control has been examined extensively within both healthy and patient populations using the Stroop task. This task involves the presentation of words such as red, green, blue, etc, written in a color different from the words' semantic meaning (Stroop, 1935; see slide presentation slides #8 to #18, during the demonstration read the color of the word out loud). The automatic response of reading the word has a "strong" stimulus-response (SR) association, so the reaction time is very quick. On the other hand, controlled processes, such as the participant's inhibition of the automatic response to read and instead state the color of the ink, have weaker SR associations and longer reaction times. Therefore, the subject has to suppress the automatic urge to read the color word (Gruber, 2002). The main difficulty in the Stroop task is caused by the competition between the two processes of word reading and color identification. Since word reading is the more automatic process, inhibiting it in order to name the color (the more controlled process) is difficult and thus prone to more errors, in both healthy and patient populations.

Patients with frontal lobe damage display poor performance on the Stroop task (Barkley et al., 1992). An fMRI study using a modified version of the Stroop task compared the performance of individuals with schizophrenia with a control group. Patients with schizophrenia showed a different pattern of activation during the performance of the task. They showed a reduced activation of the dorsolateral prefrontal, anterior cingulate, and parietal regions but a higher activation in temporal regions and posterior cingulate (Weiss et al., 2007). Such hypofrontality of the prefrontal cortex is expected in most patient populations with frontal lobe lesions as they lack control over impulsive urges. It is this lack of activation that leads to the patients' inability to suppress the automatic urge of reading the color of the word for the Stroop task.

---

[1]The presentation can be found on the accompanying CD-ROM.

11.3   Top-down and bottom-up visual attention

If there is a sudden flash that appears somewhere out in our visual field, we are likely to respond to the flash by moving our gaze in its direction. Our attention is grabbed by that particular stimulus because it is unexpected, distinctive and novel.

Saliency drives the "priority hierarchy," if you will, in the brain and determines how we will orient our attentional resources. This orientation can be led by both sensory stimulation (exogenously), and by cognition (endogenously). Both cognitive and external factors guide our visual perception in order to create a representation of what is important in our visual field (Corbetta and Shulman, 2002). Attention can be divided into two main categories: bottom-up sensory stimulation and top-down expectations with current goals. However, both systems are used systematically. We will pay more attention to certain sensory stimuli because they reflect our expectations of what it is we are going to see and what it is we want to see. This also comes into play when we think about preparatory set activity, which will be discussed in the following section.

We use our cognition, tentative plans, and goals to structure our attention as well as our actions. We need such top-down processes so that we can determine what is important to us at any given moment and during any given goal-directed activity, especially if it requires long-term planning and attention. We will need to inhibit, or ignore, these sometimes salient stimuli (i.e. the flash of light), in order to achieve our goals. This is in fact what happens during the previously discussed anti-saccade task. To complete an anti-saccade, the participant must look in the opposite direction without making a saccade to the stimulus that is more salient, unexpected and novel (Hallett, 1978). This simple task is very effective in allowing researchers to look at varying types of research questions. For example, human and nonhuman primate behavioral tasks are tested on patients with varying frontal lobe deficits and are also used to make further correlations with tasks that resemble the anti-saccade task, such as the Stroop task (Stroop, 1935).

11.4   Preparatory set

In general, we tend to be able to act in any given situation when we have intentionally prepared for what will happen. The time we spent during preparation will help us develop the appropriate action or behavior. Being prepared is important for us in all aspects of life. Whether we are anticipating a certain move during a sports game or while stopped at a red light, we need to be able to act appropriately to complete the desired task or goal (Hebb, 1972). We look to cues in the environment to prime us to behave just as experiments use certain cues to prepare the participants for action or making a response. However, an internal cue differs from an external cue, because it requires the subject to continuously monitor their response and the reward feedback.

Bilateral intraparietal (IPS) and frontal eye fields (FEF) are active during the acquisition of attentional sets. This is indeed the case for all sorts of goal-directed activities and stimulus-response selection (Mesulam, 1999). fMRI signals recorded during the time before a stimulus is presented, during anticipatory attention, usually correspond to the prestimulus anticipatory activity, or preparatory set (Corbetta and Shulman, 2002). The role of cues is to allow for more preparation for tasks (Barton et al., 2005). What you do on the first trial will affect the preparatory set for the next trial (Dorris et al., 2000). Also, the frontal cortical level of activation during the preparatory period, the time before the presentation of the stimulus, is important for how the participant will perform on the anti-saccade task in particular (DeSouza et al., 2003; Ford et al., 2005; see slide presentation slide #32).

Areas of the brain that are involved in controlling where our attention is directed are within the frontoparietal network closely integrated with the eye movement network (Corbetta et al., 1998). fMRI studies have found that during a preparatory period, a correct anti-saccade produces more activation in the frontal and parietal areas than a pro-saccade does. Also, fMRI experiments with longer preparatory periods, some up to 14 seconds, have been able to give converging results suggesting these areas show higher preparation for anti-saccade trials than pro-saccade trials (DeSouza and Everling, 2004; Ford et al., 2005; Brown et al., 2007). Results from event-related fMRI studies in humans that employed preparatory periods of 10 seconds at first seem consistent with monkey electrophysiology studies within three brain areas: SEF, FEF, DLPFC (Schlag-Rey et al., 1997; Everling and Munoz, 2000; DeSouza and Everling, 2004; Ford et al., 2005). Specifically, Ford et al. (2005) showed that a number of cortical areas exhibit differences in their BOLD signal intensity during the late preparatory period and during the S-R period between correct anti and pro and between correct anti and errors. During the late prep period, they found higher activation on anti-saccade trials than on pro-saccade ones in the DLPFC, FEF, pre-SEF, ACC, POS and IPS areas; higher activation on correct anti trials in the right DLPFC, right ACC and the pre-SEF. The correct anti-saccade, as opposed to error trials, had more activation in the DLPFC, ACC and pre-SEF. One must remember that the most important difference with fMRI studies and electrophysiology studies is the evolution of time (see DESOUZA slide presentation #82). In this slide, you see that the preparatory signal for the top panel of fMRI BOLD signal evolves over 14 seconds whereas the inset (lower figure) evolves over 100 milliseconds. Once you have taken these two points into consideration, many of the results showing preparatory signals for the anti-saccade preparation share a similar process. In conclusion, this confirms the importance of the frontal cortical areas in response suppression during the anti-saccade task. But is this response suppression related to oculomotor preparation or response suppression in general? To address this question, we have conducted an fMRI study to examine whether response suppression during the anti-saccade and Stroop task shows activation in similar frontal cortical areas (see Ovaysikia et al., 2007).

11.4.1 Is the observed activation a visual/motor response or a preparatory set?

The increased error rates of those with PFC damage may represent a top-down control signal disturbance involved in suppressing the pro-saccade and selecting the anti-saccade instead. Previous fMRI studies suggested visual or motor signals are responsible for the increased cortical activation for anti-saccades as opposed to the preparatory set signals we just discussed above (O'Driscoll et al., 1995; Sweeney et al., 1996; Connolly et al., 2000). DeSouza et al. (2003) employed a distinct methodology to separate instruction-related activity from saccade-related activity. They used a delay of 6, 10, or 14 seconds between the presentation of the instructional cue and that of the peripheral stimulus. Significant differences were found when trials were aligned on the onset of instruction in the bilateral FEF and right hemisphere DLPFC, but there were no differences when aligned with presentation of the peripheral stimulus. It was proposed that the increased activation in FEF and DLPFC for the anti-saccade task reflects the preparatory set that is necessary to suppress incorrect reflexive saccades (DeSouza et al., 2003). Thus, the increased cortical activation, which was sustained through the instruction period, appears before the saccade stimulus is presented, ruling out the possibility of visual or motor signals.

11.4.2 Reconciling higher BOLD activation with lower neural discharge rate

Single neurons show a preparatory set response during the pro- and anti-saccade tasks. Everling and Munoz (2000) recorded from identified corticotectal FEF neurons and found that saccade-related neurons showed lower discharge rates during the instruction period on anti-saccade trials compared with pro-saccade trials during periods immediately (200 ms) before cue onset. Further support for a preparatory response in frontal cortical areas come from the finding of SEF neurons that had stronger visual responses for anti-saccades showing a higher activation level on anti-saccade trials before stimulus even appears (Schlag-Rey et al., 1997).

On the other hand, using BOLD fMRI in humans, DeSouza et al. (2003) found evidence of higher activation in the FEF on anti-saccade compared with pro-saccade during the preparatory period preceding saccade stimulus presentation. While fMRI data have found higher activation in the FEF on anti-saccades, single neuron recordings have found lower discharge rates; how can such a difference be reconciled?

Logothetis et al. (2001) first compared neural discharge rate, local field potentials, and the BOLD effect. They found that the BOLD signal was slightly more correlated with local field potentials than with neural discharge rate. The fact that many others have observed a large hemodynamic response in the FEF on anti-saccade trials compared with pro-saccade trials may also indicate that the BOLD response is more highly correlated with local field potentials than action potentials and discharge rates (O'Driscoll et al., 1995; Sweeney et al., 1996; Connolly et al., 2000, 2002). It is possible that although the discharge rate is lower, a larger number of neurons have input to areas that are involved in the processing of the anti-saccade trial, leading to higher activation as measured by the fMRI. The local field potentials would reflect the activity of afferents input and interneuron activity within a cortical area rather than the action potential of neurons that form the output from that area. Therefore, the BOLD activation in the FEF found by DeSouza et al. (2003) may indicate inhibitory input into the FEF, coming from the known PFC anatomical connections to FEF and SC (Goldman and Nauta, 1976), rather than an increased output coming from the FEF on anti-saccade trials. However, it is more likely that FEF neurons convey preparatory set signals to the superior colliculus, as SC neuron activity has been shown to be correlated with preparatory set (Everling et al., 1999). The reduction of pretarget activity of FEF and SC neurons is thought to be crucial for suppressing saccades to the stimulus on anti-saccade trials (Everling et al., 1998, 1999).

11.5 Internally driven preparatory signals represent rule-dependent activity

Everling and DeSouza (2005) designed an experiment where the cue for making a pro-saccade or an anti-saccade was internally driven with the fixation cue exactly the same. They studied this by employing a switch paradigm that is, having monkeys perform "automatic" pro- and "controlled" anti-saccades in several alternating blocks. The monkeys had to acquire the current rule through trial and error based on reward feedback that was delivered at the end of each trial. After a block of 30 correct responses, the rule changed without notice. For the successful performance of this task the current mapping rule must be kept track of as no external visual cues were provided. From the analysis of 201 PFC neurons from three monkeys, 38 showed preparatory set signals, of which 63% had more activity for pro- than anti-saccades and 37% had more activity for anti- than pro-saccades. Thus, they found that there are preparatory set related neurons for internally driven saccades. This was the first study to show that neurons in the monkey lateral PFC display rule-dependent activity for pro- and anti-saccades. Moreover, the activity level of these neurons predicted the saccade response. The time epoch prior to the saccade showed that only a minority of PFC neurons were selective to stimulus location or saccade direction. The majority of PFC neurons had pre-saccade activities that depended on the interaction between location and direction, and, therefore, on the mapping rule. Recently, Johnston et al. (2007) have now compared PFC and the anterior cingulate cortex during this switch task and they found that when the cognitive task gets more difficult soon after the switch it is the cingulate cortex which shows more task selectivity than the PFC.

11.5.1 Paradoxical task switch

Task switching in general is exhausting the resources that are available to attend to and complete the tasks at hand. Such cost is even greater when one needs to switch from one rule to another rule all the while using the same stimuli (Rogers and Monsell, 1995). Along with this cost there is also an increase in the number of errors made as well as reaction time. We see this in tasks such as the Wisconsin Card sorting when the participant not only needs to figure out the rule by trial and error but must also be able to acknowledge a rule change and make the behavioral adjustments necessary to complete the new task effectively. This change in task is a change in the S-R mapping, in other words, the change in appropriate response. The appropriate response to a certain task represents the correct response given the situation (Milner, 1963).

However, such switch cost is lessened during tasks where the participants have time to prepare their response before the stimulus appearance. This suggests that preparatory set activity plays a role, when available, to help prepare the appropriate response (Meiran et al., 2000). When a task that is easy or which has been practiced extensively is performed with ample preparation time, the parietal cortex is then used (Corbetta and Shulman, 2002).

Paradoxical task switch benefit is seen in a task where the participants need to switch from making an anti-saccade to a pro-saccade or vice versa. Intuitively, one would expect that in switching from the easier, pro-saccade, to the harder, anti-saccade task, we would make more errors and have longer latencies. However, due to a type of task switch inertia (Allport et al., 1994), it is in fact much easier for subjects to switch from the pro to the anti (Fecteau, 2004; Barton et al., 2005).

In the study by Everling and DeSouza (2005), an interesting behavioral finding was that after the switch in task, subject's performance came back to baseline performance faster when switching from pro- to anti-saccade than from anti- to pro-saccade. Allport et al. (1994) also found similar results when subjects had to switch from color-naming to word-naming in a Stroop task, and as a result, proposed the Task Set Inertia (TSI) hypothesis. The TSI hypothesis posits that switch costs result from the persistent activation of previous task processes. In other words, there is a larger switch cost when changing from hard to easy task than vice versa. There is minimal activation for the easier, or automatic, task, so there is minimal persistent activation when the task must be switched to the hard, or controlled task. However, in the hard task, a more difficult rule is acquired, and the task set inertia leads to persistent activation. Thus, when there is a switch to the easy task from the hard task, more trials are required before the monkeys perform at about the 85% correct baseline level.

11.6   Visual burst

Strong activation in saccade-related areas upon presentation of visual stimulus are known as visual bursts. The superior colliculus has strong activation during reflexive saccades towards the stimulus in its receptive field (Everling et al., 1999). In agreement with this, lower discharge rates were found for saccade-related neurons in the SC and FEF during the instruction period for anti-saccades compared to pro-saccades (Everling et al., 1999, 2000). Everling et al. (1998) also found that saccade-related neurons in the SC had a higher level of preparatory activity. Furthermore, they found a strong visual burst on trials when there was a failure to suppress the reflexive saccade toward the stimulus. Prefrontal neurons also show task-dependent differences in their baseline activity (Asaad et al., 2000). This activity could provide a signal that allows conflicting sensory input registered within the PFC to be mapped on to the appropriate motor output within the SC. In accordance with this model, DeSouza and Everling (2004) hypothesized that the increased activation they found in the FEF and DLPFC on anti-saccade trials represents top-down control signals that are involved in suppressing preparatory saccade-related activity in the SC to avoid reflexive pro-saccades toward the stimulus. Their results indicate that the reduction of pretarget activity of the SC, which could come from the FEF or as more recently demonstrated by Johnston and Everling (2006) in the PFC, is predictive of errors in the anti-saccade task. Their model has the preparatory PFC response projecting down to the SC in order to suppress the visual burst signals. However, when that signal does not reach, or is not acted upon by the SC, then upon the appearance of the peripheral stimulus and subsequent visual burst, the participant makes a reflexive saccade.

11.7   Clinical populations

When conducting anti-saccade tasks on humans with frontal lobe damage, patients perform worse compared with age-matched controls (Munoz and Everling, 2004). Evidence from animal research supports this expectation as the FEF has been suggested to mediate saccades. Many clinical research studies have looked into suppression ability of patients with damage to frontal areas and schizophrenia.

In a seminal study, Guitton et al. (1985) evaluated saccade abilities in patients with frontal lobe damage using a pro-saccade and anti-saccade task. They assessed four different groups of subjects: patients who sustained unilateral removal of frontal lobe tissues, patients whose lesions ranged from islands of the cortex to complete unilateral frontal lobotomies, intact subjects, and patients with lesions to the temporal lobe. There were three significant observations made by Guitton et al. (1985). First, subjects with frontal lobe damage and temporal lobe damage had no difficulties in orienting eye movements towards a visual stimulus. However, most of them had long-term difficulties in making saccades contralateral to the visual stimulus. Second, saccades that were directed away from the cue and towards the target were usually triggered by the appearance of the target, in frontal lobe patients. Finally, latency of anti-saccade tasks was shorter when compared with pro-saccade tasks. These findings suggest the involvement of the frontal lobe in mediating regular saccades. Similarly, Fukushima et al. (1994) found a role for FEF in making saccades in patients that sustained bilateral and unilateral lesions. After conducting their experiment, researchers found that lesions to the lateral frontal lobe, which may include the FEF and portions of the prefrontal cortex, resulted in more errors than damage to other frontal areas. Furthermore, patients with frontal lobe lesions showed longer latencies in anti-saccade tasks compared with controls.

While evidence from lesion studies suggests that FEF plays a crucial role in mediating regular saccades, these findings seem to be more evident when evaluating anti-saccade tasks in patients that have schizophrenia. Schizophrenia is often associated with the enlargement of the lateral and third ventricle (Lawrie and Abukmeil, 1998) as well as basal ganglia and frontal lobe dysfunction (Buchsbaum, 1990). Since research suggests that the frontal areas and the basal ganglia may be dysfunctional in these patients, we would expect increased errors on the anti-saccade task when compared with intact subjects.

This expectation was evaluated by Fukushima et al. (1990) by assessing how well patients with schizophrenia and mild Parkinson's disease perform on anti-saccade tasks. Since prior studies with schizophrenic patients had found poor performance in anti-saccade (Fukishima et al., 1990), researchers expected similar results from their experiments. However, if patients with Parkinson's disease are successful in anti-saccade tasks, that would suggest that the FEF is mediating regular saccades in humans. Their findings showed that the patients with Parkinson's disease do not have any significant impairment in performing the anti-saccade tasks, but patients with schizophrenia do.

The anti-saccade performance in patients with schizophrenia is similar to patients with frontal lobe damage and thus such impairment may be explained by a frontal cortical dysfunction.

11.8   Neural prosthetics and beyond

The results discussed above have tried to determine the location of response inhibition or suppression. Neuroprosthetics is an emerging field that can target these areas to modify behavior. This technology is intended to replace or improve certain aspects of a damaged nervous system (Pesaran et al., 2006). The prosthetics field is an excellent example of the application of research into human thought and subsequent control of movement and purposeful behavior to improve the quality of life. Possible beneficiaries of this new and evolving technology are patients with cerebral palsy, multiple sclerosis, amyotrophic lateral sclerosis (ALS) as well as those who have been paralyzed by head or spinal cord trauma (Schwartz, 2004). A distinctive feature of neural prosthetics lies in their requisite implantation inside the human body, making them extremely mobile and adding to their practicality.

Cortical neural prosthetics work by directly recording the brain's neural activity related to the patient's thoughts (Pesaran et al., 2006), as well as those related to intended movements (Musallam et al., 2004), and decoding them to control external devices. Such external devices range from computer interfaces to robotic limbs and muscle stimulators. Cortical prosthetics for patients can be broadly classified into two types: motor and cognitive. Even though they have been categorized as two separate types of prosthetics, their signals often coexist with one another in areas such as the FEFs (Pesaran et al., 2006). Thus the distinguishing feature between cognitive and motor prosthetics lies not in the location of the recordings but rather in the type of information that is being decoded. Thus far there has not been a single prosthetic structure that has combined both cognitive-based and motor-based systems.

Brain-machine interface (BMI) technology, an application branch of neuroprosthetics, is bidirectional. BMIs have the capability to "write-in" signals to the brain, through electrical stimulation, and also "read-out" signals through recording neural activity (Andersen et al., 2004). Drawing upon the "write-in" devices, cochlear prosthetics (Loeb, 1990) and deep brain stimulation (DBS) (Follett, 2000) have been designed to treat deaf and Parkinson's disease patients respectively. In assisting paralyzed patients, "read-out" BMIs are used to record movement intentions and interpret them for using external devices.

In applying the neural prosthetic technology to vision restoration, there is still an ongoing research in further developing the design and construction of an effective BMI with the visual system neurons. In order to generate pattern vision in blind patients, the visual prosthetic interface must effectively stimulate the retinotopically organized neurons in the central visual field to elicit patterned visual percepts. It is also required that the prosthesis electrode arrays adapt to different optimal stimulus locations, stimulus patterns, and patient disease states (Cohen, 2007). Although current visual prostheses rely on electrical stimulation to excite neurons, researchers are trying more biologically compatible methods of neuron stimulation such as the use of natural brain neurotransmitters/analogs, ion channels and neuroattractive surfaces, in order to improve signal transmission across the "machine-neuron" interface (Cohen, 2007).

11.9   Concluding remarks

The goal of this chapter was to shed light on some of the executive functions performed by the prefrontal cortex, mainly its role in response selection and response suppression. We also examined the deficits in the patient population as a result of damage to the frontal areas. The ability to inhibit automatic urges may at first seem arbitrary, but its significance is quickly realized when its deficiency leads to dramatic impulsive behavior and lack of control over one's own actions. Most of the higher cognitive executive functions such as selecting and suppressing abilities are vital in our everyday lives in that they serve an adaptive function.

References

Allport, D. A., Styles, E. A. and Hsieh, S. (1994). Shifting intentional set: exploring the dynamic control of tasks. In C. Umilta and M. Moscovitch (eds.) *Attention and Performance XV*. Cambridge, MA: MIT Press, pp. 421–452.

Andersen, R. A., Musallam, S. and Pearson, B. (2004). Selecting the signals for a brain-machine interface. *Cur. Opinion Neurobiol.*, 14: 720–726.

Asaad, W. F., Rainer, G. and Miller, E. K. (2000). Task-specific neural activity in the primate prefrontal cortex. *J. Neurophysiol.*, 84: 451–459.

Barkley, R. A., Grodzinsky, G. and DuPaul, G. (1992). Frontal lobe functions in attention deficit disorder with and without hyperactivity: a review and research report. *J. Abnorm. Child Psychol.*, 20: 163–188.

Barton, J. J. S., Greenzang, C., Hefter, R., Edelman, J. and Manoach, D. S. (2005). Switching, plasticity and prediction in a saccadic task-switch paradigm. *Exp. Brain Res.*, 168: 76–87.

Brown, M. R., Vilis, T. and Everling, S. (2007). Frontoparietal activation with preparation for antisaccades. *J. Neurophysiol.*, 98: 1751–1762.

Buchsbaum, M. S. (1990). Frontal lobes, basal ganglia, temporal lobes: three sites for schizophrenia? *Schizophrenia Bull.*, 16: 379–390.

Chelazzi, L., Duncan, J., Miller, E. K. and Desimone, R. (1998). Responses of neurons in inferior temporal cortex during memory-guided visual search. *J. Neurophysiol.*, 80: 2918–2940.

Clementz, B. A., McDowell, J. E., and Zisook, S. (1994). Saccadic system functioning among schizophrenia patients and their first-degree biological relatives. *J. Abnorm. Psychol.*, 103: 277–287.

Cohen, E. D. (2007). Prosthetic interfaces with the visual system: biological issues. *J. Neural Engin.*, 4: 14–31.

Connolly, J. D., Goodale, M. A., DeSouza, J. F. X., Menon, R. S. and Vilis, T. (2000). A comparison of frontoparietal fMRI activation during anti-saccades and anti-pointing. *J. Neurophysiol.*, 84: 1645–1655.

Connolly, J. D., Goodale, M. A., Menon, R. S. and Munoz, D. P. (2002). Human fMRI evidence for the neural correlates of preparatory set. *Nature Neurosci.*, 5: 1345–1352.

Corbetta, M. and Shulman, G. L. (2002). Control of goal-directed and stimulus-driven attention in the brain. *Nature Rev. Neurosci.*, 3: 201–215.

Corbetta, M., Akbudak, E., Conturo, T. E., Snyder, A. Z., Ollinger, J. M., Drury, H. A., Linenweber, M. R., Petersen, S. E., Raichle, M. E., van Essen, D. C. and Shulman, G. L. (1998). A common network of functional areas for attention and eye movements. *Neuron*, 21: 761–773.

DeSouza, J. F. X., Menon, R. S. and Everling, S. (2003). Preparatory set associated with pro-saccades and anti-saccades in humans investigated with event-related fMRI. *J. Neurophysiol.*, 89: 1016-1023.

DeSouza, J. F. X. and Everling, S. (2004). Focused attention modulates visual responses in the primate prefrontal cortex. *J. Neurophysiol.*, 91: 855–862.

Dorris, M., Paré, M. and Munoz, D. (2000). Immediate neural plasticity shapes motor performance. *J. Neurosci.*, 20: 1–5.

Everling, S. and DeSouza, J. F. X. (2005). Rule-dependent activity for prosaccades and antisaccades in the primate prefrontal cortex. *J. Cogn. Neurosci.*, 17: 1483–1496.

Everling, S. and Munoz, D. P. (2000). Neuronal correlates for preparatory set associated with pro-saccades and anti-saccades in the primate frontal eye field. *J. Neurosci.*, 20: 387–400.

Everling, S., Dorris, M. C., Klein, R. M. and Munoz, D. P. (1999). Role of primate superior colliculus in preparation and execution of anti-saccades and pro-saccades. *J. Neurosci.*, 19: 2740–2754.

Everling S., Dorris, M. C. and Munoz, D. P. (1998). Reflex suppression in the anti-saccade task is dependent on prestimulus neural processes. *J. Neurophysiol.*, 80: 1584–1589.

Fecteau, J., Au, C., Armstrong, I. and Munoz, D. (2004). Sensory biases produce alternation advantage found in sequential saccadic eye movement tasks. *Exp. Brain Res.*, 159: 84–91.

Follett, K. A. (2000). The surgical treatment of Parkinson's disease. *Ann. Rev. Med.*, 51: 135–147.

Ford, K. A., Goltz, H. C., Brown, M. R. and Everling, S. (2005). Neural processes associated with antisaccade task performance investigated with event-related FMRI. *J. Neurophysiol.*, 94: 429–440.

Fukushima, J., Fukushima, K., Miyasaka, K. and Yamashita, I. (1994). Voluntary control of saccadic eye movement in patients with frontal cortical lesions and parkinsonian patients in comparison with that in schizophrenia. *Soc. Biol. Psychiat.*, 36: 21–30.

Fukushima, J., Fukushima, K., Morita, N. and Yamashita, I. (1990). Further analysis of the control of voluntary saccadic eye movements in schizophrenic patients. *Soc. Biol. Psychiat.*, 28: 943–958.

Fuster, J. M. (2001). The prefrontal cortex – an update: time is of the essence. *Neuron*, 30: 319–333.

Goldman, P. S. and Nauta, W. J. (1976). Autoradiographic demonstration of a projection from prefrontal association cortex to the superior colliculus in the rhesus monkey. *Brain Res.*, 116: 145–149.

Goldman-Rakic, P. S. (1992). Working memory and the mind. *Sci. Am.*, 267: 110–117.

Gruber, S. A., Rogowska, J., Holcomb, P., Soraci, S. and Yurgelun-Todd, D. (2002). Stroop performance in normal control subjects: an fMRI study. *NeuroImage*, 16: 349–360.

Guitton, D., Buchtel, H. A. and Douglas, R. M. (1985). Frontal lobe lesions in man cause difficulties in suppressing reflexive glances and in generating goal-directed saccades. *Exp. Brain Res.*, 58: 455–472.

Hallett, P. E. (1978). Primary and secondary saccades to goals defined by instructions. *Vision Res.*, 18: 1279–1296.

Hebb, D. O. (1972), *Textbook of Psychology*. Philadelphia, PA: Saunders.

Johnston, K. and Everling, S. (2006). Monkey dorsolateral prefrontal cortex sends task-selective signals directly to the superior colliculus. *J. Neurosci.*, 26: 12471–12478.

Johnston, K., Levin, H. M., Koval, M. J. and Everling, S. (2007). Top-down control-signal dynamics in anterior cingulate and prefrontal cortex neurons following task switching. *Neuron*, 53: 452–462.

Lawrie, S. M. and Abukmeil, S. S. (1998). Brain abnormalities in schizophrenia: a systematic and quantitative review of volumetric magnetic resonance imaging studies. *Brit. J. Psychiat.*, 172: 110–120.

Le Bihan, D., Jezzard, P., Haxby, J., Sadato, N., Rueckert, L. and Mattay, V. (1995). Functional magnetic resonance imaging of the brain. *Ann. Int. Med.*, 122: 296–303.

Loeb, G. E. (1990). Cochlear prosthetics. *Ann. Rev. Neurosci.*, 13: 357–371.

Logothetis, N. K., Pauls, J., Augath, M., Trinath, T. and Oeltermann, A. (2001). Neurophysiological investigation of the basis of the fMRI signal. *Nature*, 412: 150–157.

Meiran, N., Chorev, Z. and Sapir, A. (2000). Component processes in task switching. *Cogn. Psychol.*, 41: 211–253.

Mesulam, M. M. (1999). Spatial attention and neglect: parietal, frontal and singulate contributions to the mental representation and attentional targeting of salient extrapersonal events. *Philos. Trans. Roy. Soc. Lond. B Biol. Sci.*, 354: 1325–1346.

Miller, E. K., Erickson, C. A. and Desimone, R. (1996). Neural mechanisms of visual working memory in prefrontal cortex of the macaque. *J. Neurosci.*, 16: 5154–5167.

Milner, B. (1963). Effect of different brain lesions on card sorting. *Arch. Neurol.*, 9: 90–100.

Munoz, D. P. and Everling, S. (2004). Look away: the anti-saccade task and the voluntary control of eye movement. *Nat. Rev. Neurosci.*, 5: 218–228.

Musallam, S., Corneil, B. D, Greger, B., Scherberger, H. and Andersen, R. A. (2004). Cognitive control signals for neural prosthetics. *Science*, 305: 258–262.

Nobre, A. C., Coull, J. T., Frith, C. D. and Mesulam, M. M. (1999). Orbitofrontal cortex is activated during breaches of expectation in tasks of visual attention. *Nat. Neurosci.*, 2: 11–12.

O'Driscoll, G. A., Alpert, N. M., Matthysse, S. W., Levy, D. L., Rauch, S. L. and Holzman, P. S. (1995). Functional neuroanatomy of antisaccade eye movements investigated with positron emission tomography. *Proc. Nat. Acad. Sci.*, 92: 925–929.

Ovaysikia, S., Hoover, A. E. N., Chan, C. J. et al. (2007). Is the same anterior cingualte region involved in processing the supresion signals for the antisaccade and stroop tasks? Program No. 929.5. Neuroscience Meeting Planner, San Diego, CA: Society for Neuroscience. Online.

Pesaran, B., Musallam, S. and Andersen, R. A. (2006). Cognitive neural prosthetics. *Curr. Biol.*, 16: R77–R80.

Rogers, R. D. and Monsell, S. (1995). Costs of a predictible switch between simple cognitive tasks. *J. Exp. Psychol.: Gen.*, 124: 207–231.

Schall, J. D., Stuphorn, V. and Brown, J. W. (2002). Monitoring and control of action by the frontal lobes. *Neuron*, 3: 309–322.

Schlag-Rey, M., Amador, N., Sanchez, H. and Schlag, J. (1997). Antisaccade performance predicted by neuronal activity in the supplementary eye field. *Nature*, 390: 398–401.

Schwartz, A. B. (2004). Cortical neural prosthetics. *Ann. Rev. Neurosci.*, 27: 487–507.

Stroop, J. R. (1935). Studies of interference in serial verbal reactions. *J. Exp. Psychol.*, 18: 643–662.

Sowell, E. R., Thompson, P. M., Holmes, C. J., Jernigan, T. L. and Toga, A. W. (1999). In vivo evidence for post-adolescent brain maturation in frontal and striatal regions. *Nature Neurosci.*, 10: 859–861.

Sweeney, J. A., Mintun, M. A., Kwee, S., Wiseman, M. B., Brown, D. L., Rosenberg, D. R. and Carl, J. R. (1996). Positron emission tomography study of voluntary saccadic eye movements and spatial working memory. *J. Neurophysiol.*, 75: 454–468.

Walker, R., Hussain, M., Hodgson, T. L., Harrison, J. and Kennard, C. (1998). Saccadic eye movement and working memory deficits following damage to human prefrontal cortex. *Neuropsychol.*, 36: 1141–1159.

Weiss, E. M., Siedentopf, C., Golaszewski, S., Mottaghy, F. M., Hofer, A., Kremser, C., Felber, S. and Fleischhacker, W. W. (2007). Brain activation patterns during a selective attention test – a functional MRI study in healthy volunteers and unmedicated patients during an acute episode of schizophrenia. *Psychiatry Res.*, 154: 31–40.

12 Prefrontal cortex and the neurophysiology of visual knowledge: perception, action, attention, memory, strategies and goals

S. P. Wise

Some theories of prefrontal cortex hold that it contributes to only one aspect of visual knowledge, such as working memory or perception. To the contrary, neurophysiological evidence indicates that the prefrontal cortex participates in many aspects of visual cognition, including perception, the control of action, the allocation of attentional resources, the learning and application of problem-solving strategies, the selection and memory of goals, the categorization of objects, places and events, the detection of event sequences, and the updated valuation of stimuli and actions. Taken together, these and additional findings suggest that the prefrontal cortex encodes and stores behavioral knowledge for use in nonroutine situations, especially novel ones, when a subtle danger looms or an unusual opportunity knocks. In short, the function of the prefrontal cortex is knowing what, if anything, to do in an uncommon circumstance and what is likely to ensue if that is done.

12.1 Introduction

The impetus for this chapter came from session titles used at the *York Conference 2007 on Cortical Mechanisms of Vision: Cortical Mechanisms of Visual Attention*, "parietal-frontal transformations for visually guided reach," "cortical mechanisms for eye movements," "top-down influences of fronto-parietal cortex on vision," and "visual

Cortical Mechanisms of Vision, ed. M. Jenkin and L. R. Harris. Published by Cambridge University Press.
© Cambridge University Press 2009.

integration and consciousness." It struck me that although my laboratory is not known for work on attention, oculomotor control, or consciousness – we study monkeys, and whether they have any such thing as consciousness remains controversial, to say the least – just a few of our papers pertain to all of those sessions (Lebedev et al., 2001, 2004; Genovesio et al., 2005, 2006). This chapter presents the main results of those papers, all of which have something to do with high-order vision and with the activity of neurons in the prefrontal cortex.

The editors of this volume encouraged its authors "to include suitable personal and scientific anecdotes" as well as historical and scientific background, so that a non-specialist can follow and enjoy the argument and appreciate its position in the scheme of things. Accordingly, I make no attempt here at comprehensive coverage. Every finding mentioned in this chapter has been published in a peer-reviewed journal, and the details appear there. I also refrain from explaining the control tasks that provide some of the most important support for any conclusions based on neurophysiological results. And, like aging scientists from time immemorial, I simply ignore opinions and findings from others: *caveat emptor*.

As for anecdotes, the experiments summarized here all depended on advice or challenges from colleagues. These stories provide an important lesson to anyone wary of divulging his or her research plans. As Peter Medawar warned, any scientist who keeps the laboratory door closed keeps out much more than he or she keeps in. Had I not discussed far-distant experimental plans with other scientists, our experiments would not have produced what they did, and might have produced nothing at all.

The first experiment depended on a visual illusion. I had proposed a neurophysiological experiment pitting the visual guidance of movement against visual perception. My first thought was to base that experiment on a reaching task (Bridgeman, 1992). That experimental design had problems, though, from a neurophysiological perspective. Mel Goodale, who has a chapter in this book, pointed out the advantages of basing such an experiment on a little-known and infrequently cited article on eye movements (Wong and Mack, 1981). Wong and Mack showed how a visual background frame captures perception and causes a useful illusion. People report an illusory perception about which way a spot of light jumped, although they accurately move their eyes to fixate it. That is, because of the illusion they report the spot's movement incorrectly, although they move accurately in relation to it. By directing me to this paper, Goodale provided a tool for contrasting prefrontal cortex activity obtained in two conditions: perceptual reports about an object versus visually guided movements made to the same object. Here I call this tool the perception-action experiment.

The second experiment came, in part, from a challenge issued by Richard Passingham. He and his colleagues developed a task for neuroimaging research that tested the then-dominant idea that the principal (or sole) function of prefrontal cortex is working memory (Goldman-Rakic, 1987, 2000). His task pitted the maintenance of information in working memory against the selection of action, a concept Passingham came to call attentional selection (Rowe and Passingham, 2001; Rowe et al., 2002). He was convinced that the working memory theory of prefrontal cortex would fail, and – because it arose from and partly depended upon results from monkey neurophysiology – he suggested that we use his task in such an experiment. I did not think his neuroimaging task would work very well as a neurophysiological experiment, but I agreed with his purpose. So we tested the theory in a different way, which I call here the attention-memory experiment.

The third experiment stemmed from a talk, delivered by a colleague of mine, on one kind of visually guided movement: the use of symbols to instruct actions. I sometimes call this kind of visual guidance "traffic light behavior" because its most common example involves stopping a car at a red light. In this chapter, I call it symbolic mapping or arbitrary visuomotor mapping. After the talk, John Stein challenged my colleague to defend the idea that this behavior is a genuine example of visually guided movement. Stein and Glickstein (1992) had limited the concept of visual guidance to circumstances in which objects or their locations serve as targets of movement. Of course, the spatial guidance of movement is important, as many chapters in this volume indicate, but there is a lot more to visuomotor guidance than that (see Chapter 25, Section 5 in Shadmehr and Wise, 2005). Nevertheless, Stein's challenge led me to think about how general the concept of visual guidance might be. I knew that as monkeys learn arbitrary visuomotor mappings, they spontaneously adopt abstract strategies, which guide their responses to novel stimuli (Murray and Wise, 1996; Wise and Murray, 1999; Bussey et al., 2001). This behavior seemed to be visuomotor guidance at its highest level, at least for a monkey. Accordingly, we devised a task that compared prefrontal cortex activity for arbitrary visuomotor mappings with that for abstract response strategies. Here I call the main part of this task the strategy-mapping experiment, but because it revealed something about coding future and previous goals, I call another aspect of the same task the previous-future goal experiment.

The next four sections relate the tasks and main results from these experiments, in turn: perception-action, attention-memory, strategy-mapping, and previous-future goal. The final section explores whether the prefrontal cortex is a monomaniac, having an inordinate or obsessive interest in a single thing, or a polymath, encompassing great learning in many fields.

12.2   Perception versus action

The visual knowledge that we primates use results from our evolutionary history as much as from any current or previous visual inputs. Indeed, two aspects of visual knowledge – perceiving objects and reaching to them – have been central occupations of the primate mind since our inception about 60 million years ago. The former can be called vision-for-perception, the latter vision-for-action. Perceptions are hypotheses about what is out there, which can often be wrong without harmful consequences. Reaching to objects, especially food and tools, provides much less latitude for error.

Work by Goodale, Milner and their colleagues (Goodale et al., 1991; Goodale and Westwood, 2004) led to the realization that vision-for-perception had properties distinct from vision-for-action. Vision-for-action networks process visual information somewhat differently than those for visual perception (Boussaoud et al., 1990; Goodale et al., 1991; Aglioti et al., 1995). For example, subjects misperceive disks as relatively small if surrounded by large disks, but make accurate prehension movements to the edges of those disks (Aglioti et al., 1995). Similar phenomena have been observed for reaching movements (Bridgeman et al., 1994). This appears to be the opposite of a better known neurological syndrome, first described by Balint, called optic ataxia. Patients with optic ataxia seem to perceive objects and their orientation correctly, but cannot make normal movements in relation to them. A previous review elaborates these findings and related ones (Lebedev and Wise, 2002), and Goodale's chapter in this book summarizes this line of research. Here I focus on how neurophysiological analysis can identify neurons that contribute to vision-for-perception as distinct from those involved in vision-for-action (Lebedev et al., 2001).

Figure 12.1A illustrates the experimental design. The basis of this experiment was that when a small, attended object appeared on a large background frame, movements of the frame captured perception to a considerable degree. After the object and frame appeared for a period of time, both disappeared and reappeared, usually in different locations. The perception was that the light jumped: but in which direction? In the situation illustrated (Figure 12.1A, second row) people reported the small object to have moved in a direction diametrically opposed to its actual movement (Wong and Mack, 1981). This illusion occurred when the background frame jumped at the same time as the attended object, but to a larger extent in the same direction. In the example depicted in Figure 12.1A (second row), both the attended object and the background frame became visible simultaneously in an initial appearance (left). Later, both disappeared and then made a reappearance (right). Upon its reappearance, the attended object appeared farther to the left in frame-centered coordinates, but to the right in all other coordinates. (Note that the subjects did not see any vertical line within the frame, which is shown here for heuristic purposes.) In this condition, the attended object was to the right of its initial location, but because the background frame reappeared even farther to the right, subjects reported that the object had jumped left. Clearly, the frame-centered coordinate scheme had captured perception. Nevertheless, when asked to do so, the subjects made an accurate saccade to fixate the object (not illustrated). That is, they moved their eyes to the right to fixate the object, even though they had reported that the object had jumped to the left.

In the perception-action experiment, prior to recording from the prefrontal cortex, we trained a monkey to perform two versions of the task: one called the vision-for-perception task, the other called the vision-for-action task. A small light spot ("o" in Figure 12.1A) served as the attended object. An array of six similar light spots provided the background frame (depicted as the gray rectangle in Figure 12.1A). In the vision-for-perception task, the monkeys reported which direction the light spot had jumped. Of course, our monkeys did not talk and so we had to devise some way that they could make a perceptual report without words. In extensive training prior to any presentation of illusory effects, the monkey learned to report the direction of light-spot movement with a saccade to one of two report targets (Figure 12.1A, black circles): one near the left margin of the frame and the other near the right margin. Saccades (arrows) to the left report target served as left reports; saccades to the right report target counted as right reports. During the prerecording training sessions, only the veridical condition (Figure 12.1A, top row) occurred. That is, the relative movement of the background frame and light spot never sufficed to cause an illusion. After training was complete on the veridical version of the task, three additional conditions were presented, and during these sessions we monitored single-neuronal activity in the prefrontal cortex. These three new conditions were: (1) the illusion condition (second row of Figure 12.1A), (2)

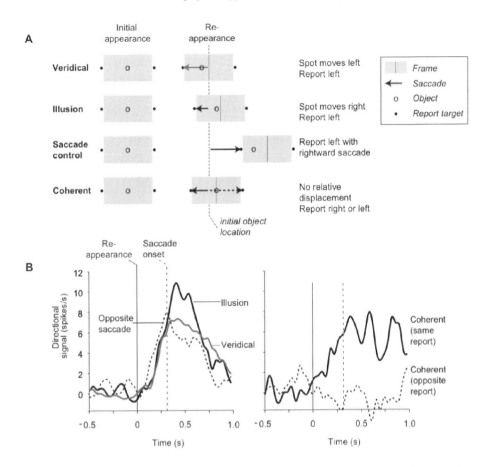

Figure 12.1. (A) Task conditions for the perception-action experiment. See text for explanation. The arrows show the saccades made to make a perceptual report about which direction, left or right, the object (o) jumped between its initial appearance and its reappearance. Note that the saccades bring fixation to one of two report targets (black circles), located to the left and right of the frame (shaded rectangle). (B) Population activity for prefrontal cortex neurons during the different task conditions.

a control for activity related to saccadic eye movements (third row), and (3) a coherent-movement condition (fourth row). The illusion condition is explained above. The frame shifted more than the light spot, in the same direction, and reliably generated the desired illusion: the monkey reported that the spot had moved in a direction opposite to what had actually occurred. In the saccade control condition, the monkey had to make a rightward saccade to report a leftward shift of the light spot (as illustrated), and vice versa. We reasoned that neurons related to eye movements would have similar activity for saccades in the same direction, and neurons related to the report would have similar activity for the same report. Finally, in the coherent-movement condition, the light spot and frame jumped by exactly the same amount. If, as assumed, the frame captured per

ception, the coherent-movement condition should have left the monkey without a cue
(and without a clue). In accord with that assumption, the monkey made both leftward
and rightward reports in this condition. Again, we reasoned that cells related to the
report would show similar activity for all four conditions, whenever the monkey made
a given report (e.g. a left report). Figure 12.1A illustrates mainly left reports (solid-line
arrows), but left and right reports occurred equally often and unpredictably. When,
in the coherent-movement condition, the monkey made a different report (dashed-line
arrow in Figure 12.1A, fourth row), the resulting activity should be very different.

Figure 12.1B shows the results of this experiment at the population level. The activity of single neurons showed the same properties as these averages, so the averages
alone can convey the results. Each curve shows the difference in activity between preferred reports and nonpreferred reports. For example, if a single neuron had its highest
discharge rate for left reports, it contributed to the average to the extent that its activity
for left reports exceeded that for right reports. In the most general terms, this was a
directional signal encoding the report. The population averages in Figure 12.1B show
these directional signals under the several conditions of the experiment. The left plot
shows the data for three of the conditions. For the veridical condition (gray curve in
the left plot), the report signal develops approximately 140 ms after the reappearance
of the stimuli, long before the initiation of the reporting saccade, which occurred at
321 ms, on average. A similar neural signal developed in the illusion condition. Cells
preferring veridical left reports also showed a preference for illusory left reports (black
curve in the left plot). Similarly, when the monkey made a rightward saccade to make a
left report (and vice versa), the individual cells and the population as a whole continued
to encode the report direction (dashed curve in the left plot). Finally, and most com-
pellingly, when the frame and spot moved coherently, the monkeys sometimes made
one report and sometimes made the other. When the report matched the preferred direction for a cell – left report, for example – the population continued to encode the
report (black curve in the right plot). However, when precisely the same visual input
appeared, but the monkey – lacking any cue – made the opposite report, the population
showed little, if any, directional signal (dashed curve in the right plot). In summary,
prefrontal cortex neurons encoded their preferred report regardless of what had actually
happened (i.e. whether the light spot had actually moved in their preferred direction)
and regardless of which saccade direction the monkey used to make the report.

As I mentioned earlier, we trained a monkey to perform two versions of the task:
the vision-for-perception task and the vision-for-action task. So far, I have discussed
only the vision-for-perception task. In the vision-for-action task, an array of light spots
appeared, disappeared, and reappeared like they did in the vision-for-perception task.
As in many studies of oculomotor control, the monkeys only had to make a saccade to
fixate the attended object. For some prefrontal cortex neurons, we could compare the
activity in the two tasks, which matched visual inputs and motor outputs very closely:
much too closely for any slight differences to have accounted for the directional signals
that we found.

We found two populations of prefrontal cortex neurons. The first showed selectivity for the vision-for-perception task, as shown in Figure 12.2A, parts 1 and 2. This
population showed a significant directional signal beginning shortly after the reappearance of the attended light spot and frame and peaking at the time of saccade onset

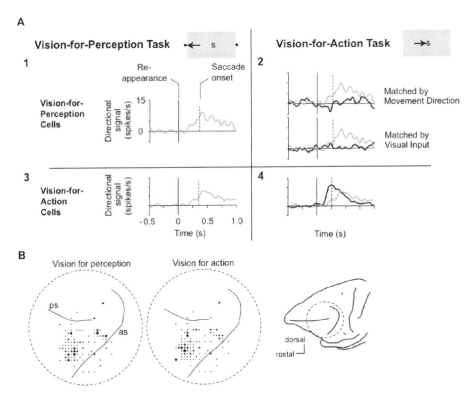

Figure 12.2. (A) Population activity for the vision-for-perception task (parts 1 and 3) and in the vision-for-action task (parts 2 and 4). Two populations are shown: cells selective for vision-for-perception (parts 1 and 2) and a separate population selective for vision-for-action (parts 3 and 4). Parts 2 and 4 copy the population average from parts 1 and 3, respectively, as gray curves. (B) Locations of vision-for-perception cells (left) and vision-for-action cells (middle) from the area encircled (dashed line) in the monkey brain (right). Top: "s" corresponds to "o" in Figure 12.1A.

(Figure 12.2A1). When we examined the activity of these cells in the vision-for-action task (black curves in Figure 12.2A2, the cells showed virtually no directional signal, regardless of whether the trials were matched for the saccade direction (top) or for visual inputs (bottom). Figure 12.2A2 directly compares the directional signal for the vision-for-perception task (gray curves, from Figure 12.2A1) and the vision-for-action task (black curves). Figure 12.2A3 and 4 show the activity of a different population of prefrontal cortex neurons, one that encoded the action rather than the report. These cells showed a small directional signal during the vision-for-perception task (Figure 12.2A3), but it was significantly smaller than the comparable signal in the vision-for-action task (black curve in Figure 12.2A4). Figure 12.2A4 shows the activity of these action-encoding cells in both the vision-for-action task (black curve) and the vision-for-perception task (gray curve, from Figure 12.2A3). This population not only had a greater signal for encoding the action (black curve) than for the report (gray curve), but the action-encoding signal peaked much earlier, during the period prior to saccade onset. The report-encoding signal peaked much later and was barely present at the time the saccade began (dashed vertical line).

Although some neuroimaging research has suggested that visual areas alone are sufficient to subserve visual perception (Tong et al., 1998; Zeki and Bartels, 1998), other evidence supports the idea that the prefrontal cortex also plays a central role in visual perception of stimuli (Crick and Koch, 1995, 1998). Indeed, the idea that prefrontal cortex subserves perception dates back at least 175 years. John Fulton (1949) wrote that the first person to make that suggestion was the French neurologist Flourens (1824), who attributed higher perceptual, associative, and executive functions to the frontal lobes (of chickens!). Like much subsequent research on prefrontal cortex, Flourens' conclusions had no validity whatsoever, yet nevertheless may have been correct.

Notwithstanding the long history of this idea or its widespread acceptance, few neurophysiological investigations have tested the hypothesis that neuronal activity in the prefrontal cortex primarily reflects perception, as opposed to lower-order functions. The perception-action experiment provided one approach to testing this idea. In contrast to the report-encoding neurons, which reflected high-order visual knowledge, the action-encoding neurons reflected plain-old saccadic eye movements to a visible target, one of the most automatic and least sophisticated visuomotor behaviors that primates perform. Yet these two kinds of neurons completely intermingled within the larger prefrontal network (Figure 12.2B), with no obvious predominance of neurons reflecting the higher-order behavior.

12.3   Attention versus memory

Ever since Carlyle Jacobsen (1935) discovered that prefrontal cortex lesions produce what appear to be memory deficits, this concept has dominated thinking about prefrontal function. Patricia Goldman-Rakic incorporated the concept of working memory into the mix when she proposed the idea that the entire prefrontal cortex was specialized for working memory (Goldman-Rakic, 1987, 2000; Levy and Goldman-Rakic, 2000). For a long period, during the 1980s and 1990s, the overwhelming majority of research papers on prefrontal cortex explored its role in working memory to the exclusion of almost everything else. Very few studies tested that hypothesis, however, and when such tests were conducted they usually obtained results that contradicted the prevailing view, beginning in the late 1990s (Rushworth et al., 1997). At the time we began the experiments summarized here, the working memory theory of prefrontal cortex was only beginning to fray (Postle et al., 2003). Specifically, neuroimaging experiments pitting aspects of attention against the maintenance of information in working memory showed a predominance of attentional functions for the dorsolateral prefrontal area (Rowe et al., 2000), and other studies also stressed attentional functions, such as monitoring items in short-term memory (Owen et al., 1996; Petrides et al., 2002). These findings intensified my doubts about neurophysiological "memory signals." Results from the published studies claiming to have observed memory signals (e.g. Funahashi et al., 1989; Romo et al., 1999; Constantinidis et al., 2001) were subject to alternative interpretations, usually because several crucial variables were neither controlled nor monitored. Yet few tests of the working memory theory had been conducted. Although it was old news that prefrontal cortex cells show sustained activity changes during memory periods (Fuster and Alexander, 1971; Kubota and Niki, 1971; Fuster, 1973), the cognitive operations going on during memory periods are complex, and this activity could reflect many different cognitive functions. The stimuli that mark a location to be remembered, for example, also attract attention. Accordingly, we designed an experiment to independently control spatial attention and spatial working memory (Lebedev et al., 2004).

Figure 12.3 shows the design for our attention-memory experiment. The monkeys began each trial by fixating a small light spot at the center of the video screen, much like in the perception-action experiment. Then a larger light spot appeared at one of four locations in the visual periphery: each a cardinal direction from the fixation point. These four potential stimulus locations are shown at far right of Figure 12.3A, in polar coordinates. After a brief stationary period at its original location, the circle began to revolve at a constant rate around the fixation point. The monkeys continued to maintain steady, central fixation during this part of each trial. Neither we nor the monkeys had any idea where the circle would stop, except that it always stopped at one of the four locations marked in Figure 12.3A (far right). The distance of the circle from the center never changed. After the circle stopped revolving, the task required that the monkeys direct considerable attentional resources to its location. The reason was that what the circle did next determined what the monkeys had to do in order to receive a reward. The monkeys still could not break central fixation. If the circle increased its brightness, which it did only by a very subtle amount, the monkeys had to made a saccadic eye movement to the original location of the circle on that trial. Nothing on the screen marked this location, at 90° in the example illustrated in Figure 12.3A (top branch). On other trials, the light spot dimmed by a small amount. This change in brightness signaled the monkeys to make a saccade to the circle's current location, which was the focus of the monkeys' attention (bottom branch of Figure 12.3A). Prior to the dimming or brightening event, the monkey could not predict which of those two possibilities would occur, so the circle's first location always had to be kept in memory. In this way, over a number of trials, we could examine the activity of prefrontal cortex neurons for selective spatial attention to any one of the four locations and also for working memory of the same locations.

Figure 12.3B shows the activity of three prefrontal cortex neurons in a compact matrix display devised by Misha Lebedev. The size of the circle in each square of the four-by-four matrix shows a cell's activity level during the delay period – the time just before the attended circle either brightened or dimmed (see Figure 12.3A) – for each combination of remembered and attended locations. During that time, the monkeys had to attend to the circle's location, while (usually) keeping a second location in memory, without breaking central fixation. The left matrix shows the activity of a cell that had a high level of activity during the delay period whenever one of the monkeys attended to the top location (90°). Regardless of the location that the monkey remembered, which varied by row, this neuron had its highest activity when the monkey directed its attention to the top location. Thus, this cell did not encode the remembered location, although the monkey did need to remember a location during the delay period. By

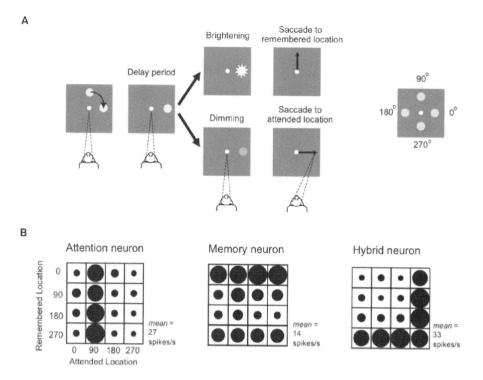

Figure 12.3. (A) Task conditions for the attention-memory experiment. The arrow shows the correct saccade to make on both kinds of trials: one requiring a saccade to the remembered location (top), the other requiring a saccade to the attended location (bottom). The dashed lines indicate the gaze angle and fixation target of the monkey. Right: the designation of all possible starting and ending locations of the stimulus, in polar coordinates. (B) Three types of neurons observed in the experiment. The size of each circle shows the mean activity during the delay period (see part A) for the designated attended locations (which vary by column) and remembered locations (which vary by row), with the overall average noted to the right of each matrix.

independently varying the attended and remembered locations, we could demonstrate that the cell encoded the attended location, not the remembered one. Had the experimental design been something simple like a spatial delayed response task (Funahashi et al., 1989), corresponding to the major diagonal of the matrix (upper left to lower right), this neuron would have been interpreted as a memory cell, with a "mnemonic field" including the top location. For this cell, that would be a misinterpretation of its activity.

Notwithstanding such misinterpretations, some cells in the prefrontal cortex did encode remembered locations. The middle matrix in Figure 12.3B shows this kind of spatial tuning, for a cell that showed its highest activity when one of the monkeys remembered the right location. Note that this property, observed by comparing rows of the matrix, did not vary with the attended location, as can be appreciated by com-

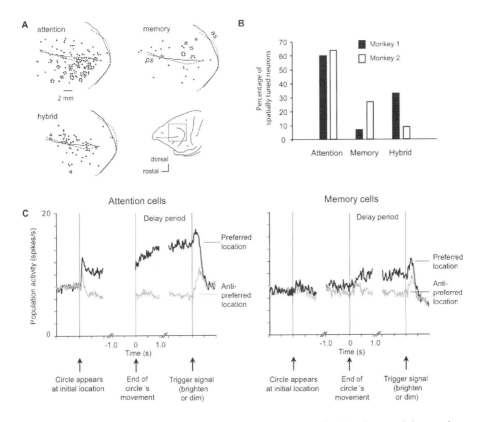

Figure 12.4. (A) Locations (black circles) of neurons selective for spatial attention, memory, or both (hybrid). Composite of two monkeys. Solid lines show one monkey's sulci, dashed lines show the other's. (B) The percentages of neurons of the three classes observed in the attention-memory experiment. (C) Population averages for attention cells (left) and memory cells (right). Each plot shows the average activity for each cells preferred location (black curves) and anti-preferred location (gray curves).

paring columns of the matrix. Yet another class of prefrontal cortex neuron showed a combination of the two kinds of spatial tuning, as shown in the right matrix.

We found that all types of spatial coding occurred: memory coding, as assumed in prior work, attention coding, as expected from other lines of research, and combinations of the two that we called hybrid tuning. The questions then were: where were these cells located and how frequent were the different types? If memory coding predominated throughout the prefrontal cortex, then the working-memory theory of prefrontal cortex function would be supported. It was not. Figure 12.4A shows that attention-coding neurons (top left) concentrate in somewhat different, although overlapping, parts of prefrontal cortex, compared with memory-coding neurons (top right). Figure 12.4B shows the relative frequency of attention, memory and hybrid neurons. Attention-coding cells, not memory-coding cells, predominated in the part of prefrontal cortex we sampled.

Beyond simply counting neurons of these types, the degree of spatial coding and the timing of the place-coding signals differed for attention- and memory-coding cells, as shown in the population averages in Figure 12.4C. The left part of the figure shows the mean activity, as a function of time, for the cells that encoded the attended location. Note that the spatial signal – the difference between the activity level for each cell's preferred location (black curve) and each cell's least preferred location (gray curve) – reached 6–8 spikes/s during the later stages of the delay period. The attention-coding signal developed very quickly after the circle first appeared and retained that level when the circle had stopped revolving, prior to its dimming or brightening. In contrast, the memory-encoding population was not only much smaller than the attention-encoding one (Figure 12.4B), but the magnitude of its spatial signal was much less (Figure 12.4C, right). Importantly, the memory signal began relatively late, as well. There was barely any memory signal as the circle revolved around the fixation point, then, once the circle stopped, a relatively weak memory signal developed, almost as if it was being read-in from somewhere else (Figure 12.4C, right). This finding was surprising because once the circle started moving, its original location needed to be stored and maintained in memory. If not, the monkey could not perform the task correctly. Because the monkeys performed the task at a very high level of accuracy, and the data presented here came from correctly executed trials only, we can be confident that the monkeys did remember the circle's original location. Yet the memory signal in the prefrontal cortex remained weak to nonexistent until long after the circle started moving and only began to develop a reliable magnitude after the circle's movement had stopped (right part of Figure 12.4C, right). This result suggests that the remembered location, which was also a potential future goal for an eye movement, was transferred to the prefrontal cortex from a neural network elsewhere that actually performs the working memory function, possibly the posterior parietal cortex.

To summarize the result of this experiment, we found that despite the task's high demand on spatial working memory, the largest proportion of prefrontal cortex neurons encode attended locations and do so early and robustly. Relatively few neurons encode remembered locations, and they do so late and weakly. These results falsify the working memory theory of prefrontal cortex, for those who allow that possibility. An analysis of other data typically brought forward in support of this theory showed, likewise, that none of it can withstand critical scrutiny (see Lebedev et al., 2004).

12.4   Strategies versus mappings

The two experiments just summarized point to a role for the primate prefrontal cortex in several aspects of vision: perception, visually guided action, attention and memory. Except for visually guided action, all of these functions are cognitive in the sense that they are not simply sensory, motor or sensorimotor. They are not particularly impressive cognitive capacities, however. Imagine that the behavior of someone was limited to remembering a place, perceiving which way a light spot moves, or attending to a location: not exactly full-professor material. There have, of course, been many neurophysiological studies of visual perception, attention, memory, and other relatively low-level cognitive functions, but very few have been devoted to more impressive, more intelligent behaviors.

The third experiment described in this chapter studied such intelligence, in a novel strategy task based on something we discovered quite by accident in what we call the arbitrary visuomotor mapping task or, more simply, the mapping task. In the mapping task, monkeys learned specific visuomotor associations. A given symbolic stimulus 1 always instructed the monkey to select a particular action or goal, whereas a stimulus 2 instructed a different action or goal (Passingham, 1993). In our experiments, there was also a stimulus 3, which instructed a third action or goal. Figure 12.5A shows an example of such associative mappings between symbols and actions (or goals), which must be learned by trial-and-error. In our mapping experiment (Figure 12.5A), the monkey saw three potential goals on each trial (as illustrated at the top of Figure 12.5B). Cue 1 mapped to the top goal, cue 2 mapped to the right one, and cue 3 mapped to the left one. With extensive experience at learning such mappings, each time with a novel set of three cues, our monkeys could learn new visuomotor mappings very quickly. Nevertheless, the only way to learn them is through trial-and-error experience with particular exemplars, memorized in a list-wise manner.

In the 1990s we found that as monkeys learn arbitrary visuomotor mappings, many adopt certain response strategies that can be applied to novel stimuli, independent of any experience with those particular stimuli (Murray and Wise, 1996; Wise and Murray, 1999). Figure 12.5C shows what we discovered or, to be more precise, it shows what the monkeys discovered. They noticed, long before we did, that the task as we constructed it had two types of trials (Figure 12.5B). One-third of the time, the symbolic cue repeated from the previous trials (the left branch of Figure 12.5B, as time runs from top to bottom); two-thirds of the time it changed (right branch). We call the former kind of trial repeat trials, the latter change trials. The monkeys learned that it paid off to stay with their previous response on repeat trials. On change trials, they recognized that since the cue had changed, so too should their goal. We call the strategy used on repeat trials the repeat-stay strategy and that used on change trials the change-shift strategy, although it is as reasonable to consider them together as a single repeat-stay/change-shift strategy.

Figure 12.5C shows the performance benefits gained by four monkeys as they employed the repeat-stay strategy while attempting to learn arbitrary visuomotor mappings. Early in a block of trials, when all three of the cues were novel, performance on repeat trials (black curve) exceeded that on change trials (gray curve). Right from the start of their attempt to learn the associative mappings (Figure 12.5A), the monkeys made intelligent decisions about what to do when faced with novel stimuli. When the stimulus repeated from the previous trial, even though they had not yet learned the visuomotor mapping, they knew to stay with their previous goal. Likewise, when the cue changed, they knew to reject their previous goal in favor of one of the two alternatives. Applied perfectly in the context of our experiment, these strategies double the monkeys' success rate prior to learning any of the visuomotor mappings. The monkeys did not apply the repeat-stay strategy perfectly, however. If they had, they would have made no errors on repeat trials. Nevertheless, they made very few errors on those trials, many fewer than would have occurred by chance, which was a 67% error rate. The monkeys' performance of the change-shift strategy is not illustrated here, but many (not all) of the

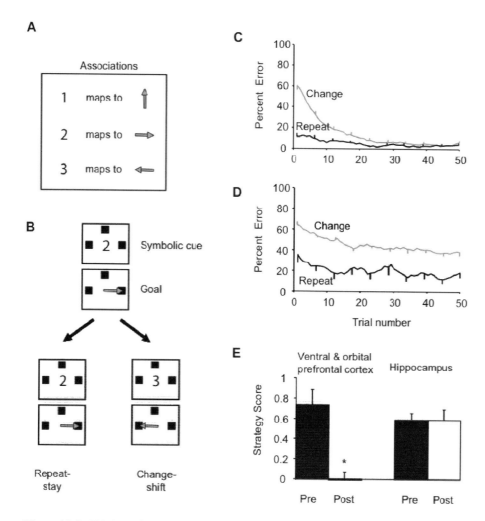

Figure 12.5. (A) Associative mappings between cues and goal. Cue 1 maps to the top of three goals, arranged as shown in part B (black squares), etc. (B) The two trials types in the strategy task. The white rectangles represent the video screen at two times during each trial: when the cue appears and when the monkey makes a saccade to fixation on of the three potential goals. The left branch, reading from top to bottom, shows a repeat trial and the repeat-stay strategy. The right branch shows a change trial and the change-shift strategy. (C) Learning curves for four monkeys divided by trial type. Each curve shows a grand mean composed of 40 three-stimulus sets (such as depicted in part A) from each monkey, with each stimulus novel at the beginning of a block of 50 trials. (D) Learning curves for the same four monkeys after bilateral ablations of the hippocampus and nearby structures. (E) A measure of strategy implementation, with 1 indicating perfect application, before (Pre) and after (Post) bilateral lesions of the brain structure noted at the top. The asterisk denotes a statistically significant difference of a pre–post pair. Error bars show SEM in parts C, D and E.

monkeys reduced their error rate on change trials from chance level (67%) to near the theoretical limit of the strategy (50%). Complete, bilateral lesions of the hippocampus (plus some additional structures near it), had no effect on the application of either the repeat-stay or change-shift strategy (Murray and Wise, 1996; Wise and Murray, 1999). After the lesion, the monkeys learned the visuomotor mappings much more slowly, as evidenced by the higher error rates in Figure 12.5D compared with Figure 12.5C, but they continued to employ the strategies that helped them in the initial stages of learning prior to the lesion (Figure 12.5C). Figure 12.5E (right) compares the monkeys' ability to apply the strategies before (Pre) and after (Post) the hippocampal lesions, using a strategy score. A score of 1 would indicate that the monkeys had obtained the maximal benefit of the strategies. In accord with Figure 12.5D, hippocampal lesions had no effect. In contrast to this negative result, bilateral lesions of the ventral and orbital parts of the prefrontal cortex (Figure 12.5E, left) completely eliminated the monkeys' ability to use the repeat-stay and change-shift strategies (Bussey et al., 2001).

The monkeys' discovery of the repeat and change trials, and their intelligent approach to novel stimuli, served as the background for the strategy-mapping experiment. In the strategy task, we trained different monkeys to perform the strategies that the previous monkeys had spontaneously adopted. As shown in Figure 12.5C, the monkeys quickly dispensed with the need to use the strategies as they learned the visuomotor mappings. Within 20–25 trials, on average, the monkeys made so few errors that it became impossible to measure the benefits gained by employing the repeat-stay (or change-shift) strategy. Accordingly, we devised a new task that required them to employ strategies in the absence of learning visuomotor mappings (Genovesio et al., 2005). Specifically, monkeys were trained to respond to initially novel symbolic cues according to the repeat-stay and change-shift strategies. As illustrated in Figure 12.6A, if the cue had repeated from the previous trial, monkeys needed to choose the same goal as on the previous trial; if the cue had changed, they needed to reject the previous goal in favor of one of the two remaining ones. A couple of examples show how the task worked. Take for granted that each trial ended in the choice of a goal that produced a reward. (We gave the monkeys an unlimited number of "second chances" to ensure that this was always the case.) In Figure 12.6A, the cue illustrated as 2 appeared on the previous trial (left), and the monkey chose the goal to the right. The monkey indicated its choice by making a saccade from the original, central fixation point to the goal and maintaining fixation there for 1.5 s. On repeat trials (the top branch of the figure), cue 2 appeared again on the current trial (right). As in the visuomotor mapping task, repeats occurred on one-third of the trials. The correct goal, in this example, is shown at the top: the monkey chose the rightmost goal again, and this produced another reward. Any other choice, such as the choice of the left goal, constituted a strategic error, which never produced a reward. On change trials (the bottom branch of the figure), cue 2 did not appear. The example shows cue 3. The monkey could then make either of two strategically correct choices, in this example either the left or top goals. To match the situation in the mapping task, only one of these choices produced a reward. Staying with the previous goal, illustrated at the bottom of Figure 12.5A, was a strategic error that produced no reward.

Figure 12.6B shows why the monkeys could not learn any visuomotor mappings in the strategy task. In a sequence of possible trials at the beginning of a recording

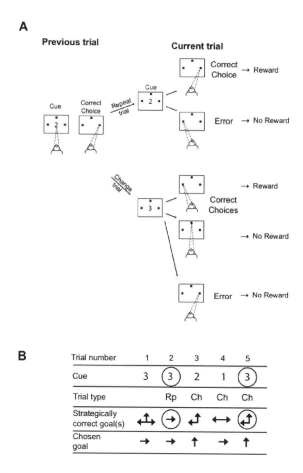

Figure 12.6. (A) The two trial types in the strategy task: repeat trials (top branch) and change trials (bottom branch). Each pair of rectangles is in the format of Figure 12.5B. (B) A possible five-trial sequence of cues and goal choices in the strategy task. Circles mark the cues and choices for key trials discussed in the text.

session, cue 3 appeared three times in the first five trials: on the first, second, and fifth trials. To receive a reward on the second trial, the monkey must have chosen the rightmost goal. To have any chance of receiving a reward on the fifth trial, however, the monkey could not have chosen the rightmost goal. In this way, over the course of dozens of trials, no single mapping between cue and goal remained consistent for any significant number of trials.

We compared activity for the strategy task (Figure 12.6A) and the arbitrary visuo-motor mapping task (Figure 12.5A), with trials matched for identical stimuli and responses. Of the prefrontal cortex neurons that showed significant activity modulations during the task, nearly half showed a significant difference between the strategy and mapping tasks. Obviously, neither the stimulus nor the movement could account for such differences, and separate analyses and control conditions ruled out reward antici-

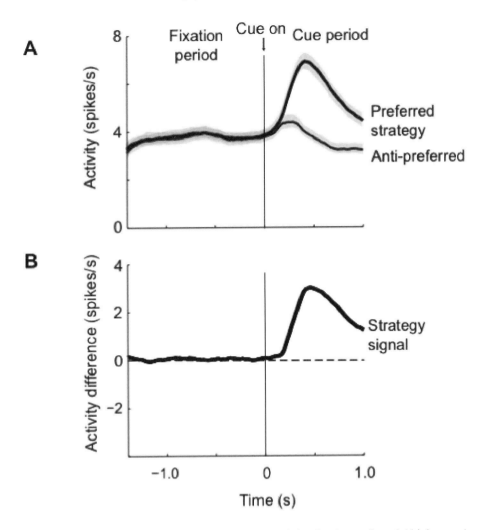

Figure 12.7. (A) Population averages showing activity for the preferred (thick curve) and anti-preferred (thin curve) strategies in the prefrontal cortex. For strategically correct trials only. Shading shows SEM. (B) The difference between the two curves in part A: the strategy signal.

pation or reward prediction for a majority of these cells. Cells preferring the mapping task outnumbered those preferring the strategy task by a ratio of approximately 2:1. For cells preferring the strategy task, selectivity for the repeat-stay and change-shift strategies were equally common (Figure 12.8B).

We also examined whether the activity of prefrontal cortex neurons differed significantly according to the strategy used. Figure 12.7A shows the average activity of the prefrontal cortex population that preferred the strategy task. As with the perception-

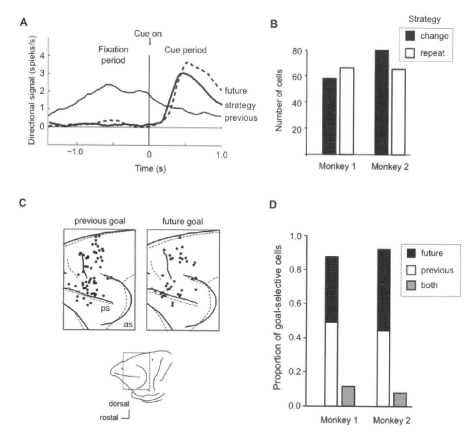

Figure 12.8. (A) Neural signals, in the format of Figure 12.7B, for future-goal, previous-goal, and strategy-selective populations of prefrontal cortex neurons. (B) The numbers of cells preferring the repeat-stay and change-shift strategies in the strategy task. (C) Locations of previous- and future-goal cells. Composite of two monkeys. Format as in Figure 12.4A. (D) Proportion of future-goal and previous-goal cells, and cells that encode both types of goal. The previous- and future-goal cells are shown stacked in order to contrast the large proportion encoding one of the two spatial variables versus the small proportion encoding both.

action experiment, the population average captures the single-cell activity quite well, so averages can illustrate the results. Figure 12.7A shows the average activity of the population for each cell's preferred strategy (i.e. the strategy associated with the highest discharge rate). It also shows the average of each cell's activity for the other strategy, called the anti-preferred strategy. If, for example, a cell preferred the repeat-stay strategy, the anti-preferred strategy was change-shift. After cue presentation, the population increased its activity for both strategies at first, but after 237 ms the activity during the preferred strategy exceeded that during the anti-preferred one. Figure 12.7B shows the strategy signal, defined as the difference between the two curves in Figure 12.7A. The strategy signal decayed during the period that the stimulus was present (a minimum of 1 s), but remained present throughout.

Implementation of the repeat-stay and change-shift strategies required five cognitive processes: memory for the cue presented on the previous trial, memory for the goal chosen on the previous trial, use of cue memory to evaluate repeats and changes of the cue (Wallis and Miller, 2003; Muhammad et al., 2006), use of the goal memory to reject or repeat the previous goal, and memory of the future goal until the go signal arrived as much as 2 s after the cue appeared. We did not find any cells that reflected the previous cue during the period running up to cue presentation. Some prefrontal neurons were selective for either the repeat-stay or change-shift strategy, but showed no selectivity for the particular response chosen. These cells probably contributed to the evaluation of stimulus repetition or change or selection of the correct strategy. Other cells were specific for the cue upon which the strategy was based or for the goal selected on the basis of the strategy. These cells could contribute to the implementation of the strategy (see Genovesio and Wise, 2007).

12.5   Previous versus future goals

In addition to the cells described above for the strategy task, many prefrontal cortex neurons encoded either the previous or the future goal (Genovesio et al., 2006). Some of these were the mixed effect cells mentioned above as having activity specific for the goal selected on the basis of a given strategy. Other prefrontal cortex neurons encoded the previous or future goals without reflecting a strategy.

In the behavioral design used for the strategy-mapping experiment (Figure 12.6A), the monkeys had to use their knowledge of previous goals, along with other information, to select their future goals according to a strategy. Figure 12.8 shows the neural signals in these two populations (Figure 12.8A), the distribution of these two cell types in the prefrontal cortex (Figure 12.8C), and their relative frequency (Figure 12.8D). As with the perception and action neurons illustrated in Figure 12.2B, the future- and previous-goal encoding neurons appeared to be completely intermingled within the sampled regions of prefrontal cortex (Figure 12.8C). Of special interest was the finding, shown in Figure 12.8D, that the vast majority of prefrontal cells encoded either the previous goal (white bars) or the future goal (black bars), but only rarely both (gray bars).

Maintaining the distinction between accomplished goals and pending ones is another fundamental aspect of intelligent behavior. Although the experiment we performed involved spatial goals, it seems likely that the neural separation of previous- and future goal representations applies generally. When an accomplished goal is misrepresented as a pending, this mistake is likely to cause an inability to recognize that a goal has been achieved. We proposed that a problem of this kind could underlie compulsive checking symptoms in obsessive-compulsive disorder and response perseveration (Genovesio et al., 2006). If a goal or task cannot be classified by the neural network as accomplished, then the chances are good that another attempt will be made to achieve that goal or accomplish that task. Conversely, when pending goals are misrepresented as already accomplished, then important activities – both physical and intellectual – will be omitted, which is one of the problems seen in patients with dementia.

Figure 12.8A shows the time course of the previous- and future-goal signals. The fixation period occurs for 1 s prior to the appearance of the symbolic cue in the strategy task. Then, once the cue appears, the previous-goal signal (thin curve) decreases roughly as the future-goal signal (dashed curve) increases. The strategy signal (thick curve), taken from Figure 12.7B, closely follows the future-goal signal. These data accord with the idea that the previous goal becomes less relevant once the monkey selects the future goal on the basis of the strategy. Also, once the monkey selects its future goal, the strategy becomes less important, although both the goal selected and the strategy used have continued importance for monitoring once feedback occurs.

12.6   Prefrontal cortex: polymath or monomaniac

In *The Hitchhiker's Guide to the Galaxy* by Douglas Adams, a computer named Deep Thought churned for 7.5 million years to answer the Great Question of Life, the Universe and Everything. The answer turned out to be forty-two, and as Deep Thought surmised, the people did not like it. Our question is simple enough, and probably more closely related to the Great Question than we can appreciate: What does the prefrontal cortex do? Can we tolerate the conclusion that it does nearly everything? Put somewhat differently, can we accept the primate prefrontal cortex as the brain's paramount polymath, or is it really a monomaniac at heart?

In the results summarized in this chapter, the perception-action experiment yielded one population of prefrontal cortex neurons that reflected perceptual reports about a visual cue, whereas the activity of an intermingled population reflected actions aimed at that cue. In the attention-memory experiment, some prefrontal cortex activity was related to working memory, but most reflected the allocation of visual attention, instead. In the strategy-mapping task, some prefrontal neurons exhibited activity that reflected arbitrary visuomotor mappings, whereas others reflected which strategy a monkey used to choose a goal. In the future-previous goal experiment, the activity of one neuronal population encoded future goals, and a largely distinct yet intermingled population encoded previous goals. The picture that emerges from these results is that the prefrontal cortex seems to "care about" each of these aspects of visual knowledge, and results from other laboratories point to additional processes and knowledge, such as categorization (Freedman et al., 2002; Shima et al., 2007), predictive coding (Rainer et al., 1999), rules (Hoshi et al., 1998; White and Wise, 1999; Asaad et al., 2000; Wallis et al., 2001; Wallis and Miller, 2003), behavioral inhibition and preparatory set (Fuster, 1989), and the detection and generation of event sequences across time (Quintana and Fuster, 1999; Averbeck et al., 2002; Ninokura et al., 2003; Hoshi and Tanji, 2004), sometimes termed cross-temporal contingencies (Fuster et al., 2000). Can we stand for such a long list, the mark of a true polymath?

Like forty-two, some answers are fundamentally unsatisfying. We all would like a synthetic theory of prefrontal cortex, rather than a list of functions related to each other in complex ways. It would be tempting, for example, to simply accept the idea that the principal function of prefrontal cortex is working memory (Goldman-Rakic,

1987, 2000; Levy and Goldman-Rakic, 2000). Yet in the attention-memory experiment, the activity of most prefrontal cortex cells correlated better with the allocation of visual attention than with visual working memory. Thus, the neurophysiological evidence shows that prefrontal cortex functions extend far beyond working memory. The prefrontal cortex is not a mnemonic monomaniac.

Perhaps we could find a simple synthesis of prefrontal cortex function along a different dimension. One possibility is that the prefrontal cortex is specialized for perceptual processes, in contrast to the motor and premotor areas, which control actions. In the perception-action experiment, however, the activity of one neuronal population reflected perceptual reports about a visual stimulus, whereas the activity of an intermingled population reflected actions aimed at that stimulus. The perception-action experiment provides reason to believe that there is nothing too automatic for the prefrontal cortex to encode, including the most direct visually guided movements to a target. The prefrontal cortex is also not a perceptual monomaniac.

At a different level of explanation, another possibility is that the prefrontal cortex functions specifically in high-order reason, as opposed to knowledge based on accumulated experience with relatively low-level exemplars. Pinker (1999) pointed out that this dichotomy maps onto empiricism and rationalism, respectively. Does the prefrontal cortex specialize for one aspect of this dichotomy? It would be satisfying, for example, to attribute only the highest brain functions to the prefrontal cortex, much as Flourens did nearly two centuries ago. Unfortunately, the results of the strategy-mapping experiment fail to provide any support for this idea. Approximately twice as many prefrontal neurons preferred the mapping task, which requires the empirical memorization of experienced exemplars, compared with the strategy task, which requires the rational application of abstract strategies for responding to novel visual symbols. The prefrontal cortex does not seem to be a monomaniacal rationalist, either.

Perhaps the key dimension involves predictions, with the prefrontal cortex functioning as the brain's oracle. In the future-previous goal experiment, however, the activity of one neuronal population encoded future goals, and a largely distinct population encoded previous goals. The number of cells encoding the future goal did not exceed that encoding the previous goal. So the prefrontal cortex does not appear to have a monomania for the future at the expense of the past.

To sum up, two common themes have emerged from the experiments summarized in this chapter. First, even when more-or-less completely intermingled, populations of prefrontal neurons tend to specialize in one kind of knowledge when contrasted with another. And second, no single cognitive process predominates prefrontal cortex function. Accordingly, our findings militate against a single cognitive process, such as working memory, attention, or perception, as the basis for a simple synthesis of prefrontal cortex function. The prefrontal cortex appears to be more polymath than monomaniac. Or is it?

12.7   *E pluribus unum*

The strategy-mapping experiment might help us approach that question. The strategy task required several cognitive functions, including working memory (of the cue and goal from the previous trials), a rule-based decision about whether the cue on the current trial matched that on the previous one, and a selection of a goal under demanding circumstances. The strategy task thus required the processes invoked in several theories of prefrontal cortex: the maintenance of working memories (Goldman-Rakic, 1987, 2000; Levy and Goldman-Rakic, 2000), adaptive coding – the ability to guide behavior whenever problems exceed routine levels of difficulty (Duncan et al., 1996; Duncan and Owen, 2000) – and attentional selection (Rowe and Passingham, 2001; Rowe et al., 2002), including the monitoring of items in working memory (Owen et al., 1996; Petrides et al., 2002). Perhaps all of these functions have their greatest biological importance when applied to the learning and use of abstract response strategies and similar functions. Behavioral strategies typically require a large number of coordinated processes, including top-down attention, categorization, selecting goals based on context and predicted outcomes, and maintaining choices and goals in memory, prospectively, along with alternatives – discarded for the moment, but not forever. It seems likely that the prefrontal cortex contributes to all of these processes, and all of them are necessary for the selection and implementation of abstract response strategies. Thus, it is not surprising that neurophysiological studies, each focused on one or a few of these processes, would find evidence for all of them.

Out of the long list of neural processes mentioned thus far – and others could, of course, be added – might there nevertheless be the strain of monomania in prefrontal cortex function that would provide a satisfying synthesis? My answer *du jour* uses an analogy. It is now generally accepted that the inferior temporal and perirhinal areas of cortex encode and store knowledge about objects (Buckley and Gaffan, 1998; Bussey et al., 2003; Murray et al., 2007). By analogy, it appears that the prefrontal cortex encodes and stores knowledge about behavior (Wood and Grafman, 2003). This knowledge contributes to attention, memory, strategies, rules, valuations, and perceptions, as well as the selection, maintenance, and monitoring of goals and their achievement. A unified theory along these lines would subsume the traditional notions of response selection, decisions and choice, as championed by animal learning theorists and contemporary neuroeconomists, but it would do so from a more comprehensive, cognitive perspective. From such a perspective, the various parts of the prefrontal cortex appear, collectively, to contribute to all of the behaviors important in the life of primates. There is a long list of prefrontal cortex functions, but perhaps they all contribute to "knowing what to do" and "knowing what will happen if that is done," especially in extraordinary situations, when a subtle danger looms or a exceptional opportunity arises.

Acknowledgments

I thank my co-authors on the papers reviewed here, in the order of presentation: Misha Lebedev, Sohie Moody Lee, Diana Douglass, Adam Messinger, Jay Kralik, Peter Brasted, Aldo Genovesio, Andy Mitz, and Satoshi Tsujimoto. This research was supported by the Intramural Research Program of the National Institutes of Health, NIMH (Z01MH-01092).

References

Aglioti, S., DeSouza, J. F. X. and Goodale, M. A. (1995). Size-contrast illusions deceive the eye but not the hand. *Curr. Biol.*, 5: 679–685.

Asaad, W. F., Rainer, G. and Miller, E. K. (2000). Task-specific neural activity in the primate prefrontal cortex. *J. Neurophysiol*, 84: 451–459.

Averbeck, B. B., Chafee, M. V., Crowe, D. A. and Georgopoulos, A. P. (2002). Parallel processing of serial movements in prefrontal cortex. *Proc. Nat. Acad. Sci. USA*, 99: 13172–13177.

Boussaoud, D., Ungerleider, L. G. and Desimone, R. (1990). Pathways for motion analysis: cortical connections of the medial superior temporal and fundus of the superior temporal visual areas in the macaque. *J. Comp. Neurol.* 296: 462–495.

Bridgeman, B. (1992). Conscious vs. unconscious processes. *Theory Psychol.*, 2: 73–88.

Bridgeman, B., Vanderheijden, A. H. C. and Velichkovsky, B. M. (1994). A theory of visual stability across saccadic eye movements. *Behav. Brain Sci.* 17: 247–292.

Buckley, M. J. and Gaffan, D. (1998). Perirhinal cortex ablation impairs visual object identification. *J. Neurosci.*, 18: 2268–2275.

Bussey, T. J., Saksida, L. M. and Murray, E. A. (2003). Impairments in visual discrimination after perirhinal cortex lesions: testing 'declarative' vs. 'perceptual-mnemonic' views of perirhinal cortex function. *Eur. J. Neurosci.*, 17: 649–660.

Bussey, T. J., Wise, S. P. and Murray, E. A. (2001). The role of ventral and orbital prefrontal cortex in conditional visuomotor learning and strategy use in rhesus monkeys. *Behav. Neurosci.*, 115: 971–982.

Constantinidis, C., Franowicz, M. N. and Goldman-Rakic, P. S. (2001). The sensory nature of mnemonic representation in the primate prefrontal cortex. *Nat. Neurosci.*, 4: 311–316.

Crick, F. and Koch, C. (1995). Are we aware of neural activity in primary visual cortex? *Nature*, 375: 121–123.

Crick, F. and Koch, C. (1998). Consciousness and neuroscience. *Cereb. Cortex*, 8: 97–107.

Duncan, J. and Owen, A. M. (2000). Common regions of the human frontal lobe recruited by diverse cognitive demands. *Trends Neurosci.*, 23: 475–483.

Duncan, J., Emslie, H., Williams, P., Johnson, R. and Freer, C. (1996). Intelligence and the frontal lobe: the organization of goal-directed behavior. *Cogn. Psychol.*, 30: 257–303.

Flourens, P. (1824). *Recherches expérimentales sur les propriétés et les fonctions du système nerveux dans les animaux vertébrés*. Paris: Chez Crevot.

Freedman, D. J., Riesenhuber, M., Poggio, T. and Miller, E. K. (2002). Visual categorization and the primate prefrontal cortex: Neurophysiology and behavior. *J. Neurophysiol.*, 88: 929–941.

Fulton, J. F. (1949). *Physiology of the Nervous System.* New York: Oxford University Press.

Funahashi, S., Bruce, C. J. and Goldman-Rakic, P. S. (1989). Mnemonic coding of visual space in the monkey's dorsolateral prefrontal cortex. *J. Neurophysiol.*, 61: 331–349.

Fuster, J. M. (1973). Unit activity in prefrontal cortex during delayed-response performance: neuronal correlated of transient memory. *J. Neurophysiol.*, 36: 61–78.

Fuster, J. M. (1989). *The Prefrontal Cortex: Anatomy, Physiology and Neuropsychology of the Frontal Lobe.* New York: Raven Press.

Fuster, J. M. and Alexander, G. E. (1971). Neuron activity related to short-term memory. *Science*, 173: 652–654.

Fuster, J. M., Bodner, M. and Kroger, J. K. (2000). Cross-modal and cross-temporal association in neurons of frontal cortex. *Nature*, 405: 347–351.

Genovesio, A. and Wise, S. P. (2007). The neurophysiology of abstract strategies. In S. A. Bunge and J. D. Wallis (eds.), *Rule Guided Behavior*. New York: Oxford University Press, pp. 81–105.

Genovesio, A., Brasted, P. J., Mitz, A. R. and Wise, S. P. (2005). Prefrontal cortex activity related to abstract response strategies. *Neuron*, 47: 307–320.

Genovesio, A., Brasted, P. J. and Wise, S. P. (2006). Representation of future and previous spatial goals by separate neural populations in prefrontal cortex. *J. Neurosci.*, 26: 7281–7292.

Goldman-Rakic, P. (1987). Circuitry of primate prefrontal cortex and regulation of behaviour by representational memory. In F. Plum and V. B. Mountcastle (eds.), *Handbook of Physiology: The Nervous System, Vol. 5*. Bethesda, MD: American Physiological Society, pp. 373–417.

Goldman-Rakic, P. (2000). Localization of function all over again. *NeuroImage*, 11: 451–457.

Goodale, M. A. and Westwood, D. A. (2004). An evolving view of duplex vision: Separate but interacting cortical pathways for perception and action. *Curr. Opin. Neurobiol.*, 14: 203–211.

Goodale, M. A., Milner, A. D., Jakobson, L. S. and Carey, D. P. (1991). A neurological dissociation between perceiving objects and grasping them. *Nature*, 349: 154–156. cortex. *J. Neurophysiol.*, 80: 3392–3397.

Hoshi, E. and Tanji, J. (2004). Area-selective neuronal activity in the dorsolateral prefrontal cortex for information retrieval and action planning. *J. Neurophysiol.*, 91: 2707–2722.

Hoshi, E., Shima, K. and Tanji, J. (1998). Task-dependent selectivity of movement-related neuronal activity in the primate prefrontal

Jacobsen, C. F. (1935). Functions of the frontal association cortex in primates. *Archiv. Neurol. Psychiat.*, 33: 558–569.

Kubota, K. and Niki, H. (1971). Prefrontal cortical unit activity and delayed alternation performance in monkeys. *J. Neurophysiol,*, 34: 337–347.

Lebedev, M. A. and Wise, S. P. (2002). Insights into seeing and grasping: distinguishing the neural correlates of perception and action. *Behav. Cogn. Neurosci. Rev.*, 1: 108–129.

Lebedev, M. A., Douglass, D. K., Moody, S. L. and Wise, S. P. (2001). Prefrontal cortex neurons reflecting reports of a visual illusion. *J. Neurophysiol.*, 85: 1395–1411.

Lebedev, M. A., Messinger, A., Kralik, J. D. and Wise, S. P. (2004). Representation of attended versus remembered locations in prefrontal cortex. *PLoS, Biology*, 2: 1919–1935.

Levy, R. and Goldman-Rakic, P. S. (2000). Segregation of working memory functions within the dorsolateral prefrontal cortex. *Exp. Brain Res.*, 133: 23–32.

Muhammad, R., Wallis, J. D. and Miller, E. K. (2006). A comparison of abstract rules in the prefrontal cortex, premotor cortex, inferior temporal cortex, and striatum. *J. Cogn. Neurosci.*, 18: 974–989.

Murray, E. A. and Wise, S. P. (1996). Role of the hippocampus plus subjacent cortex but not amygdala in visuomotor conditional learning in rhesus monkeys. *Behav. Neurosci.*, 110: 1261–1270.

Murray, E. A., Bussey, T. J. and Saksida, L. M. (2007). Visual perception and memory: a new view of medial temporal lobe function in primates and rodents. *Ann. Rev. Neurosci.*, 30: 99–122.

Ninokura, Y., Mushiake, H. and Tanji, J. (2003). Representation of the temporal order of visual objects in the primate lateral prefrontal cortex. *J. Neurophysiol.*, 89: 2868–2873.

Owen, A. M., Evans, A. C. and Petrides, M. (1996). Evidence for a two-stage model of spatial working memory processing within the lateral frontal cortex: a positron emission tomography study. *Cereb. Cortex*, 6: 31–38.

Passingham, R. E. (1993). *The Frontal Lobes and Voluntary Action*. Oxford, UK: Oxford University Press.

Petrides, M., Alivisatos, B. and Frey, S. (2002). Differential activation of the human orbital, midventrolateral, and mid-dorsolateral prefrontal cortex during the processing of visual stimuli. *Proc. Nat. Acad. Sci. USA*, 99: 5649–5654.

Pinker, S. (1999). *Word and Rules*. New York: Basic Books.

Postle, B. R., Druzgal, T. J. and D'Esposito, M. (2003). Seeking the neural substrates of visual working memory storage. *Cortex*, 39: 927–946.

Quintana, J. and Fuster, J. M. (1999). From perception to action: temporal integrative functions of prefrontal and parietal neurons. *Cereb. Cortex*, 9: 213–221.

Rainer, G., Rao, S. C. and Miller, E. K. (1999). Prospective coding for objects in primate prefrontal cortex. *J. Neurosci.*, 19: 5493–5505.

Romo, R., Brody, C. D., Hernandez, A. and Lemus, L. (1999). Neuronal correlates of parametric working memory in the prefrontal cortex. *Nature*, 399: 470–473.

Rowe, J., Friston, K., Frackowiak, R. and Passingham, R. (2002). Attention to action: specific modulation of corticocortical interactions in humans. *NeuroImage*, 17: 988–998.

Rowe, J. B. and Passingham, R. E. (2001). Working memory for location and time: activity in prefrontal area 46 relates to selection rather than maintenance in memory. *NeuroImage*, 14: 77–86.

Rowe, J. B., Toni, I., Josephs, O., Frackowiak, R. S. and Passingham, R. E. (2000). The prefrontal cortex: response selection or maintenance within working memory? *Science*, 288: 1656–1660.

Rushworth, M. F. S., Nixon, P. D., Eacott, M. J. and Passingham, R. E. (1997). Ventral prefrontal cortex is not essential for working memory. *J. Neurosci.*, 17: 4829–4838.

Shadmehr, R. and Wise, S. P. (2005). *The Computational Neurobiology of Reaching and Pointing: A Foundation for Motor Learning*. Cambridge, MA: MIT Press.

Shima, K., Isoda, M., Mushiake, H. and Tanji, J. (2007). Categorization of behavioural sequences in the prefrontal cortex. *Nature*, 445: 315–318.

Stein, J. F. and Glickstein, M. (1992). Role of the cerebellum in visual guidance of movement. *Physiol. Rev.*, 72: 967–1017.

Tong, F., Nakayama, K., Vaughan, J. T. and Kanwisher, N. (1998). Binocular rivalry and visual awareness in human extrastriate cortex. *Neuron*, 21: 753–759.

Wallis, J. D., Anderson, K. C. and Miller, E. K. (2001). Single neurons in prefrontal cortex encode abstract rules. *Nature*, 411: 953–956.

Wallis, J. D. and Miller, E. K. (2003). From rule to response: neuronal processes in the premotor and prefrontal cortex. *J. Neurophysiol.*, 90: 1790–1806.

White, I. M. and Wise, S. P. (1999). Rule-dependent neuronal activity in the prefrontal cortex. *Exp. Brain Res.*, 126: 315–335.

Wise, S. P. and Murray, E. A. (1999). Role of the hippocampal system in conditional motor learning: mapping antecedents to action. *Hippocampus* 9: 101–117.

Wong, E. and Mack, A. (1981). Saccadic programming and perceived location. *Acta Psychol.*, 48: 123–131.

Wood, J. N. and Grafman, J. (2003). Human prefrontal cortex: processing and representational perspectives. *Nature Rev. Neurosci.*, 4: 139–147.

Zeki, S. and Bartels, A. (1998). The asynchrony of consciousness. *Proc. Roy. Soc. Lond. Ser. B*, 265: 1583–1585.

13 Saccade target selection in unconstrained visual search

M. Paré, N. W. D. Thomas and K. Shen

Our visual system is regularly faced with more information than it can process at once. As a result, our visual experience generally arises from the sequential sampling of visual details by overtly shifting perceptual resources through reorienting the fovea with saccadic eye movements. An emerging view is that this natural visual behavior can be promoted in visual search tasks that do not emphasize accuracy over speed. Here we review recent neurophysiological findings, which were obtained with such an approach, showing that the process of selecting a saccade target involves neurons within the dorsal "vision-for-action" processing stream of the cerebral cortex of monkeys. The visual responses of these posterior parietal cortex neurons evolve to signal both where the search target is located and when the targeting saccade will be made. Consistent with the involvement of attentional processes in saccade target selection, the magnitude of the enhancement of parietal activity in advance of a search saccade parallels what has been reported in neurons within the ventral "object-recognition" pathway when attention is covertly allocated.

13.1 Introduction

We see the world by shifting our perceptual resources either covertly by allocating visual attention to peripheral locations or overtly by reorienting the fovea with saccadic eye movements. Although these two processes can operate independently – it is undeniable that we can mentally scan a visual scene without moving our eyes (e.g. Sperling and Melchner, 1978) – experimental evidence suggests that they may be functionally coupled: shifting attention covertly to a spatial location facilitates the processing of saccades directed to that location, whereas planning a saccade to a spatial location facilitates perceptual processing of objects at that location (Hoffman and Subramaniam, 1995; Kowler et al., 1995; Deubel and Schneider, 1996). Furthermore, the high rate of

Cortical Mechanisms of Vision, ed. M. Jenkin and L. R. Harris. Published by Cambridge University Press.
ⓒ Cambridge University Press 2009.

saccades in natural tasks such as visual search, text reading and scene perception suggests that there are few attentional shifts besides those associated with the execution of saccades when the eyes are free to move (for a review see Findlay and Gilchrist, 2003). The current view that has emerged from these studies is that covert orienting may only assist overt orienting by analyzing the visual periphery during fixation intervals and contributing to the selection of the goal of each saccade (see Henderson, 1992; Schneider, 1995). Such a functional coupling between covert and overt shifts of attention may result from the overlapping of their respective neural circuits (Nobre et al., 1997; Corbetta et al., 1998) and from the massive connections between brain areas with visual and oculomotor functions (Schall et al., 1995a). Consistent with this interconnectivity, voluntary shifts in visual attention are associated with enhanced neural activity not only in visual cortical areas but also in the brain regions essential for saccade production: the frontal eye field (FEF) and the superior colliculus (SC) (see for review Moore et al., 2003; Awh et al., 2006).

A different picture has, however, emerged from studies that examined this coupling with controlled tasks that promote natural visual behavior, such as the visual search paradigm. Neurophysiological findings in FEF and SC studies with monkeys performing various visual search tasks suggest a dissociation of covert and overt processes. First, the activity of visually responsive neurons reflects the process of selecting a salient stimulus even when monkeys withhold directing their gaze to it (FEF: Schall et al., 1995b; Thompson et al., 1997, 2005a, b) or direct their gaze away from it (FEF: Murthy et al., 2001; Sato et al., 2001; Sato and Schall, 2003; SC: Shen and Paré, 2007). Second, the allocation of visual attention to the target and the subsequent planning of the saccade appear to correspond to the selective activity of distinct neuronal populations within both the FEF (Thompson et al., 1996; Sato and Schall, 2003) and the SC (McPeek and Keller, 2002). Although these findings are very valuable, as they inform us about the neural signatures of the sequential unfolding of decision processing stages that experimental psychology has long identified (e.g. Theios, 1975; Allport, 1987; LaBerge and Brown, 1989; Schall and Thompson, 1999), they are difficult to reconcile with the idea that covert attention only assists overt orienting during free viewing of visual scenes.

It is reasonable to presume that this uncoupling of covert and overt processes in the above studies is an outcome of the constrained nature of the visual search tasks that were used. Given their emphasis on accuracy, these tasks explicitly enforced the strategy to withhold the rapid orienting behavior that is frequently observed in response to the presentation of visual search displays (Findlay, 1997; Williams et al., 1997; Maioli et al., 2001). In sum, the very different response times observed in discrimination tasks when accuracy versus speed is emphasized must reflect different strategies and increased accuracy demands may require extensive training that can modify the neural substrate of the behavior. Here we review recent studies from our laboratory, as well as others, that have investigated the brain mechanisms underlying saccade target selection in visual search tasks that are less constrained than in previous monkey studies.

13.2   Automatic responses during visual search

The visual search paradigm has been developed to study the deployment of visual attention in humans (see for review Wolfe and Horowitz, 2004). This approach requires subjects to indicate the presence of a search target within a multistimulus display with a manual response without them being instructed to foveate that target, but several studies have also monitored where subjects look while performing this task (e.g. Binello et al., 1995; Zelinsky and Sheinberg, 1995; Williams et al., 1997; Scialfa and Joffe, 1998; Maioli et al., 2001). Generally, the number of saccades is highly correlated with the time it takes to report the presence of the search target. The latency of the initial response to the search display, however, does not necessarily vary with task difficulty. In contrast, previous monkey studies have required the explicit foveation of the search target after a single saccade and they have reported longer response times with increasing task difficulty (Bichot and Schall, 1999; Buracas and Albright, 1999; Sato et al., 2001; Thompson et al., 2005a; but see Motter and Belky, 1998).

To study the processes underlying the deployment of visual attention and the guidance of saccades during natural visual behavior, and to reconcile the differences between the human and monkey visual search literature, Shen and Paré (2006) examined the gaze behavior of monkeys trained to perform visual search tasks more akin to the human studies. These experiments did not demand high immediate performance accuracy and thus required relatively little training. Monkeys had to foveate a target stimulus and they received a full liquid reward (and a reinforcement tone) if their first saccade landed on that stimulus. Nevertheless, they were granted a generous length of time (>2 s) to freely visit whichever stimuli they wished to examine. In those trials, in which they foveated the target after several saccades, they received a partial reward, which amounted practically to only the reinforcement tone. In all tasks, the target was identified either solely by color (Figure 13.1A) or by a conjunction of color and shape (Figure 13.1B).

Human attention studies have shown that the search for a target stimulus defined by a conjunction of features is typically less efficient than when that target is defined by a single feature and performance is usually impaired by the addition of distractors, as if the display stimuli were being processed serially (Treisman and Gelade, 1980). In line with these previous observations from human subjects, Shen and Paré (2006) found that monkey's search time – the total amount of time needed to foveate the target – was longer during conjunction search and lengthened with increasing display size, whereas it remained unchanged by display size in feature search (Figure 13.2A). Correspondingly, the accuracy of the first saccades during feature search did not vary with increasing display size, but it was significantly less during conjunction search and gradually fell with increasing display size (Figure 13.2B). The latency of these first correct saccades, however, varied with neither the number of visual stimuli nor the difficulty of the search task (Figure 13.2C); the average response time was 167 ms. The independence of these initial responses from the visual context of the search displays demonstrates that the visual behavior of these monkeys was less constrained than in previous monkey studies, and it suggests that these responses were largely independent of voluntary control (Jonides et al., 1985). Consequently, the monkey's decision about where and when to make a saccade to a visual stimulus within the search display

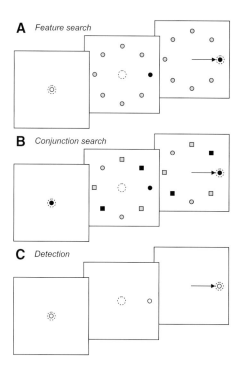

Figure 13.1. All behavioral tasks were initiated by the fixation of a central spot. After monkeys maintained fixation for 500–800 ms, the fixation spot disappeared simultaneously with the appearance of a saccade target at one of eight locations. In the visual feature search task (A), the saccade target was identified solely by color (red or green). In the visual conjunction search task (B), the target was identified by a conjunction of color (red or green) and shape (circle or square). In the visual detection task (C), the target was presented singly. Monkeys had to generate a targeting saccade within 500 ms. If their first saccade failed to land on target, they were given an additional 2 s to foveate the target. The dotted circle and arrow indicate current gaze position and saccade vector, respectively.

was presumably based on limited processing of the available visual information. This was further evidenced by the uniformly distributed landing positions of the erroneous first saccades made in the more difficult visual (conjunction) search task as well as by the lack of significant differences in response time between correct and incorrect trials (Shen and Paré, 2006). Such an imperfect decision process was also observed by Ludwig et al. (2005) in human subjects, whose response times were best accounted for by a temporal filter model that integrates only the earliest visual information (first 100 ms) following the search display onset. Altogether, it appears that attentional resources beyond those recruited for regulating saccades are not required when subjects are "free" to search.

Although the visual search tasks of Shen and Paré (2006) did not stress accuracy as much as in previous monkey studies, the probability that the first saccade correctly

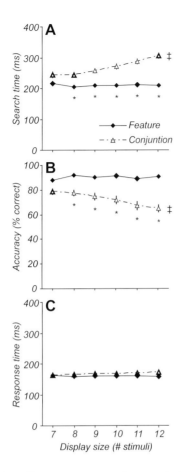

Figure 13.2. Behavioral performance across feature (solid line) and conjunction (dashed line) search tasks. Average search time (A), accuracy of the first saccade (B), and response time of correct saccades (C) are plotted as a function of display size. Data were obtained from three monkeys, each performing a total of eight conjunction search sessions (30,804 trials) and three feature search sessions (10,632 trials). Statistical differences within each task (display size effect) were assessed with one-way ANOVA tests, whereas between-task differences at each display size (task effect) were assessed with pairwise rank sum tests ($p = 0.0083$ after correction). *, significant task effect; ‡, significant display size effect. Error bars, SE.

landed on target was high (>0.80). While all the above visual search tasks involved explicit target foveation, the difference in reward contingency appears to be significant enough to promote different search strategies. Eliminating all reward contingency on saccade production (as it was done by Ipata and colleagues, in a study discussed below) may not be necessary to promote in monkeys the natural rapid and invariant responses usually observed in humans performing visual search tasks.

13.3 Visual processing during visual search

Most previous studies of saccade target selection in visual search were conducted either in saccade executive centers (FEF: Schall and Hanes, 1993; Schall et al., 1995b; Thompson et al., 1996; Bichot and Schall, 1999; SC: McPeek and Keller, 2002; Shen and Paré, 2007) or in visual cortical areas (area V4: Chelazzi et al., 2001; Mazer and Gallant, 2003; Ogawa and Komatsu, 2004, 2006; Bichot et al., 2005; area TEO: Chelazzi et al., 1993). A comprehensive understanding of saccade target selection is, however, still wanting because little is known about the selection mechanisms operating at the interface between visual and saccade processes. Thomas and Paré (2007) recently addressed this need by examining the activity of visually responsive neurons within the posterior parietal cortex of monkeys performing the unconstrained visual feature search task described above (Figure 13.1A). Specifically, single neurons were recorded in the lateral intraparietal (LIP) area, a key area in the dorsal "vision-for-action" stream, where neurons can integrate a variety of visual signals from converging inputs from visual cortical areas (Andersen et al., 1990; Baizer et al., 1991) and influence saccade production via direct projections to saccade executive centers (Paré and Wurtz, 1997; Ferraina et al., 2002). The posterior parietal cortex in general and area LIP in particular are ideally positioned to participate in the process of selecting saccade targets during visual search. Human imaging studies have provided considerable evidence in support of this hypothesis (Corbetta et al., 1993; Donner et al., 2000, 2002), and human attention studies have shown that visual search depends on the integrity of the posterior parietal cortex (Riddoch and Humphreys, 1987; Eglin et al., 1989; Arguin et al., 1993; Ashbridge et al., 1997). In the monkey, several studies using instructed delayed saccade tasks have implicated area LIP in selective visual attention (see for review Goldberg et al., 2006) and saccade planning (see for review Andersen and Buneo, 2002), two processes closely associated with visual search. Furthermore, Wardak and colleagues (2002) have reported that visual search behavior is particularly impaired when area LIP is pharmacologically inactivated. Despite this body of evidence, the contribution of LIP neuronal activity to the active process underlying saccade target selection in visual search had not been directly investigated.

To study the visual processing of multistimulus search displays in area LIP, Thomas and Paré (2007) examined the initial activation of LIP neurons while two of the monkeys studied in Shen and Paré (2006) performed a feature search task (Figure 13.1A and Figure 13.3, top), in which the target was identified by color, and a single-stimulus detection task (Figure 13.1C and Figure 13.3, bottom). With receptive fields restricted to the contralateral visual hemifield, these neurons had visually evoked responses significantly tuned with respect to target location in the detection task. In the search task, these responses were independent of whether the stimulus presented in their receptive fields was a target or a distractor (Figure 13.4A, solid symbols), suggesting that area LIP does not initially represent stimulus identity. In any given trial, the search target could be either green or red and the sensitivity to local stimulus irregularities found in visual cortical neurons (e.g. Knierim and Van Essen, 1992) could serve to locate the conspicuous stimuli in those displays. To test for feature selectivity in LIP neurons, Thomas and Paré (2007) examined whether their responses were modulated by the target color. Only 6% (3/50) neurons had some color selectivity, suggesting that

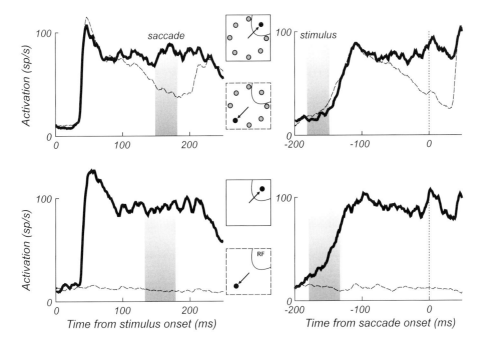

Figure 13.3. Representative LIP neuronal activity in visual feature search (top) and detection (bottom) trials, in which the target appeared in one neuron's receptive field (solid line) or in a diametrically opposite position (dashed line). Average activity of one neuron is depicted as spike density functions computed from data aligned with the presentation of the stimulus (left) or the onset of the targeting saccade (right). Spike density functions were constructed by convolving spike trains with a combination of growth (1-ms time constant) and decay (20-ms time constant) exponential functions that resembled a postsynaptic potential (see Thompson et al., 1996).

area LIP is virtually featureless. An influence of visual context was also observed, as the visually evoked responses in the search task were attenuated by 28% from what was observed in the detection task (Figure 13.4B, solid symbols). Surprisingly, this attenuation subsided until the saccade was initiated (Figure 13.4B, open symbols), even though there was no significant difference between the saccades produced in the two tasks; the changes in LIP pre-saccade activity between tasks was related neither to changes in saccade amplitude nor peak velocity. These results suggest that significant visual processing continues to take place until saccade initiation, thus questioning a direct contribution of area LIP to saccade production.

LIP neuronal activation eventually evolved to signal the presence of the search target in a neuron's receptive field in advance of correct targeting saccades: activity associated with the target became enhanced and that associated with distractors became suppressed (Figure 13.3, top). Unlike their visually evoked responses, the pre-saccade activity of LIP neurons was tuned to target location, being significantly greater in target trials compared with distractor trials (Figure 13.4A, open symbols). To estimate the

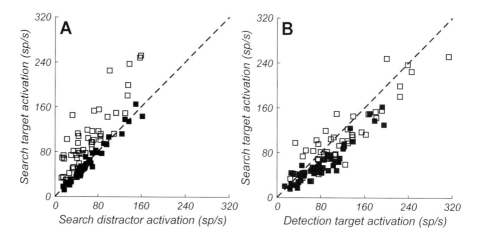

Figure 13.4. Scatterplot of LIP neuronal activation between target and distractor trials in the feature search task (A) and in target trials between feature search and detection tasks (B). Data from 50 neurons. Solid symbols: visually evoked responses (first 25 ms of significant activation after stimulus onset). Open symbols: pre-saccade activity (last 25 ms of activation before saccade initiation).

time at which LIP neuronal activity became significantly greater in target trials than in distractor trials, Thomas and Paré (2007) applied successive *rank-sum tests* on this activity starting from the onset of the search display (Figure 13.5, top). Nearly all LIP neurons (92%, 46/50) were found to have statistically significant discriminating activity before saccade initiation (Figure 13.6A). These neurons reached a significant discrimination, on average, 132 ms (range 105–180 ms) after the search display onset and 34 ms before saccade initiation.

To permit a direct comparison with previous visual search studies in FEF (Thompson et al., 1996) and SC (McPeek and Keller, 2002), Thomas and Paré (2007) also used Signal Detection Theory (Green and Swets, 1966) to determine the time course of how well an ideal observer (or postsynaptic neurons) of LIP neuronal activity can discriminate the target from distractors by estimating the separation between the distribution of activity in correct target and distractor trials from the area under receiver operating characteristic (ROC) curves (Figure 13.5, bottom). According to this *ideal observer analysis*, the probability of discriminating the target from distractor stimuli for many of these neurons grew from chance level (0.5) during the initial activation to an asymptotic magnitude that fell short of perfect discrimination (1.0), which would indicate distinctly greater activity in target trials. The discrimination magnitude of LIP neurons averaged 0.81, and it exceeded the standard criterion of 0.75 in 60% (30/50) of the neurons at a time that did not exceed the mean response time of the monkeys (Figure 13.6B). The discrimination time (DT) of these 30 neurons occurred, on average, 138 ms (range 108–170 ms) after the search display onset and 32 ms before saccade initiation (Figure 13.6C). Figure 13.6D shows that the estimate of LIP discrimination

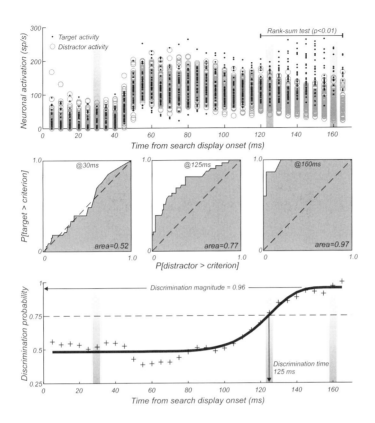

Figure 13.5. Estimation of LIP neuronal discrimination time. The activity of one neu-ron associated with target (•) and distractor (○) trials was compared every 5 ms (top) with the nonparametric *rank-sum test* to determine when the rate of activity in target trials became significantly greater ($p < 0.01$) than that in distractor trials. In the ideal observer analysis, the same activity was compared to determine the probability that the rate of neuronal activity when a target fell within the receptive field is greater than a criterion rate as a function of the probability that the rate of neuronal activity associated with distractor trials is greater than that same criterion (middle). The area under the ROC curves was then plotted (+) as a function of time (bottom) and fit with a Weibull function (solid line) to describe the time course of neural discrimination. The point at which the best-fit Weibull function reached a criterion value of 0.75 represents the *discrimination time*. Functions were calculated only with activity occurring before sac-cade initiation and terminated when there were less than five target or distractor trials; the ranges of saccade response times for the two sets of trials were matched. Dis-crimination magnitude was defined by the upper limit of the best-fit Weibull function and represents the strength of discrimination. See Thompson et al. (1996) for further details.

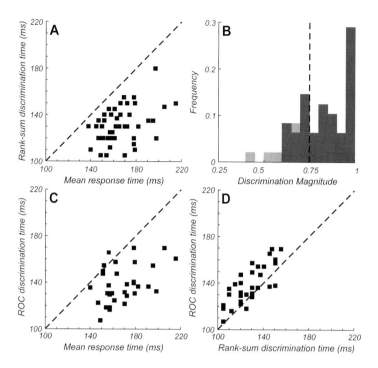

Figure 13.6. (A) Relationship between LIP discrimination time and saccade response time in visual feature search; estimate of discrimination time was obtained by determining when each neuron's activity in target trials first became significantly greater than in distractor trials with a *rank-sum test* applied on successive 5-ms intervals from the onset of the search display (n = 46). (B) Distribution of discrimination magnitude for the sample of LIP neurons (n=50), as estimated with the *ideal observer analysis* (see Figure 13.5 for details); black, statistically significant discrimination (rank-sum test, $p < 0.01$). (C) Relationship between LIP discrimination time and saccade response time in visual feature search; estimate of discrimination time was defined as when the best-fit function across the ROC curves calculated from each neuron's activity in target and distractor trials first exceeded the standard criterion of 0.75 (see Figure 13.5 for details). Data from 32 neurons, two of which showing discrimination times that lagged the mean response time. (D) Scatterplot of LIP discrimination times estimated with the ROC analysis against those estimated with the rank-sum test analysis (n = 32).

time obtained with the *ideal observer analysis* was closely related to that obtained with the *rank-sum test* ($R^2 = 0.60$), the former lagging by 11 ms on average.

The direct comparison afforded by the common *ideal observer analysis* used in the LIP, FEF and SC studies reveals that neurons across these brain regions reliably discriminate target from distractors with similar timing relative to the search display presentation (FEF: 140 ms, Thompson et al. 1996 (their Table 1); SC: 138 ms, McPeek and Keller, 2002 (exact figures graciously provided by R. M. McPeek); LIP: 138 ms) (see also Schall et al., 2007). However, FEF and SC neurons appear to discriminate in greater proportion and at earlier times with respect to saccade initiation (FEF: 78% and 53 ms; SC: 98% and 45 ms; LIP: 60% and 26 ms). These proportion and timing differences could be due to the shorter response times that were observed in the LIP study (FEF: 192 ms; SC: 189 ms; LIP: 169 ms), which could have provided insufficient time for neurons to reach criterion. Alternatively, these differences could indicate a slower, less efficient selection process in LIP. Despite these comparative differences, the finding that nearly all LIP neurons had statistically significant discriminating activity indicates that LIP neurons do have activity patterns sufficient to contribute to the active process of selecting saccade targets in visual search, albeit perhaps only in its early stage.

Previous evidence that LIP neuronal activity evolves to discriminate visual stimuli was obtained with instructed, delayed saccade tasks (Platt and Glimcher, 1997; Paré and Wurtz, 2001; Toth and Assad, 2002). The observation of Thomas and Paré (2007) that LIP activity represents all visual stimuli until a saccade goal is selected is consistent with these reports and adds to these previous investigations of area LIP by documenting the time course of this selection process during an active visual search task, in which the saccade target is specified by conspicuity. A similar time course was also reported by another recently published study (Ipata et al., 2006a) describing LIP activity in a free-viewing visual search task, which did not require foveation of the search target. In this study, two monkeys were presented with a display containing a single character – right side up ($\top$) or upside down ($\bot$) – among seven distractors (+) and they were rewarded for indicating the orientation of the unique target character by releasing a lever in either the right or left hand. Although the monkeys eventually foveated the target stimulus in the great majority of trials (88–99% per session), they correctly selected and foveated the search target with a single saccade in only 56% and 44% of the trials (Ipata et al., 2006b). This lower saccade accuracy is not surprising given that saccades were not rewarded directly, but it suggests that the process of saccade target selection was only partially or infrequently completed. Nevertheless, LIP activity evolved to signal the location of the saccade target. Unfortunately, the different analysis of LIP discrimination time used by the authors of this study does not permit a direct comparison with FEF and SC data.

Another recent publication by Buschman and Miller (2007) describes LIP neuronal activity in feature and conjunction search tasks that emphasized accuracy over speed, as in previous monkey studies. Activity from neurons in FEF and lateral prefrontal cortex was also simultaneously recorded, but the discrimination time of all neuronal samples was estimated on a neuron-by-neuron basis with a method based on Information Theory (Shannon and Weaver, 1949), instead of Signal Detection Theory. Comparison with other studies of LIP with visual search tasks as well as with the previous FEF and SC studies is thus limited. Furthermore, serious difficulties with this study have been pointed out (Schall et al., 2007). First, the very early discrimination of LIP neurons found by Buschman and Miller (approximately 50 ms after the feature search display onset) is inconsistent with the observations made by Thomas and Paré (2007) that area LIP never discriminates before at least 100 ms after the onset of the search display as well as with the general finding that the initial activation of visually responsive neurons throughout the visual and oculomotor circuits is indiscriminant (e.g. Schall and Thompson, 1999). Second, the majority of neurons in the samples of Buschman and

Miller (2007), especially in the more difficult conjunction search task, did not discriminate before the initiation of the targeting saccades. This low proportion of discriminating neurons is again inconsistent with other LIP studies (Ipata et al., 2006a; Thomas
and Paré, 2007) and it may be related to either heterogeneous sampling, because neurons were not selected on visual responsiveness, or suboptimal activation of neurons,
because the visual stimuli were not centered in their receptive fields. That these non-
discriminating neurons could contribute to behavior is certainly unlikely and to include
them in a sample is highly questionable, especially because only a minority of LIP
neurons projecting to either FEF or SC has been found to have properties unrelated to
sensory-motor processing (Paré and Wurtz, 1997; Ferraina et al., 2002). The impact
of the paper of Buschman and Miller (2007) on our understanding of the neural mechanisms underlying saccade target selection, particularly at the vision–action interface,
appears to be marginal.

13.4   Attentional processing during visual search

Covert visual attention has been suggested to underlie the process of saccade target
selection (e.g. Henderson, 1992; Schneider, 1995), and it may explain the enhanced
activation of LIP neurons observed in visual search. Attention-related enhancement
has been observed in neurons in several extrastriate areas (see for review Maunsell
and Treue, 2006) as well as in posterior parietal cortex (see for review Constantinidis,
2006; Goldberg et al., 2006). Furthermore, visual attention is easily captured by the
appearance of a salient stimulus (Yantis, 1996), such as the conspicuous target in our
feature search task, and this attentional capture has been shown to drive both covert
(Theeuwes, 1991) and overt (Theeuwes et al., 1998) selection.

   To determine the relationship between LIP neuronal selection and visual attention,
we conducted an analysis introduced by Reynolds et al. (1999) to quantify the effect of
attention on neuronal responses to multiple stimuli presented within the receptive fields
of extrastriate neurons. This analysis examines how well responses to multiple stimuli
are predicted by a weighted average of the responses to each single stimulus. The receptive fields of LIP neurons generally encompass three of the eight stimuli presented
in the visual search task. Using the results obtained in the detection trials, a neuron's
selectivity for a given stimulus (presented either in the very center of the receptive field
or in its periphery) was quantified by subtracting the neuron's responses to that stimulus from the responses elicited by the other stimulus. The impact of the additional
stimuli presented simultaneously in the search trials on a neuron's responses to each of
the stimuli considered above was then quantified by computing the interaction between
that neuron's response to the stimulus together with the other stimuli (search trials)
and that to the stimulus alone (detection trials); this was calculated by subtracting the
neuron's responses in detection trials from the responses in search trials. In this analysis, if the responses to each of the stimuli presented in a neuron's receptive field were
equally weighted during search trials, the relationship between stimulus selectivity and
interaction should be positive with a slope of 0.5. Alternatively, if a stimulus were
attended, its weight should increase (Moran and Desimone, 1985) and the selectivity
and interaction relationship have a slope greater than 0.5.

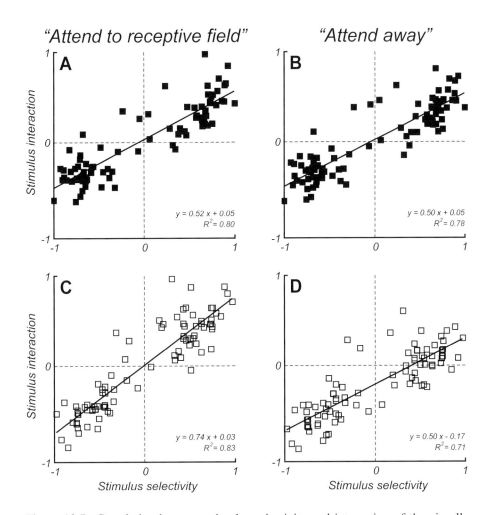

Figure 13.7. Correlation between stimulus selectivity and interaction of the visually evoked responses (A,B) and pre-saccade activity (C,D) of 50 LIP neurons for trials in which the search target appeared either within (A,C) or opposite to (B,D) the neurons' receptive fields. A neuron's selectivity for a given stimulus was quantified by subtracting the neuron's responses to that stimulus from the responses elicited by the other stimulus; this analysis considered the responses to the stimulus presented in the very center of the receptive field in detection trials and the average responses to the stimuli presented 45 degrees off that position; that is, near the margin of the receptive field. The interaction between a neuron's responses to each stimulus presented alone in detection trials and its responses to the combined presentation of the stimuli in search trials was quantified by subtracting the neuron's responses in detection trials from the responses in search trials. Each neuron's responses were normalized by dividing them by the highest discharge rate observed for that neuron in any of the conditions.

Figure 13.7 shows the results of our analysis of the LIP neurons recorded by Thomas and Paré (2007) during visual search. Linear regressions between stimulus selectivity and interaction of LIP neurons computed from their initial visually evoked responses (Figure 13.7A, B) showed significant correlations with slopes near 0.5 and intercepts near zero ($R^2 > 0.77$, $p < 0.001$). This was true whether we considered search trials in which the target stimulus was presented within the neuron's receptive field (Figure 13.7A) – when visual attention would have been directed toward it – or at the diametrically opposite position (Figure 13.7B) – when visual attention would then have been directed away. We conclude from these results that the initial LIP responses to the stimuli are averaged with equal weight during visual search, a finding consistent with the observation that these responses do not discriminate stimulus identity (cf. Figure 13.4A, solid symbols).

When we considered the pre-saccade activity of the same LIP neurons, the slope of the linear fit between stimulus selectivity and interaction was 0.74 ($R^2 = 0.83$, $p < 0.001$), which was significantly greater than 0.5 (t-test, $p < 0.001$). This relationship was observed when the search target stimulus fell in the neuron's receptive field (Figure 13.7C), as if the overall neuronal responses were driven toward the responses associated with the appearance of the target stimulus alone. Most interestingly, the weight of this stimulus in driving the neuronal responses to the search display (given by the relationship's slope) was increased by as much as that observed in V4 neurons with voluntary shifts in covert visual attention (Reynolds et al., 1999), thereby suggesting that the enhancement of the LIP representation of the search target is also driven by covert attention. When the search target stimulus fell outside the neuron's receptive field (Figure 13.7D) – and attention was presumably directed away from that receptive field – the slope of the linear fit between stimulus selectivity and interaction was 0.5 ($R^2 = 0.71$, $p < 0.001$), indicating that stimuli exerted approximately equal influence over the responses in visual search. However, the large and significantly less than zero (t-test, $p < 0.001$) intercept of this regression reveals that the simultaneous presence of stimuli within the receptive field caused a reduction in mean response, indicating that the LIP representations of these distractor stimuli were suppressed. Altogether, these findings suggest that the modulation of the interaction between multiple stimulus representations prescribed by the "biased-competition model" of attention (Desimone and Duncan, 1995) is a plausible mechanism underlying saccade target selection within area LIP.

13.5   Saccade processing during visual search

Even though the latency of the first saccades made by monkeys during unconstrained visual search appears independent of the search difficulty (Shen and Paré, 2006), it shows a trial-by-trial variability within a given search task. Such response variability has long been attributed to decision processes (see for review Smith and Ratcliff, 2004) whose nature is still being investigated. The temporal relationship between the discriminating activity of LIP neurons and saccade initiation can address this issue and shed light on the nature of the processing occurring within this cortical area. On the one hand, LIP discriminating activity could be involved in the decision about both where

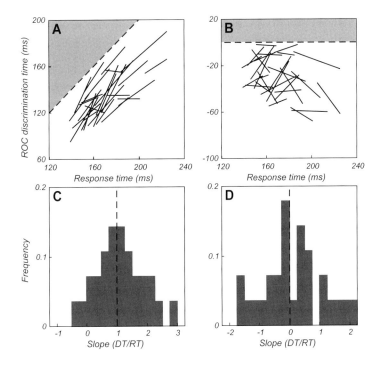

Figure 13.8. Plots of LIP discrimination times of short and long response time groups for activity aligned on stimulus onset (A) and saccade onset (B); shaded areas indicate time after saccade initiation. Distribution of the slopes of the relationships between ROC discrimination times and response times for activity aligned on stimulus onset (C) and saccade onset (D). Data are from neurons with discrimination magnitude exceeding 0.75 in both response time groups ($n = 28$).

and when to make a saccade, in which case it would be closely related to the programming of the saccade and thus correlated with saccade initiation. On the other hand, it could strictly signal where (not when) to make a saccade, in which case it would occur irrespective of saccade initiation and perhaps reflect the aforementioned attentional process hypothesized to underlie the selection of the search target.

To test these alternatives, Thomas and Paré (2007) segregated their visual search trials into two equal-sized groups according to their response times (RT) and computed the discrimination time (DT) separately for short and long RT group (Figure 13.8A, B). The slope of the curve connecting each paired DT/RT value was then used to quantify the relationship between these two variables (Figure 13.8C, D). When the neural data were aligned on the search display onset, the distribution of these DT/RT slopes was unimodal and not significantly different from unity (Figure 13.8C) but it was significantly different from zero. Consistent with LIP discriminating activity predicting saccade initiation, the distribution of DT/RT slopes calculated from neural data aligned on the time of saccade initiation (Figure 13.8D) was not significantly different from zero, but it was significantly different from unity.

Previous studies reported bimodal distributions of DT/RT slopes in FEF (Thompson et al., 1996; Sato and Schall, 2003) and SC (McPeek and Keller, 2002), which were interpreted as evidence that the selection of the search target (invariant DT) and targeting saccade (DT predictive of RT) are instantiated by distinct populations of neurons. The neuronal sample of Thomas and Paré (2007) is presumably composed of infragranular pyramidal neurons, because their recordings were largely confined to regions within the lateral bank of the intraparietal sulcus at which LIP neurons were antidromically activated by SC stimulation (Paré and Wurtz, 1997). Since these neurons preferentially project to SC (Ferraina et al., 2002) and that many SC neurons have DT/RT slopes close to unity (McPeek and Keller, 2002), it may not be surprising that LIP discriminating activity shows a similar relationship with saccade initiation. This hypothesis is, however, at odds with the finding of Paré and Wurtz (1997, 2001) that LIP neurons projecting to the SC do not have functionally distinct properties that are shared with SC neurons. The same prediction should apply to FEF, but the results in the FEF studies are in disagreement (Thompson et al., 1996; Sato and Schall, 2003). Interestingly, Thompson and Schall (2000) reported that the majority of anatomically localized FEF neurons from the sample of neurons studied by Thompson et al. (1996) were supragranular pyramidal neurons potentially providing feedback to visual cortical areas. The higher proportion of corticocortical neurons recorded in the FEF studies could thus explain why this cortical area appeared predominantly involved in a visual selection process in contrast to area LIP, which appears more concerned with the selection of the targeting saccade perhaps because corticofugal neurons were primarily recorded in this area.

Ipata et al. (2006a) obtained similar results to Thomas and Paré (2007), thereby providing additional support for the hypothesis that the role of area LIP in active visual search is limited to the selection of saccades. This hypothesis is, however, difficult to reconcile with previous findings that LIP activity discriminates visual stimuli substantially in advance of saccade initiation in instructed, delayed saccade tasks (Platt and Glimcher, 1997; Paré and Wurtz, 2001; Toth and Assad, 2002). Instead, the dependence of LIP pre-saccade activity on the presence of additional stimuli within the search array suggests that LIP neuronal activity reflects both visual and saccade processing during visual search. The difference between visual search tasks may explain why the results obtained in the FEF (and SC) studies were not replicated in the studies of Thomas and Paré (2007) and Ipata et al. (2006a), whose "free-viewing" task did not emphasize accuracy over speed. It is our contention that visual and saccade selection processes are not distinguishable in natural situations, in which saccades are not associated directly with a reward or punishment. This hypothesis is consistent with the idea that the selective deployment of visual attention is not temporally distinct from the selection of the next saccade during free-viewing behavior.

13.6   Conclusion

We reviewed recent neurophysiological evidence that the process of selecting a saccade target involves neurons within the dorsal "vision-for-action" processing stream of the cerebral cortex of monkeys when they "freely" search for a visual target among distractor stimuli. The initial visual responses of these posterior parietal cortex neurons are neither feature selective nor do they represent whether a stimulus will later be selected, but their activity evolves to reflect this selection process as well as to predict when the targeting saccade is initiated. These results suggest that, during natural visual behavior, visual attention is shifted concomitantly with saccade planning. Consistent with this hypothesis, the enhancement of parietal activity in advance of a search saccade parallels what has been observed in neurons within the ventral "object-recognition" pathway when attention is covertly allocated.

Acknowledgments

The Canadian Institutes of Health Research, the EJLB Foundation, and the J. P. Bickell Foundation supported this work. M. P. was supported by a New Investigator Award from the Canadian Institutes of Health Research and an Early Researcher Award from the Ontario Ministry of Research and Innovation. K. Shen was supported by an Ontario Graduate Scholarship and a postgraduate scholarship from the Natural Sciences and Engineering Council of Canada.

References

Allport, A. (1987). Selection for action: some behavioral and neurophysiological considerations of attention and action. In H. Heuer and A. Sanders (eds.) *Perspectives on Perception and Action*. Hillsdale, NJ: Laurence Erlbaum, pp. 395–419.

Andersen, R. A., Asanuma, C., Essick, G. and Siegel, R. M. (1990). Corticocortical connections of anatomically and physiologically defined subdivisions within the inferior parietal lobule. *J. Comp. Neurol.*, 296: 65–113.

Andersen, R. A. and Buneo, C. A. (2002) Intentional maps in posterior parietal cortex. *Ann. Rev. Neurosci.*, 25: 189–220.

Arguin, M., Joanette, Y. and Cavanagh, P. (1993). Visual search for feature and conjunction targets with an attention deficit. *J. Cogn. Neurosci.*, 5: 436–452.

Ashbridge, E., Walsh, V. and Cowey, A. (1997). Temporal aspects of visual search studied by transcranial magnetic stimulation. *Neuropsychologia*, 35: 1121–1131.

Awh, E., Armstrong, K. M. and Moore, T. (2006). Visual and oculomotor selection: links, causes and implications for spatial attention. *Trends Cogn. Sci.*, 10: 124–130.

Baizer, J. S., Ungerleider, L. G. and Desimone, R. (1991). Organization of visual inputs to the inferior temporal and posterior parietal cortex in macaques. *J. Neurosci.*, 11: 168–190.

Bichot, N. P. and Schall, J. D. (1999). Saccade target selection in macaque during feature and conjunction visual search. *Visual Neurosci.*, 16: 81–89.

Bichot, N. P., Rossi, A. F. and Desimone, R. (2005). Parallel and serial neural mechanisms for visual search in macaque area V4. *Science*, 308: 529–534.

Binello, A., Mannan, S. and Ruddock, K. H. (1995). The characteristics of eye movements made during visual search with multi-element stimuli. *Spatial Vis.*, 9: 343–362.

Buracas, G. T. and Albright, T. D. (1999). Covert visual search: a comparison of performance by humans and macaques (macaca mulatta). *Behav. Neurosci.*, 113: 451–464.

Buschman, T. J. and Miller, E. K. (2007). Top-down versus bottom-up control of attention in the prefrontal and posterior parietal cortices. *Science*, 315: 1860–1862.

Chelazzi, L., Miller, E. K., Duncan, J. and Desimone, R. (1993). A neural basis for visual search in inferior temporal cortex. *Nature*, 363: 345–347.

Chelazzi, L., Miller, E. K., Duncan, J. and Desimone, R. (2001). Responses of neurons in macaque area V4 during memory-guided visual search. *Cereb. Cortex*, 11: 761–772.

Constantinidis, C. (2006). Posterior parietal mechanisms of visual attention. *Rev. Neurosci.*, 17: 415–427.

Corbetta, M., Akbudak, E., Conturo, T. E., Snyder, A. Z., Ollinger, J. M., Drury, H. A., Linenweber, M. R., Petersen, S. E., Raichle, M. E., Van Essen, D. C. and Shulman, G. L. (1998). A common network of functional areas for attention and eye movements. *Neuron*, 21: 761–773.

Corbetta, M., Miezin, F. M., Shulman, G. L. and Petersen, S. E. (1993). A PET study of visuospatial attention. *J. Neurosci.*, 13: 1202–1226.

Desimone, R. and Duncan, J. (1995). Neural mechanisms of selective visual attention. *Ann. Rev. Neurosci.*, 18: 193–222.

Deubel, H. and Schneider, W. X. (1996). Saccade target selection and object recognition: evidence for a common attentional mechanism. *Vision Res.*, 36: 1827–1837.

Donner, T., Kettermann, A., Diesch, E., Ostendorf, F., Villringer, A. and Brandt, S. A. (2000). Involvement of the human frontal eye field and multiple parietal areas in covert visual selection during conjunction search. *Eur. J. Neurosci.*, 12: 3407–3414.

Donner, T. H., Kettermann, A., Diesch, E., Ostendorf, F., Villringer, A. and Brandt, S. A. (2002). Visual feature and conjunction searches of equal difficulty engage only partially overlapping frontoparietal networks. *NeuroImage*, 15: 16–25.

Eglin, M., Roberson, L. and Knight, R. (1989). Visual search performance in the neglect syndrome. *J. Cogn. Neurosci.*, 1: 372–385.

Ferraina, S., Paré, M. and Wurtz, R. H. (2002). Comparison of cortico-cortical and cortico-collicular signals for the generation of saccadic eye movements. *J. Neurophysiol.*, 87: 845–858.

Findlay, J. M. (1997) Saccade target selection during visual search. *Vision Res.*, 37: 617–631.

Findlay, J. M. and Gilchrist, I. D. (2003). *Active Vision: The Psychology of Looking and Seeing*, New York, NY: Oxford University Press.

Goldberg, M. E., Bisley, J. W., Powell, K. D. and Gottlieb, J. (2006). Saccades, salience and attention: the role of the lateral intraparietal area in visual behavior. *Prog. Brain Res.*, 155: 157–175.

Green, D. M. and Swets, J. A. (1966). *Signal Detection Theory and Psychophysics.* New York, NY: Wiley.

Henderson, J. (1992). Visual attention and eye movement control during reading and picture viewing. In K. Rayner (ed.) *Eye Movements and Visual Cognition.* Berlin: Springer, pp. 261–283.

Hoffman, J. E. and Subramaniam, B. (1995). The role of visual attention in saccadic eye movements. *Percept. Psychophys.*, 57: 787–795.

Ipata, A. E., Gee, A. L., Goldberg, M. E. and Bisley, J. W. (2006a). Activity in the lateral intraparietal area predicts the goal and latency of saccades in a free-viewing visual search task. *J. Neurosci.*, 26: 3656–3661.

Ipata, A. E., Gee, A. L., Gottlieb, J., Bisley, J. W. and Goldberg, M. E. (2006b). LIP responses to a popout stimulus are reduced if it is overtly ignored. *Nature Neurosci.*, 9: 1071–1076.

Jonides, J., Naveh-Benjamin, M. and Palmer, J. (1985). Assessing automaticity. *Acta Psychologica*, 60: 157–171.

Knierim, J. J. and Van Essen, D. C. (1992). Neuronal responses to static texture patterns in area V1 of the alert macaque monkey. *J. Neurophysiol.*, 67: 961–980.

Kowler, E., Anderson, E., Dosher, B. and Blaser, E. (1995). The role of attention in the programming of saccades. *Vision Res.*, 35: 1897–1916.

LaBerge, D. and Brown, V. (1989). Theory of attentional operations in shape identification. *Psycholog. Rev.*, 96: 101–124.

Ludwig, C. J., Gilchrist, I. D., McSorley, E. and Baddeley, R. J. (2005). The temporal impulse response underlying saccadic decisions. *J. Neurosci.*, 25: 9907–9912.

Maioli, C., Benaglio, I., Siri, S., Sosta. K. and Cappa, S. (2001). The integration of parallel and serial processing mechanisms in visual search: evidence from eye movement recording. *Eur. J. Neurosci.*, 13: 364–372.

Maunsell, J. H. and Treue, S. (2006). Feature-based attention in visual cortex. *Trends Neurosci.*, 29: 317–322.

Mazer, J. A. and Gallant, J. L. (2003). Goal-related activity in V4 during free viewing visual search: evidence for a ventral stream visual salience map. *Neuron*, 40: 1241–1250.

McPeek, R. M. and Keller, E. L. (2002). Saccade target selection in the superior colliculus during a visual search task. *J. Neurophysiol.*, 88: 2019–2034.

Moore, T. (2006) The neurobiology of visual attention: Finding sources. *Curr. Opin. Neurobiol.*, 16: 159–165.

Moore, T., Armstrong, K. M. and Fallah, M. (2003). Visuomotor origins of covert spatial attention. *Neuron*, 40: 671–683.

Moran, J. and Desimone, R. (1985). Selective attention gates visual processing in the extrastriate cortex. *Science*, 229: 782–784.

Motter, B. C. and Belky, E. J. (1998). The zone of focal attention during active visual search. *Vision Res.*, 38: 1007–1022.

Murthy, A., Thompson, K. G. and Schall, J. D. (2001). Dynamic dissociation of visual selection from saccade programming in frontal eye field. *J. Neurophysiol.*, 86: 2634–2637.

Nobre, A. C., Sebestyen, G. N., Gitelman, D. R., Mesulam, M. M., Frackowiak, R. S. and Frith, C. D. (1997). Functional localization of the system for visuospatial attention using positron emission tomography. *Brain*, 120: 515–533.

Ogawa, T. and Komatsu, H. (2004). Target selection in area V4 during a multidimensional visual search task. *J. Neurosci.*, 24: 6371–6382.

Ogawa, T. and Komatsu, H. (2006). Neuronal dynamics of bottom-up and top-down processes in area V4 of macaque monkeys performing a visual search. *Exp. Brain Res.*, 173: 1–13.

Paré, M. and Wurtz, R. H. (1997). Monkey posterior parietal cortex neurons antidromically activated from superior colliculus. *J. Neurophysiol.*, 78: 3493–3497.

Paré, M. and Wurtz, R. H. (2001). Progression in neuronal processing for saccadic eye movements from parietal cortex area lip to superior colliculus. *J. Neurophysiol.*, 85: 2545–2562.

Platt, M. L. and Glimcher, P. W. (1997). Responses of intraparietal neurons to saccadic targets and visual distractors. *J. Neurophysiol.*, 78: 1574–1589.

Reynolds, J. H., Chelazzi, L. and Desimone, R. (1999). Competitive mechanisms subserve attention in macaque areas V2 and V4. *J. Neurosci.*, 19: 1736–1753.

Riddoch, M. J. and Humphreys, G. W. (1987). A case of integrative visual agnosia. *Brain*, 110: 1431–1462.

Sato, T., Murthy, A., Thompson, K. G. and Schall, J. D. (2001). Search efficiency but not response interference affects visual selection in frontal eye field. *Neuron*, 30: 583–591.

Sato, T. R. and Schall, J. D. (2003). Effects of stimulus-response compatibility on neural selection in frontal eye field. *Neuron*, 38: 637–648.

Schall, J. D. and Hanes, D. P. (1993). Neural basis of saccade target selection in frontal eye field during visual search. *Nature*, 366: 467–469.

Schall, J. D. and Thompson, K. G. (1999). Neural selection and control of visually guided eye movements. *Ann. Rev. Neurosci.*, 22: 241–259.

Schall, J. D., Morel, A., King, D. J. and Bullier, J. (1995a). Topography of visual cortex connections with frontal eye field in macaque: convergence and segregation of processing streams. *J. Neurosci.*, 15: 4464–4487.

Schall, J. D., Hanes, D. P., Thompson, K. G. and King, D. J. (1995b). Saccade target selection in frontal eye field of macaque. I. Visual and premovement activation. *J. Neurosci.*, 15: 6905–6918.

Schall, J. D., Paré, M. and Woodman, G. F. (2007). Comment on "top-down versus bottom-up control of attention in the prefrontal and posterior parietal cortices". *Science*, 318: 44a-b.

Schneider, W. (1995). VAM: a neuro-cognitive model for visual attention control of segmentation, object recognition and space-based motor action. *Visual Cogn.*, 2: 331–376.

Scialfa, C. T. and Joffe, K. M. (1998). Response times and eye movements in feature and conjunction search as a function of target eccentricity. *Percept. Psychophys.*, 60: 1067–1082.

Shannon, C. and Weaver, W. (1949). *The Mathematical Theory of Communication.* Urbana, IL: University of Illinois.

Shen, K. and Paré, M. (2006). Guidance of eye movements during visual conjunction search: local and global contextual effects on target discriminability. *J. Neurophysiol.*, 95: 2845–2855.

Shen, K. and Paré, M. (2007). Neuronal activity in superior colliculus signals both stimulus identity and saccade goals during visual conjunction search. *J. Vision*, 7: 15, 1–13.

Smith, P. L. and Ratcliff, R. (2004). Psychology and neurobiology of simple decisions. *Trends Neurosci.*, 27: 161–168.

Sperling, G. and Melchner, M. J. (1978). The attention operating characteristic: examples from visual search. *Science*, 202: 315–318.

Theeuwes, J. (1991). Exogenous and endogenous control of attention: the effect of visual onsets and offsets. *Percept. Psychophys.*, 49: 83–90.

Theeuwes, J., Kramer, A., Hahn, S. and Irwin, D. (1998). Our eyes do not always go where we want them to go: capture of the eyes by new objects. *Psycholog. Sci.*, 9: 379–395.

Theios, J. (1975). The components of response latency in simple human information processing tasks. In P. Rabbitt and S. Dornic (eds.) *Attention and Performance V.* London: Academic Press, pp. 418–440.

Thomas, N. W. D. and Paré, M. (2007). Temporal processing of saccade targets in parietal cortex area LIP during visual search. *J. Neurophysiol.*, 97: 942–947.

Thompson, K. G. and Schall, J. D. (2000). Antecedents and correlates of visual detection and awareness in macaque prefrontal cortex. *Vision Res.*, 40: 1523–1538.

Thompson, K. G., Bichot, N. P. and Schall, J. D. (1997). Dissociation of visual discrimination from saccade programming in macaque frontal eye field. *J. Neurophysiol.*, 77. 1046–1030.

Thompson, K. G., Bichot, N. P. and Sato, T. R. (2005a). Frontal eye field activity before visual search errors reveals the integration of bottom-up and top-down salience. *J. Neurophysiol.*, 93: 337–351.

Thompson, K. G., Biscoe, K. L. and Sato, T. R. (2005b). Neuronal basis of covert spatial attention in the frontal eye field. *J. Neurosci.*, 25: 9479–9487.

Thompson, K. G., Hanes, D. P., Bichot, N. P. and Schall, J. D. (1996). Perceptual and motor processing stages identified in the activity of macaque frontal eye field neurons during visual search. *J. Neurophysiol.*, 76: 4040–4055.

Toth, L. J. and Assad, J. A. (2002). Dynamic coding of behaviourally relevant stimuli in parietal cortex. *Nature*, 415: 165-168.

Treisman, A. M. and Gelade, G. (1980). A feature-integration theory of attention. *Cogn. Psychol.*, 12: 97–136.

Wardak, C., Olivier, E. and Duhamel, J. R. (2002). Saccadic target selection deficits after lateral intraparietal area inactivation in monkeys. *J. Neurosci.*, 22: 9877–9884.

Williams, D. E., Reingold, E. M., Moscovitch, M. and Behrmann, M. (1997). Patterns of eye movements during parallel and serial visual search tasks. *Can. J. Exp. Psychol.*, 51: 151–164.

Wolfe, J. M. and Horowitz, T. S. (2004). What attributes guide the deployment of visual attention and how do they do it? *Nature Rev. Neurosci.*, 5: 1–7.

Yantis, S. (1996). Attentional capture in vision. In A. Kramer A, M. Coles and G. Logan (eds.) *Converging Operations in the Study of Selective Visual Attention*. Washington, DC: American Psychological Association, pp. 45–76.

Zelinsky, G. and Sheinberg, D. (1995). Why some search tasks take longer than others: using eye movements to redefine reaction times. In J. M. Findlay, R. Walker and R. W. Kentridge (eds.) *Eye Movement Research: Mechanisms, Processes and Applications*. New York, NY: Elsevier, pp. 325–336.

14 Oculomotor control of spatial attention

M. Fallah and H. Jordan

14.1 Introduction

Something that abruptly appears or disappears in the environment might be the hall-mark of a predator to be wary of, or prey to capture for one's own benefit. When something unexpected occurs in your surroundings, selective attention is automatically oriented to the region, initiating a cascade of processing designed to determine as quickly as possible, whether it should have consequences for future behavior. Alternatively, attention can be voluntarily directed to a location. Commonly, attention and eye movements are oriented to the same location, bringing the image of the event onto the fovea, the region of the retina with highest acuity. However, the eyes can be held at one location, while still allowing (covert) attentional allocation to a different spatial location. This can be much to the chagrin of many school children as their teacher watches them "from the corner of her eye."

Although covert orienting is not visible to the observer, the benefits of spatial attention allocation an external event are seen behaviorally, in the form of faster or more accurate processing of visual stimuli at the attended location (Posner et al., 1978, 1980; Posner, 1980; Jonides, 1981). Valid cues result in facilitation, or a benefit in performance, at the attended location. Invalid cues result in a cost, or impaired performance, at unattended locations. Spatial attention allocation results in preferential processing of visual stimuli at the attended location in the visual field (Posner et al., 1978, 1980; Posner, 1980; Jonides, 1981) and modulates the responses of neurons in the visual system whose receptive fields coincide with the attended location in the visual field (Moran and Desimone, 1988; Spitzer et al., 1988; Luck et al., 1997; Reynolds et al., 1999; Ress et al., 2000). The focus of this chapter is elucidating the mechanism that deploys spatial attention.

Cortical Mechanisms of Vision, ed. M. Jenkin and L. R. Harris. Published by Cambridge University Press.
© Cambridge University Press 2009.

14.2   Spatial attention

In the laboratory, studies of the deployment of spatial attention use one of two strategies to direct attention to a particular location: endogenous and exogenous cueing (Jonides, 1981). Spatial attention can be automatically drawn to the location of an external peripheral event, such as the onset of a visual stimulus or an abrupt luminance change in a currently presented stimulus. This is described as an exogenous cue capturing spatial attention (Posner, 1980). In contrast to automatic capture by exogenous cues, spatial attention can be intentionally allocated to a region under volitional control. Endogenous cueing is induced by a stimulus which indicates the probable location of the subsequent target to the participant. Commonly in the laboratory, the endogenous cue is a central symbolic cue, such as an arrow presented at the fixation point, which directs attention to the probable location of the target (Posner, 1980; Posner et al., 1980; Jonides, 1981). An endogenous cue does not have to be predictive. When the fixation point is a representation of a face, a shift of the eyes to a possible target location directs spatial attention along the line of gaze (Driver et al., 1999; Hietanen, 1999; Langton and Bruce, 1999). From an evolutionary standpoint, this may provide a social benefit as the ability to orient to nonverbal signals would benefit personal and group survival.

14.3   Control of spatial attention

Imaging studies have shown a network of cortical areas that are active during the allocation of spatial attention, which include the frontal lobe and posterior parietal cortex (Corbetta et al., 1998, 2000; Coull and Nobre, 1998; Perry and Zeki, 2000; Hopfinger et al., 2000). The network of frontoparietal areas that are activated with covert shifts of spatial attention involves the precentral sulcus, including the frontal eye fields (FEF) and the dorsolateral prefrontal cortex (DLPFC), and the posterior parietal cortex, including the lateral intraparietal sulcus (LIP). One common feature of these areas is that they have individually been implicated in the control of eye movements. In fact, the same fMRI activation pattern is seen in the frontal eye fields regardless of whether the subjects orient attention towards the target in association with (overt) or without (covert) eye movements (Corbetta et al, 1998). This observation is not altogether surprising – there is an important functional relationship between attention and eye movements. In general, when you attend to a target, you generally also perform an eye movement, to bring the image of the attended region onto the fovea. However it is possible to deploy attention in the absence of an eye movement. Given the close functional relationship between these systems, it makes sense that there is some overlap in the cortical areas that are involved in deploying spatial attention and eye movements. While these studies demonstrate a correlation in activity between spatial attention mechanisms and structures which are responsible for oculomotor behavior, they do not have the ability to identify the nature of this relationship.

Attention certainly affects eye movements. When you attend to a target, you normally follow that up with an eye movement, although you can suppress the gaze shift if you wish. Visual stimuli that capture spatial attention also decrease the latency of eye movements to their locations (Shepherd et al., 1986; Theeuwes et al., 1999). This suggests that spatial attention can prime eye movements. Conversely, eye movements affect spatial attention. Spatial attention is deployed to the target location of a saccade prior to the initiation of the saccade (Hoffman and Subramaniam, 1995; Deubel and Schneider, 1996), even when the participant is instructed to attend to a different location (Hoffman and Subramaniam, 1995). In fact, just planning a saccade shifts attention to that spatial location (Posner, 1980; Posner et al., 1982; Shepherd et al., 1986; Rafal et al., 1989; Sheliga et al., 1994). These findings show that attention is automatically deployed to the spatial location of an eye movement prior to the eye movement, regardless of whether the saccade is carried out. It is impossible to make an eye movement without a preceding shift of spatial attention.

There are two main classes of theories which describe the relationship between spatial attention and the oculomotor system. The first category is characterized by the assumption that there is a division between sensory and motor functions in the brain, and that spatial attention mechanisms are separate from the oculomotor system (e.g. Remington, 1980; Klein and Pontefract, 1994; Hoffman and Subramaniam, 1995). This approach conceptualizes spatial attention as a sensory phenomenon, purely involving preferential processing of sensory stimuli. Only after attention has influenced processing, sensory information is fed forward into the motor system. This contrasts with the other class of theories which suggest that the oculomotor system plays a causal role in deploying spatial attention (Rizzolatti et al., 1987, 1988; Moore and Fallah, 2001, 2004). These theories postulate that a motor plan, that is, the intention to perform an eye movement, results in preferential sensory processing at the gaze endpoint, either because the target of the movement is now behaviorally relevant or to better guide the movement.

The second oculomotor approach has gained increasing support as motor areas are being shown to have cognitive properties, suggesting a continuum between purely sensory areas and motor output. Because attention precedes a saccadic eye movement, it is possible that covert shifts of attention are oculomotor plans for saccadic eye movements that are just not carried out. Consistent with this hypothesis, shifts of spatial attention have metrics similar to that of actual saccadic eye movements. The velocity and duration of spatial attention shifts are similar to the velocity and duration of eye movements of the same amplitude (Duncan et al., 1994; Crowe et al., 2000).

Further evidence comes from studies of saccade trajectories during covert orienting of spatial attention. It has been shown that during attentional fixation, saccades electrically evoked from the frontal eye fields are reduced in amplitude and velocity (Goldberg et al., 1986). Therefore, it appears that attending to the fixation point results in suppression of the oculomotor system. Actively attending to the fixation point suggests that the monkey is not allocating attention to a peripheral location. Thus, the reduction in the evoked saccade could be due to a bias towards the attended location, in this case, the fixation point. Supporting this hypothesis, another study showed that when human subjects are cued to covertly attend to a location in the visual field while making a voluntary saccade orthogonal to their attention, the saccade deviates away from the location of spatial attention (Sheliga et al., 1995). Covert orienting of spatial attention affected the oculomotor plans.

The effect of spatial attention on eye movements is even greater when the saccades are electrically evoked. When monkeys attend to a location in the visual field, and a saccadic eye movement is evoked by electrical stimulation of the superior colliculus, the actual saccade produced is an average of a saccade to the attended location and the saccade that would have been evoked by stimulation alone (Kustov and Robinson, 1996). These studies suggest that spatial attention and oculomotor mechanisms share a common neural basis. Imaging studies have corroborated this idea, showing that covert orientation of spatial attention has the same activation pattern as oculomotor planning (Corbetta et al., 1998; Coull and Nobre, 1998).

But the question of the functional relationship between spatial attention and eye movements remains. One proposal is that spatial attention is a separate mechanism that can drive the oculomotor system, predisposing it to eye movements towards the attended location (e.g. Remington, 1980; Hoffman and Subramaniam, 1995; Kustov and Robinson, 1996). An alternative explanation is that the oculomotor system drives the spatial attention mechanisms (e.g. Klein, 1980; Shepherd et al., 1986; Rizzolatti et al.,1987). A third explanation is that the two systems share a common neural basis, in which case both of the other two explanations would be true.

14.4   Frontal eye fields (FEF)

Ferrier discovered the frontal eye fields in 1874. When he electrically stimulated a region of the frontal lobe, the monkey made saccades into the contralateral visual field. Thus, FEF plays a role in initiating eye movements. However, the frontal eye fields are not necessary for producing saccades. In the brainstem, the brainstem saccade generator controls the oculomotor muscles that produce eye movements. Several oculomotor areas can initiate saccades.

The areas and connections of the oculomotor system are depicted in Figure 14.1. The brainstem saccade generator produces eye movements. Saccadic eye movements are probably controlled by the superior colliculus (SC) sending signals to the brainstem saccade generator. These oculomotor plans either originate in the superior colliculus itself, or in the cortical oculomotor areas that connect to the superior colliculus. Both the frontal eye fields and the lateral intraparietal area have reciprocal connections with the superior colliculus and with each other. Both of these cortical areas evoke saccades when electrically stimulated.

14.5   Anatomy of the frontal eye fields

The frontal eye field is a cortical region in the anterior bank of the arcuate sulcus extending over the prearcuate cortical surface, as illustrated in Figure 14.2. FEF is not well defined by architecture as it crosses Brodmann's areas 6 and 8. Rather, it is delineated by saccade-related functional properties, with electrical stimulation of FEF eliciting eye movements (Bruce and Goldberg, 1985). The cortical areas around FEF have rather different functional properties. Premotor cortex, posterior to FEF, has both

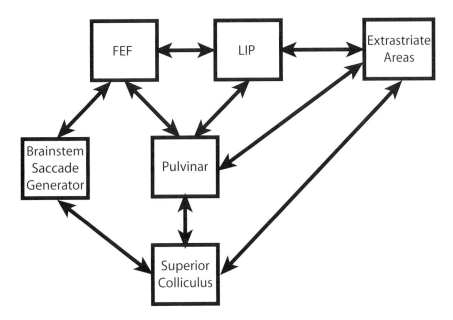

Figure 14.1. Depiction of oculomotor circuitry. The saccade generator in the brainstem controls the oculomotor muscles. The superior colliculus and the frontal eye fields can directly program these saccades. Other cortical areas can affect the oculomotor plans and be affected by them via reciprocal connections.

tactile receptive fields and limb motor responses, and bimodal visual-tactile responses are observed in the region posterior to the fundus of the arcuate sulcus (Graziano and Gandhi, 2000). Neurons in the principal sulcus, anterior to FEF, have visual properties and are involved in spatial working memory but lesions of the area do not affect the metrics of saccades (Funahashi et al., 1993). Furthermore, stimulation of neurons in the principal sulcus does not evoke eye movements.

FEF has widespread reciprocal connections to many cortical areas. As shown in Figure 14.1, FEF is directly connected with the brainstem saccade generator and reciprocally connected with the superior colliculus (Sommer and Wurtz, 2000). The arrows in Figure 14.3 show connections possibly relevant to the role of FEF neurons in spatial attention. FEF is reciprocally connected with posterior visual areas (Huerta et al., 1987) and the effects of spatial attention are observed in these posterior visual areas. Neurons in these areas show changes in response rates and selectivity, when attention is allocated towards or away from their receptive fields (Moran and Desimone, 1985; Richmond and Sato, 1987; Spitzer et al., 1988; Luck et al., 1997; McAdams and Maunsell, 1999, 2000; Reynolds et al., 1999; Seidemann and Newsome, 1999; Treue and Maunsell, 1996, 1999; Recanzone and Wurtz, 2000; Yeshurun and Carrasco, 2000). Therefore, if FEF is involved in allocating spatial attention, the connections from FEF to the posterior visual areas could directly modulate neurons in those visual areas.

FEF is also reciprocally connected with the parietal lobe (Huerta et al., 1987). Posterior parietal cortex is involved in spatial representations (Gross and Graziano, 1995)

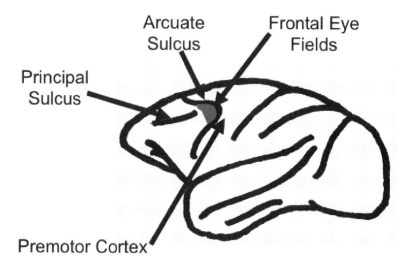

Figure 14.2. Location of FEF in the primate brain. FEF lies on the anterior bank of the arcuate sulcus. It is posterior to the principal sulcus and anterior to premotor cortex.

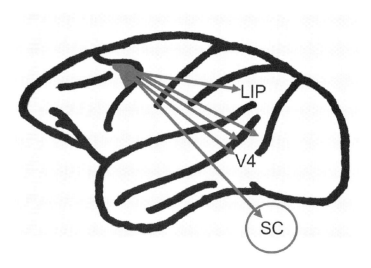

Figure 14.3. FEF projections. Arrows represent connections possibly relevant to the role of FEF neurons in spatial attention. FEF is reciprocally connected with posterior visual areas, such as area V4 whose neurons show the effects of spatial attention.

and damage results in a variety of spatial and attentional deficits, including neglect and extinction (Weinstein and Friedland, 1977; Lynch and McLaren, 1989; Làdavas et al., 1998; Vuilleumier and Rafal, 2000). Furthermore, right parietal damage patients are impaired in deploying spatial attention to the contralesional hemifield (Posner et al., 1982).

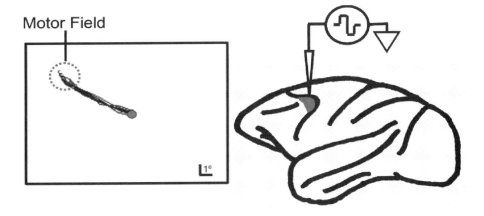

Figure 14.4. Motor field of an FEF site. When an FEF site is stimulated suprathreshold, a fixed vector saccade is produced. Left panel shows a series of 10 stimulation-evoked saccades. The endpoints of the saccades are clustered within a spatial region. That region is termed the motor field.

14.6 Single unit activity

A subset of FEF neurons have visual receptive fields (Bichot et al., 1996). These neurons respond to visual stimuli placed within the contralateral visual field. Other neurons in FEF are motor neurons that evoke saccadic eye movements. The visual receptive fields follow the oculomotor map within FEF. Neurons in this region are associated with voluntary saccadic eye movements (Bruce et al., 1985). Due to the correspondence between the visual and motor properties of FEF neurons, they can be considered to have "motor fields." As shown in Figure 14.4, a neuron's motor field is the region of the visual field that contains the termination points of saccades evoked from that neuron.

An FEF neuron's response to a visual stimulus in its motor field is increased when the stimulus is the target of a saccade (Goldberg and Bushnell, 1981). Furthermore, the neurons show an increase in firing rate leading up to and time-locked to a saccade, termed pre-saccadic activity (Bruce et al., 1985; Goldberg and Bushnell, 1981). The neurons start building up this pre-saccadic activity 150 ms prior to the saccade (Segraves and Park, 1993).

Both the visual responses and pre-saccadic activity of FEF neurons are modulated by spatial attention (Kodaka et al., 1997). Spatial attention modulates the firing rate; increasing if the motor field is the attended location and decreasing if another location is attended instead.

14.7 Lesion studies

After unilateral FEF lesions, monkeys are impaired at making voluntary and reflexive saccades into the contralateral hemifield, although progressive recovery occurs after a number of weeks (Crowne et al., 1981). However, lesions of both FEF and the superior colliculus permanently impair saccadic eye movements (Schiller et al., 1979). Humans with FEF lesions show an increase in latency for saccades made into the contralateral hemifield (Rivaud et al., 1994). Therefore, the FEFs are involved in the production of saccadic eye movements, but are not necessary for producing saccades.

Lesions of the FEF in monkeys also result in visual neglect, where the contralateral hemifield is ignored and the monkeys appear to be unaware of stimuli presented therein (Schiller et al., 1979), though recovery does occur with time. It has been suggested that visual neglect is an attentional deficit, resulting from an impairment of directing spatial attention to the contralateral hemifield. Supporting a role for this region being involved in spatial attention, humans with frontal lobe damage are impaired at maintaining spatial attention on a target in the presence of distractors (Grueninger and Pribram, 1969), although this damage is not confined to the FEF.

14.8   Oculomotor map

FEF has three distinct zones for three different types of eye movements, illustrated in Figure 14.5, elucidated by stimulation of neurons. There is a zone deep in the fundus of the arcuate sulcus that upon stimulation elicits ipsiversive smooth pursuit eye movements (Gottlieb et al., 1993). This zone is surrounded by the majority of the periarcuate region, whose stimulation evokes saccadic eye movements (Bruce et al., 1985). The third zone is the portion of FEF directly opposite the posterior end of the principal sulcus. Stimulation of neurons in this zone evokes vergence eye movements (Gamlin and Yoon, 2000).

Within the saccadic eye movement zone of FEF, there is a representation of oculomotor space, illustrated in Figure 14.6. FEF in each cerebral hemisphere elicits saccadic eye movements into the contralateral visual field. Moving along the periarcuate region from the superior branch to the inferior branch results in saccades of decreasing amplitudes. The largest saccades are elicited from the medial portion of FEF, and the smallest saccades are elicited from the lateral portion (Robinson and Fuchs, 1969). The direction of the saccade vector changes systematically with depth (Bruce et al., 1985). Representation of these two components, amplitude and direction, allow fixed-vector saccades to be made to any location in the contralateral visual field.

14.9   Stimulation

To electrically evoke saccades from FEF, currents of 10–200 microamps are necessary, although commonly less than 50 microamps is required (Bruce et al., 1985). The current required to evoke saccades 50% of the time is termed the movement threshold current. Currents that evoke saccades reliably, in 100% of cases, are defined as suprathreshold currents. Currents so low that they do not evoke any saccades are defined as subthreshold currents. These threshold levels are modulated by task demands (Tehovnik et al., 1999). If the task requires the monkey to maintain fixation, the thresholds are many times greater than those observed during free viewing or saccade tasks.

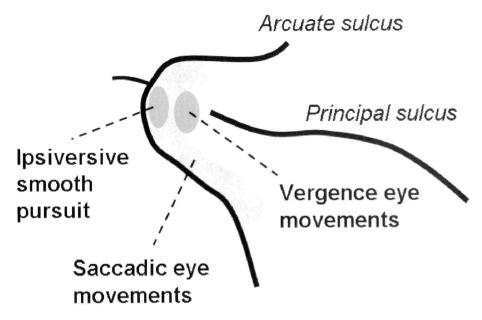

Figure 14.5. Zones within the frontal eye fields. Three zones within FEF are distinguished by the types of eye movements elicited with electrical stimulation. Saccadic eye movements are most often associated with FEF studies.

Therefore, the threshold current levels for an FEF site must be empirically determined for a given task.

Saccades are considered fixed-vector because the vectors do not change with the eye's position in the orbit. Furthermore, if the length of stimulation time is increased, staircase saccades occur. After one saccade is completed, another saccade occurs, which results in a characteristic staircase pattern observed when monitoring either the horizontal or vertical component of the eye position. There are two limitations to fixed-vector saccades. The first is that the vectors do shorten as the eye reaches its oculomotor limit, the absolute physical extent it can shift in the orbit. The second limitation is that when the head is not fixed in a single position, combined head and eye movements occur (Tu and Keating, 2000).

14.10   Rationale

Previously, studies of the relationship between spatial attention and eye movement mechanisms have all used a correlational approach, and generally conclude that the two mechanisms are closely linked (Posner, 1980; Posner et al., 1982; Shepherd et al., 1986; Rafal et al., 1989; Sheliga et al., 1994; Hoffman and Subramaniam, 1995). However, correlational studies cannot by nature determine causality. Testing the causal relationship requires activating neurons directly, under experimental control.

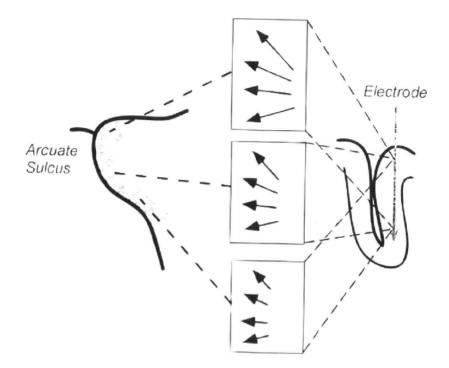

Figure 14.6. Oculomotor map within the frontal eye fields. Saccade amplitude decreases medial-laterally. Saccade direction changes methodically from the cortical surface down into the arcuate sulcus.

Spatial attention has been modulated by the systemic injection of cholinergic drugs into the subjects (Witte et al., 1997; O'Neill et al., 1999; Davidson and Marrocco, 2000). In effect these studies have injected chemicals to alter neuronal activity and measure the effects on spatial attention. However, systemic injections are nonspecific and do not localize functions to areas. With electrical stimulation, the injection of current was localized in space (approximately 0.5 mm spread, under 50 μA) and in time (e.g. Tehovnik, 1996). This stimulation is not identical to physiological neuronal activity, due to its stable frequency. However, the electrical stimulation modulates neuronal activity, in the same way as drug infusions. In essence, electrical stimulation is a better paradigm for modulating neuronal activity because it is localized both in time and the area of effect. Furthermore, it can be performed on a trial-by-trial basis, something that is not possible with either systemic injections or microdialysis.

The first study to use microstimulation of oculomotor areas to explicitly test the causal relationship between oculomotor mechanisms and spatial attention was performed by Moore and Fallah (2001). In this study, the authors injected an oculomotor signal by electrically stimulating cortical sites in the FEF. The microstimulation was applied at subthreshold current levels – current levels below the levels that initiate saccadic eye movements. The goal was to determine if oculomotor mechanisms deploy spatial attention, in the absence of a motor response. If these oculomotor signals direct attentional signals, then subthreshold stimulation may result in covert attentional shifts, in the absence of an eye movement. Subthreshold stimulation would mimic pre-saccadic build-up activity. This increased activation may be equivalent to setting up an oculomotor plan to saccade to a target location, but not carrying out the motor action. If this activity at an FEF cortical site either is the spatial attention signal or directs it, subthreshold microstimulation to a specific motor field should simulate the effect of cueing that location.

One method of observing the effects of spatial attention is to measure changes in psychophysical thresholds as a result of the attentional manipulation. The architecture of the visual system determines measurable physical thresholds for detecting visual stimuli or changes in visual stimuli. However, by adjusting the viewing conditions, the task can be made more difficult, and instead of reaching the physical threshold, the less optimal psychophysical threshold is determined (Mulligan and MacLeod, 1988; Blackwell, 1998). The psychophysical threshold is the threshold under particular task demands, and is never better than the physical threshold.

Detection of a luminance change in a target depends on the targets starting luminance, size, the luminance of the surrounding background area, and the overall light level in the viewing environment. The luminance change threshold is the smallest luminance change detectable under those conditions. The psychophysical threshold can be modulated by the effects of spatial attention. For example, if the subject knows the probable location of the target, the psychophysical luminance detection threshold is lower, meaning the participant detects an even smaller luminance change from the starting luminance. However, if the target appears at an unexpected location outside the cued location, the threshold is higher, meaning the target needs to have a larger luminance change from the starting luminance to be detected. Thus, if an oculomotor signal acts as a signal for spatial attention, then the sensitivity to detect luminance changes should increase.

Therefore, Moore and Fallah measured the psychophysical threshold for detecting a luminance change with and without subthreshold microstimulation. Subthreshold microstimulation involves injecting an electrical current into an FEF site, but the current level is lower than the current required to initiate a stimulation-evoked saccade. By using subthreshold microstimulation, the oculomotor system is activated, without a saccade response. If the oculomotor system directs spatial attention or shares a common neural basis with spatial attention, then the animals should detect a smaller luminance change threshold in the microstimulation condition versus the control condition where no microstimulation occurs.

This increased sensitivity should occur when the target is placed within the motor field of the FEF stimulation site, but not when the target is placed at a location outside the motor field. As per cueing studies of spatial attention, facilitation occurs within the cued location, in this case inside the motor field, and there is often a cost, or at least no benefit, at unattended locations outside the motor field.

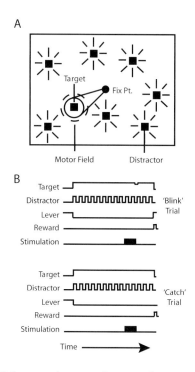

Figure 14.7. Diagram of the attention paradigm used to measure the effects of stimulation. (A) display used in the spatial attention task. In the task, the monkey attends to a peripheral target (indicated by searchlight) while maintaining central fixation and signals a transient dimming of the target with a lever release. During the task, a distractor is flashed in rapid succession at random locations throughout the display. The distractor is shown as scattered throughout the display to convey its appearance due to visual persistence. To test the effect of frontal eye field stimulation on attention, the target was placed at the location to which suprathreshold stimulation would shift the monkey's gaze, the motor field (MF). (B) timing of events in the spatial attention task. Top: sequence of events on trials in which the target dims (blink trial), the monkey correctly releases the lever and a reward is delivered. Bottom: the same, but for trials in which the target does not dim (catch trial) and the monkey is rewarded for holding down the lever. When testing the effect of FEF stimulation on task performance, stimulation occurred before the target change, or at random times during catch trials. (Taken from Moore and Fallah, 2004; used with permission.)

14.11   Attention task

The monkey was placed in a primate chair and head restrained. A computer monitor was placed 57 cm in front of the monkey. As illustrated in Figure 14.7, the monkey fixated a 0.5 degree red fixation point and maintained fixation throughout the trial. Eye position was monitored via a scleral search coil.

The monkey initiated the trial by fixating and depressing a lever that was placed within reach but out of the field of view of the monitor. Appearing at this point was the target stimulus, a white square with dimensions of 0.25–1.25 deg^2 based upon eccentricity, with a luminance of 26 cd/m^2. Since there was only a single target at a known location, spatial attention could be allocated to that location, depicted as the cone radiating from the fixation point. At a random point in the trial, between 500 and 1800 ms after target stimulus onset, the target stimulus decreased in luminance for 40 ms and then returned to its original luminance. The monkey had to respond within 800 ms, by releasing the lever to indicate he detected the luminance change, at which time he would get a juice reward. These are called "blink trials," as the stimulus appeared to blink, or transiently dim. On one-third of the trials, the target stimulus never changed luminance, called "catch trials." On these trials, the monkey needed to keep the lever pressed for the full time period (up to 2300 ms), including the response window, for a correct response and juice reward. The addition of catch trials was used to measure the rate of false alarms; that is, the proportion of trials in which the monkey released the lever, without the blink event having occurred.

The task described thus far would not be very sensitive to spatial attention effects. There is only a single target whose location is known prior to the blink event. Single targets alone do not show much modulation by spatial attention, because there is no competition for attentional resources. In order for the task to be more sensitive to the effects of spatial attention, we added a visual distractor to the task. The appearance and disappearance of a distractor was intended to draw attention away from the target stimulus (Remington et al., 1992). The distractor was similar in shape and brightness to the target. It was presented at a random location for 16 ms and then removed from the display for 16 ms before being replotted. The location of the distractor was restricted by some constraints. It was not plotted within 1.0° of the central fixation spot to aid the monkey in maintaining fixation. It was also not plotted in the region near the target stimulus, to avoid flanker (Miller, 1991; Castiello et al., 1999) or masking effects (Snowden and Hammett, 1998). These effects occur when nearby stimuli interfere with judgments of the target stimulus, possibly through local effects or lateral inhibition. In the case of this experimental paradigm, these effects would increase the threshold, if the distractor were plotted near the target stimulus at the time the blink even occurs. Thus, the distractor was not plotted within 3.5° of the center of the target stimulus.

To determine the detectable luminance decrement threshold, a staircase design was used. The initial luminance decrement was set to an arbitrary level above the expected psychophysical threshold. A block of trials consisted of two blink trials and one catch trial. If the monkey responded correctly to at least one of the blink trials and also responded correctly to the catch trial, the luminance decrement of the blink was decreased slightly, making it harder to detect. If the monkey missed both blink trials or released the lever on the catch trial, then the luminance decrement of the blink was increased, making it easier to detect. The amount of increase or decrease for a single step of the staircase was held constant throughout a series of blocks. During the experimental session, the luminance decrement was adjusted via steps in the staircase until it reached threshold.

Estimating the luminance decrement threshold was done in two stages. First, the raw staircase data were interpolated by computing the running average of steps (y)

across blocks (x), where i is the block number:

$$x = (x_i + x_{i+1})/2$$
$$y = (y_i + y_{i+1})/2$$

This interpolation provides a better fit, as by definition at threshold the monkey is alternating between two step values, e.g. 30%, 35%, 30%, 35%. The next stage in estimating the threshold was done using a least-squares fit of the interpolated staircase data with an asymptotic function:

$$y = a(a/x^{x/b})$$

where a is the asymptotic luminance change threshold and b is the block number at asymptote. Sensitivity is the reciprocal of the threshold.

14.12   Distractor effect

While evidence suggested that the addition of a distractor would affect the psychophysical threshold thus making the task attentionally demanding, we tested this idea explicitly. In this preliminary experiment, the target was 1° square and placed at 5° along the horizontal meridian. The distractors were squares varying in size from 0.1 to 1.0° per side between experimental sessions. Two conditions were interleaved in a simultaneous staircase procedure. In the distractor condition the target was accompanied by a distractor stimulus, whereas in the no distractor condition, the target appeared alone. This allowed for a paired comparison of the effect of the distractor and an analysis of the effect of increasing distractor size. We hypothesized that the distractor condition would result in a larger luminance decrement threshold than the no distractor condition. We also expected that increasing distractor size would increase the effect of the distractor and thus further increase the luminance decrement threshold.

One monkey ran this task in 17 experimental sessions. The data from one session (Figure 14.8) show a larger threshold in the distractor condition. Combining the sessions results in the distractor thresholds being significantly worse than the no distractor thresholds (paired t-test, $p < 0.01$). Detection of the blink event was impaired with the addition of a distractor. In addition, as distractor size increased, the effect of the distractor increased (Figure 14.9).

The effects of spatial attention are often measured along the same axes as these impairments. That is, spatial attention results in smaller detection thresholds, faster reaction times and increased accuracy when the target is in the attended versus the unattended location. Abrupt onsets and offsets of visual stimuli capture spatial attention (Yantis and Jonides, 1984). Increasing distractor density increases psychophysical thresholds when the distractor and the target share a similarity in features (Caputo and Guerra, 1998). Therefore, the results seen are likely due to the distractor competing for spatial attention. Thus, the distractor was having the intended effect of pulling spatial attention away from the target. Now the ability of oculomotor mechanisms to guide and deploy spatial attention can be tested, since allocation of spatial attention to the target would counteract the effects of the distractor, and thus result in a better luminance decrement threshold.

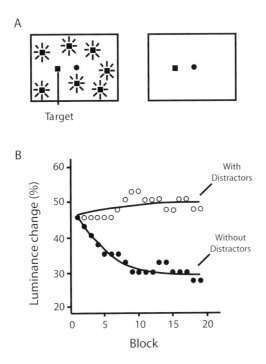

Figure 14.8. Effect of removing the distractor on detection of target luminance change. Example of thresholds obtained during blocks of trials in which the monkey had to detect a target luminance change in the presence of the flashing distractor (open symbols) or without the distractor (filled symbols) during interleaved trials. (a) display as viewed by the monkey and the presence (left) or absence of the distractor (right). (B) Plot shows the interpolated staircase data obtained during 20 blocks of trials in each condition. (Taken from Moore and Fallah, 2004; used with permission.)

14.13 Microstimulation task

In each session, a cortical site in the frontal eye fields was first found, based on its location and properties as described previously. The motor field was mapped out with suprathreshold stimulation and the microstimulation threshold was determined in a simple fixation task. A preliminary study (Figure 14.10) showed that higher currents, between 70 and 90% of the movement threshold, did not initiate saccades during the fixation task, but caused saccades during the spatial attention task.

This may have been due to the monkeys allocating spatial attention to the target, which could add to the effect of stimulation or lower the movement threshold. Either way, a saccade could be generated. Thus currents below 50% of the movement threshold were used. The distribution of test currents used is shown in Figure 14.11.

Once the motor field and subthreshold current were determined, the attention task was run. The target was placed within the motor field. Microstimulation at two stimulation onset asynchronies (one short: 30–175 ms and one long: 275–525 ms, see Fig-

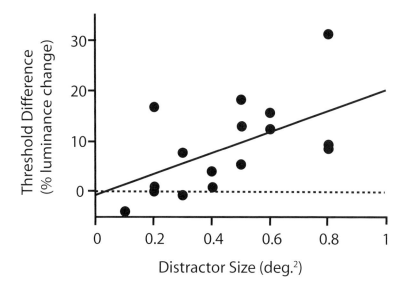

Figure 14.9. Effect of distractor size on luminance detection thresholds. Threshold difference is: Threshold No Dist – Threshold Dist. Increasing the size of the distractor decreases sensitivity to detect the target change. This is seen as an increase in the difference between the threshold with no distractors and the threshold with distractors. Threshold Difference $= -0.7 + 20.6 *$ Distractor Size ($R^2 = 0.4$).

ure 14.12) and no microstimulation conditions were interleaved in a triple simultaneous staircase procedure. This prevented the microstimulation from presenting a timing cue for when the target luminance decrement was going to occur. In the microstimulation conditions, a 100 ms microstimulation train started prior to the target event. On microstimulation catch trials, the time for the target event was randomly determined as per a blink trial, but no blink actually occurred. Instead, this set the time for the microstimulation to occur.

For a subset of the FEF sites that were tested with the target inside the motor field, the monkeys performed the same task again, except the target was placed at a location outside the motor field. The target was placed at a location approximately 90° away from the motor field vector, at the same eccentricity and within the same hemifield.

14.14 Effects of microstimulation: inside the motor field

Figure 14.13 depicts an example of the effects of subthreshold FEF microstimulation on the attention task. In Figure 14.13A, upper panel, stimulation at 25 μA produced saccades that allowed for mapping the motor field. In Figure 14.13A, lower panel, the effect of stimulation current on the production of saccades is shown. The arrow shows the subthreshold current used for this site. Figure 14.13B, upper panel, shows that the target was placed within the motor field. Figure 14.13B, lower panel, shows the luminance change during the staircase procedure for no stimulation (open circles) and

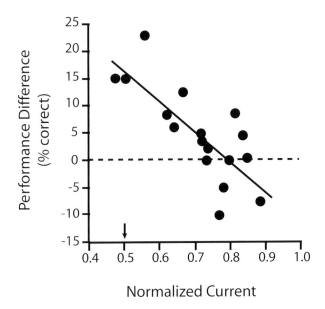

Figure 14.10. Effect of FEF stimulation on attention task performance (% correct) during initial experiments in which the stimulation current varied with respect to the current threshold. Points represent the difference between stimulation and control task performance (stimulation – control) across varying current. Current is shown normalized to the movement threshold (i.e. current used/threshold current). Mean difference in performance was significantly greater than 0, but this difference depended on the current used relative to the threshold current. Subsequent experiments were therefore carried out using current at ∼50% of threshold current (arrow). (Taken from Moore and Fallah, 2004; used with permission.)

stimulation trials (closed circles). At this site, stimulation raised the relative sensitivity by 37%. Across the population of 59 experiments, there was a significant 12% increase in relative sensitivity (Figure 14.14A).

Aside from the psychophysical threshold being directly affected via spatial attention mechanisms, it is possible that the threshold difference could be due to a change in response rate in the blink or catch trials. If the subthreshold stimulation affected lever releases, but did not affect the psychophysical threshold, the thresholds measured in this task could still be altered. Granted, the stimulation is in a cortical oculomotor area and the response is via a manual lever release, so it is not likely that the stimulation would affect the response directly. A two (stimulation condition: stimulation, no stimulation) by two (display condition: blink, catch) repeated measures analysis of variance was carried out on the proportion of correct responses for targets appearing within the FEF motor field for each monkey. This indicated a reliable main effect for display condition with a higher proportion of accurate responses in the catch compared with the blink trials ($p < 0.01$). This is expected as the staircase method for determining a threshold depends upon a predefined performance level. In this case, the staircase

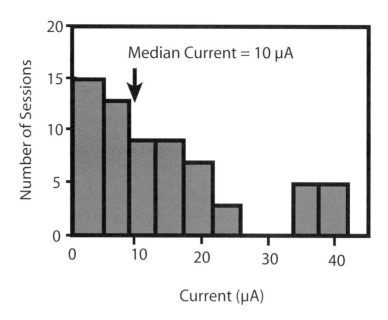

Figure 14.11. Distribution of test current used. Median current was 10 μA, range 1–42 μA.

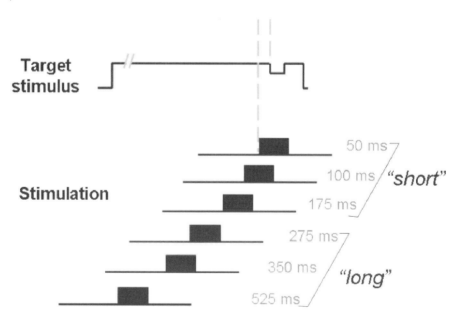

Figure 14.12. Stimulus onset asynchronies (SOAs) used in the study. One short and one long SOA were paired in each experimental session as follows: 50 ms and 275 ms, 100 ms and 350 ms, 175 ms and 525 ms. As can be seen, the 50 ms SOA completely overlapped the blink event.

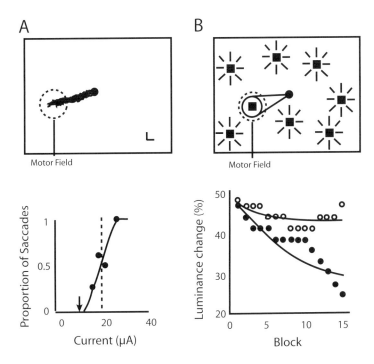

Figure 14.13. Illustration of a typical experiment and the effect of stimulation on psychophysical performance. (A) Top: Individual saccade vectors obtained during suprathreshold stimulation of an FEF site illustrating how the MF was mapped. Vector traces show 8 saccades evoked on 8 trials at a (suprathreshold) current of 25 μA. Calibration bar indicates 2°, vertical and horizontal. Bottom: Proportion of evoked saccades measured at different current levels to determine the current threshold. Open arrowhead indicates the subthreshold current (9 μA) used during the spatial attention task. (B) Top: Depiction of the attention task performed with the target positioned in the MF. Bottom: Staircase functions used to obtain target change thresholds (% Michaelson contrast from background) with (filled symbols) and without microstimulation (open symbols). Each set of points is fitted with an asymptotic function to estimate threshold. (Taken from Moore and Fallah, 2004; used with permission.)

compared performance on two blink trials with one catch trial. There was no main effect for stimulation conditions which shows that the stimulation did not result in a response bias towards releasing or not releasing the lever. The interaction between these factors was also not reliable which shows that stimulation did not result in a criterion shift, which would have had opposing effects on blink trial and catch trial performance. Thus, subthreshold stimulation of cortical sites within the frontal eye fields affected the psychophysical thresholds.

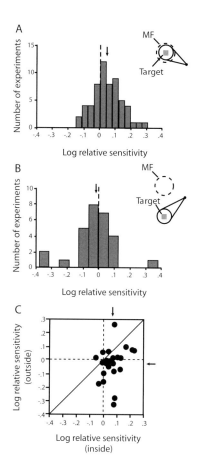

Figure 14.14.   Effect of microstimulation on sensitivity to target luminance changes.   (A) Histogram shows distribution of the log relative sensitivity (log[sensitivity$_{stimulation}$/sensitivity$_{control}$]). Distribution shows data obtained during 59 experiments in which the task was performed with the target in the MF (icon on right). A lack of an effect of stimulation would result in a distribution centered on 0. The distribution of relative sensitivity shown has a mean at 0.048 (arrow) signifying a 12% increase in sensitivity to the target change with stimulation. (B) Effect of stimulation when the target was positioned outside of the MF. Distribution of relative sensitivity values for 28 experiments in which the target was positioned outside of the MF. Distribution is centered on 0, illustrating no significant effect of stimulation. (C) Comparison of effects of stimulation on relative sensitivity when the target was either positioned inside or outside of the MF. Scatter plot shows the relative sensitivity values obtained from experiments with the target inside the MF (abscissa) and those obtained outside of the MF (ordinate) when both experiments were performed at the same FEF site (n = 26). Arrows on the right and top indicate the mean inside and outside values. (Taken from Moore and Fallah, 2004; used with permission.)

14.15 Effects of microstimulation: outside the motor field

Was the improvement in psychophysical thresholds with stimulation nothing more than a tap-on-the-shoulder effect? If someone receives a tap on the shoulder indicating that the target event is about to occur, then they would be more alert and ready and thus perform better on the task. Arousal is just such a general increase in alertness, which results in facilitation in many cognitive processes. Arousal is not spatial attention, since it results in improved performance throughout the visual field. To determine that the effect of FEF microstimulation was the deployment of spatial attention to the motor field, the experiment was repeated while placing the stimulus at a location outside of the motor field. When the target was placed outside of the motor field, stimulation did not improve the psychophysical thresholds (Figure 14.14B). Figure 14.14C compares the effects of microstimulation when the target was inside versus outside of the motor field for each stimulation site. Thus, there was a spatial extent to the facilitation effect of microstimulation. Cortical sites within the frontal eye fields that can give rise to saccadic eye movements can also facilitate detection of luminance changes in a visual target within their motor fields.

The effects of spatial attention are often seen as a cost or impaired performance, at unattended locations (Posner, 1980; Posner et al., 1980; Jonides, 1981). There was no significant cost seen when the target was placed outside the motor field. However, when the target was outside of the motor field, there was no visual stimulus in the motor field. The strength of the oculomotor signal may be modulated by the presence or absence of a visual target (e.g. Tehovnik, 1996). This hypothesis assumes that the strength of the modulation by spatial attention is based on the strength of the oculomotor signal.

14.16 Timing

When the allocation of visual attention to a cued spatial location is driven by a transient peripheral visual event, exogenous cueing, a biphasic cueing pattern is observed: facilitation occurs at short stimulus onset asynchrony (SOA) and is replaced by impaired processing, called inhibition of return (IOR) at longer SOAs (Posner, 1980; Maylor, 1985). The effect of varying the SOA from 50 to 525 ms when the target was inside the motor field is shown in Figure 14.15. While microstimulation did produce analogous facilitatory cueing effects, there was no evidence of IOR being induced by microstimulation at longer SOAs. Rather, observation of an attentional facilitatory effect with short SOAs without the subsequent inhibitory effect with longer SOAs resembles the behavioral pattern observed with endogenous cueing.

The difference between exogenous and endogenous cueing is the presentation of a visual stimulus at the peripheral location to be attended. The visual stimulus presented at that location is processed by the visual system and its location is the target location for the allocation of spatial attention. On the other hand, an endogenous cue is a symbolic cue. It represents the target location for the allocation of spatial attention, but its own location is irrelevant. It has previously been suggested that the locus of influence of location-based (spatial) IOR is within subcortical structures, specifically the supe-

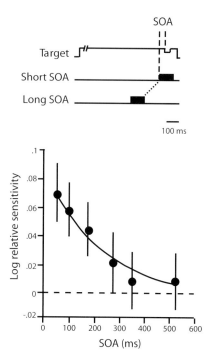

Figure 14.15. Comparison of the effects of stimulation at different stimulation onset asynchronies (SOAs). On stimulation trials, the interval between the onset of the stimulation train and the target luminance change was either short or long (top). (Bottom) Effects of specific SOAs on mean relative sensitivity. Higher three SOAs represent the long SOAs and lower three represent the short SOAs. Effect of stimulation increased as the SOA approached 0 and peaked at 0.073 or 18% above control. (Taken from Moore and Fallah, 2004; used with permission.)

rior colliculus (Rafal et al., 1988; Sapir et al., 1999). Therefore, the IOR effect could be mediated by the location of the peripheral cue as it is processed by the superior colliculus through direct connections from the retina. If this hypothesis is true, then it is not surprising that neither purely symbolic cueing nor microstimulation of an FEF site results in IOR, though both can result in facilitation.

14.17   Pathways

By what pathways could microstimulation of FEF affect visual processing? The attentional modulation has to reach the early visual areas to have any perceptual and behavioral effects on the visual stimulus. Single unit recording studies have shown that neurons in the visual system are modulated by spatial attention (Moran and Desimone, 1985; Richmond and Sato, 1987; Spitzer et al., 1988; Treue and Maunsell, 1996, 1999; Luck et al., 1997; McAdams and Maunsell, 1999, 2000; Reynolds et al., 1999; Seidemann and Newsome, 1999; Recanzone and Wurtz, 2000; Yeshurun and Carrasco, 2000). These neurons are then the target sites of action for spatial attention, in that spatial attention modulated their responses. One possible pathway for microstimulation to modulate neurons in posterior visual areas is through FEF's direct connections to those posterior visual areas. This pathway has been investigated by stimulating sites within the FEF while recording from neurons in area V4 (Moore and Armstrong, 2003, 2007). These studies have shown that FEF microstimulation enhances responses of V4 neurons whose receptive fields are at the same location as the motor field of the stimulation site. More importantly, FEF microstimulation improved V4 neuronal discrimination of stimuli. Such an improvement in visual discrimination is one of the hallmarks of spatial attention. Additionally, FEF is part of an oculomotor network that includes the superior colliculus (SC) and posterior parietal cortex and it could be that FEF microstimulation works through one of those areas to deploy spatial attention. In support of that, a similar study of SC microstimulation also showed behavioral improvements in visual discrimination albeit for motion discrimination (Müller et al., 2005). Also, area LIP has been shown to be involved in spatial attention (Bisley and Goldberg, 2003, 2006). To determine which areas are necessary and which pathways are used will require microstimulation of one area combined with inactivation of others.

14.18 Methodology for future studies of spatial attention

Previously, studies have had to direct spatial attention through behavioral means such as exogenous or endogenous cueing. Inherent in those designs is the requirement that a cue be processed. An exogenous visual cue also activates inhibition of return, whereas an endogenous symbolic cue requires cognitive processing. Furthermore in animal studies of spatial attention, the animals are often trained to attend to the target. Long-term training may affect the systems being studied (Grunewald et al., 1999). However, microstimulation of FEF sites can be used as a way of directing spatial attention to a specific peripheral location, in the absence of these other processes.

14.19 Conclusions

Spatial attention has long been linked to eye movements. In fact, it is the oculomotor system that deploys visual spatial attention. Which areas within the oculomotor network are involved is still unknown. Subthreshold microstimulation activates oculomotor neurons at rates below their saccadic threshold. This activation is similar to a motor plan, where the intention to move is represented by increased neuronal firing. Thus the brain is found to once again be efficient. A single system, the oculomotor system, can be activated to deploy covert spatial attention, and when the strength increases above threshold the eyes move, deploying overt spatial attention. Still to be determined is if similar systems work for other modalities, such as auditory and somatosensory spatial attention.

References

Armstrong, K. M., Moore, T. (2007). Rapid enhancement of visual cortical response discriminability by microstimulation of the frontal eye field. *Proc. Nat. Acad. Sci. USA*, 104: 9499–9504.

Bichot, N. P., Schall, J. D. and Thompson, K. G. (1996). Visual feature selectivity in frontal eye fields induced by experience in mature macaques. *Nature*, 381: 697–699.

Bisley, J. W. and Goldberg, M. E. (2003). Neuronal activity in the lateral intraparietal area and spatial attention. *Science*, 299: 81–86.

Bisley, J. W. and Goldberg, M. E. (2006). Neural correlates of attention and distractibility in the lateral intraparietal area. *J. Neurophysiol.*, 95: 1696–1717.

Blackwell, K. T. (1998). The effect of white and filtered noise on contrast detection thresholds. *Vision Res.*, 38: 267–280.

Bruce, C. J. and Goldberg, M. E. (1985). Primate frontal eye fields. I. Single neurons discharging before saccades. *J. Neurophysiol.*, 53: 603–635.

Bruce, C. J., Goldberg, M. E., Bushnell, M. C. and Stanton, G. B. (1985). Primate frontal eye fields. II. Physiological and anatomical correlates of electrically evoked eye-movements. *J. Neurophysiol.*, 54; 714–734.

Caputo, G. and Guerra, S. (1998). Attentional selection by distractor suppression. *Vision Res.*, 38: 669–689.

Castiello, U., Badcock, D. R. and Bennett, K. M. B. (1999). Sudden and gradual presentation of distractor objects: differential interference effects. *Exp. Brain Res.*, 128: 550–556.

Corbetta, M., Akbudak, E., Conturo, T. E., Snyder, A. Z., Ollinger, J. M., Drury, H. A., Linenweber, M. R., Petersen, S. E., Raichle, M. E., Van Essen, D. C. and Shulman, G. L. (1998). A common network of functional areas for attention and eye movements. *Neuron*, 21: 761–773.

Corbetta, M., Kincade, J. M., Ollinger, J. M., McAvoy, M. P. and Shulman, G. L. (2000). Voluntary orienting is dissociated from target detection in human posterior parietal cortex. *Nature Neurosci.*, 3: 292–297.

Coull, J. T. and Nobre, A. C. (1998). Where and when to pay attention: the neural systems for directing attention to spatial locations and to time intervals as revealed by both PET and fMRI. *J. Neurosci.*, 18: 7426–7435.

Crowe, D. A., Averbeck, B. B., Chafee, M. V., Anderson, J. H. and Georgopoulos, A. P. (2000). Mental maze solving. *J. Cogn. Neurosci.*, 12: 813–827.

Crowne, D. P., Yeo, C. H. and Russell, I. S. (1981). The effects of unilateral frontal eye field lesions in the monkey: visual-motor guidance and avoidance behaviour. *Behav. Brain Res.*, 2: 165–187.

Davidson, M. C. and Marrocco, R. T. (2000). Local infusion of scopolamine into intraparietal cortex slows covert orienting in rhesus monkeys. *J. Neurophysiol.*, 83: 1536–1549.

Deubel, H. and Schneider, W. X. (1996). Saccade target selection and object recognition: evidence for a common attentional mechanism. *Vision Res.*, 36: 1827–1837.

Driver, J., Davis, G., Ricciardelli, P., Kidd, P., Maxwell, E. and Baron-Cohen, S. (1999). Gaze perception triggers reflexive visuospatial orienting. *Visual Cogn.* 6: 509–540.

Duncan, J., Ward, R. and Shapiro, K. L. (1994). Direct measurement of attentional dwell time in human vision. *Nature*, 369: 313–315.

Funahashi, S., Bruce, C. J. and Goldman-Rakic, P. S. (1993). Dorsolateral prefrontal lesions and oculomotor delayed-response performance: evidence for mnemonic "scotomas." *J. Neurosci.*, 13: 1479–1497.

Gamlin, P. D. and Yoon, K. (2000). An area for vergence eye movement in primate frontal cortex. *Nature*, 407: 1003–1007.

Goldberg, M. E. and Bushnell, M. C. (1981). Behavioral enhancement of visual responses in monkey cerebral-cortex. 2. Modulation in frontal eye fields specifically related to saccades. *J. Neurophysiol.*, 46: 773–787.

Goldberg, M. E., Bushnell, M. C. and Bruce, C. J. (1986). The effect of attentive fixation on eye-movements evoked by electrical-stimulation of the frontal eye fields. *Exp. Brain Res.*, 61: 579–584.

Gottlieb, J. P., Bruce, C. J. and MacAvoy, M. G. (1993). Smooth eye movements elicited by microstimulation in the primate frontal eye field. *J. Neurophysiol.*, 69: 786–799.

Graziano, M. S. A. and Gandhi, S. (2000). Location of the polysensory zone in the precentral gyrus of anesthetized monkeys. *Exp. Brain Res.*, 135: 259–266.

Gross, C. G. and Graziano, M. S. A. (1995). Multiple representations of space in the brain. *Neuroscientist*, 1: 43–50.

Grueninger, W. E. and Pribram, K. H. (1969). Effects of spatial and nonspatial distractors on performance latency of monkeys with frontal lesions. *J. Comp. Physiol. Psychol.*, 68: 203–209.

Grunewald, A., Linden, J. F. and Andersen, R. A. (1999). Responses to auditory stimuli in macaque lateral intraparietal area. I. Effects of training. *J. Neurophysiol.*, 82: 330–342.

Hietanen, J. K. (1999). Does your gaze direction and head orientation shift my visual attention? *NeuroReport*, 10: 3443–3447.

Hoffman, J. E. and Subramaniam, B. (1995). The role of visual-attention in saccadic eye-movements. *Percept. Psychophys.*, 57: 787–795.

Hopfinger, J. B., Buonocore, M. H. and Mangun, G. R. (2000). The neural mechanisms of top-down attentional control. *Nature Neurosci.* 3: 284–291.

Huerta, M. F., Krubitzer, L. A. and Kaas, J. H. (1987). Frontal eye fields as defined by intracortical microstimulation in squirrel monkeys, owl monkeys, and macaque monkeys: II. Cortical connections. *J. Comp. Neurol.* 265: 332–361.

Jonides, J. (1981). Voluntary versus automatic control over the mind's eye's movement. In J. B. Long and A. D. Baddleley (eds.), *Attention and Performance IX*. Hillsdale, NJ: Lawrence Erlbaum, pp. 187-203.

Klein, R. M. (1980). Does oculomotor readiness mediate cognitive control of visual attention. In R. Nickerson (ed.) *Attention and Performance VIII*. Hillsdale, NJ: Erlbaum, pp. 259–276.

Klein, R. M. and Pontefract, A. (1994). *Does Oculomotor Readiness Mediate Cognitive Control of Visual Attention? Revisited!*. Cambridge, MA: MIT Press.

Kodaka, Y., Mikami, A. and Kubota, K. (1997). Neuronal activity in the frontal eye field of the monkey is modulated while attention is focused on to a stimulus in the peripheral visual field, irrespective of eye movement. *Neurosci. Res.*, 28: 291–298.

Kustov, A. A. and Robinson, D. L. (1996). Shared neural control of attentional shifts and eye movements. *Nature*, 384: 74–77.

Làdavas, E., di Pellegrino, G., Farnè, A. and Zeloni, G. (1998). Neuropsychological evidence of an integrated visuotactile representation of peripersonal space in humans. *J. Cogn. Neurosci.*, 10: 581–589.

Langton, S. R. H. and Bruce, V. (1999). Reflexive visual orienting in response to the social attention of others. *Visual Cogn.*, 6: 541–567.

Luck, S. J., Chelazzi, L., Hillyard, S. A. and Desimone, R. (1997). Neural mechanisms of spatial selective attention in areas V1, V2, and V4 of macaque visual cortex. *J. Neurophysiol.*, 77: 24–42.

Lynch, J. C. and McLaren, J. W. (1989). Deficits of visual attention and saccadic eye movements after lesions of parietooccipital cortex in monkeys. *J. Neurophysiol.*, 61: 74–90.

Maylor, E. A. (1985). Facilitatory and inhibitory components of orienting in visual space. In M. I. Posner and O. S. M. Marin (eds.), *Attention and Performance, XI*. Hillsdale, NJ: Lawrence Erlbaum, pp. 701–711.

McAdams, C. J. and Maunsell, J. H. R. (1999). Effects of attention on orientation-tuning functions of single neurons in macaque cortical area V4. *J. Neurosci.*, 19: 431–441.

McAdams, C. J. and Maunsell, J. H. R. (2000). Attention to both space and feature modulates neuronal responses in macaque area V4. *J. Neurophysiol.*, 83: 1751–1755.

Miller, J. (1991). The flanker compatibility effect as a function of visual angle, attentional focus, visual transients, and perceptual load: a search for boundary conditions. *Percept. Psychophys.*, 49: 270–288.

Moore, T. and Armstrong, K. M. (2003). Selective gating of visual signals by microstimulation of frontal cortex. *Nature*, 421: 370–373.

Moore, T. and Fallah, M. (2001). Control of eye movements and spatial attention. *Proc. Nat. Acad. Sci.*, 98: 1273–1276.

Moore, T. and Fallah, M. (2004). Microstimulation of the frontal eye field and its effects on covert spatial attention. *J. Neurophysiol.*, 91: 152–162.

Moran, J. and Desimone, R. (1985). Selective attention gates visual processing in the extrastriate cortex. *Science*, 229: 782–784.

Müller, J. R., Philiastides, M. G. and Newsome, W. T. (2005). Microstimulation of the superior colliculus focuses attention without moving the eyes. *Proc. Nat. Acad. Sci. USA*, 102: 524–529.

Mulligan, J. B. and MacLeod, D. I. A. (1988). Reciprocity between luminance and dot density in the perception of brightness. *Vision Res.*, 28: 503–519.

O'Neill, J., Fitten, L. J., Siembieda, D. W., Crawford, K. C., Halgren, E., Fisher, A. and Refai, D. (1999). Divided attention-enhancing effects of AF102B and THA in aging monkeys. *Psychopharmacol.*, 143: 123–130.

Perry, R. J. and Zeki, S. (2000). The neurology of saccades and covert shifts in spatial attention: an event-related fMRI study. *Brain*, 123: 2273–2288.

Posner, M. I. (1980). Orienting of attention. *Quart. J. Exp. Psychol.*, 23: 3–25.

Posner, M. I., Cohen, Y. and Rafal, R. D. (1982). Neural systems control of spatial orienting. *Phil. Trans. Roy. Soc. (Lond.) B*, 298: 187–198.

Posner, M. I., Nissen, M. J. and Ogden, W. C. (1978). Attended and unattended processing modes: the role of set of spatial location. In N. H. L. Pick and I. J. Saltzman (eds.) *Modes of Perceiving and Processing Information*. Hillsdale, NJ: Erlbaum, pp. 137–157.

Posner, M. I., Snyder, C. R. R. and Davidson, B. J. (1980). Attention and the detection of signals. *J. Exp. Psychol.: Gen.*, 109: 160–174.

Rafal, R. D., Calabresi, P. A., Brennan, C. W. and Sciolto, T. K. (1989). Saccade preparation inhibits reorienting to recently attended locations. *J. Exp. Psychol.: Hum. Percept. Perf.*, 15: 673–685.

Rafal, R. D., Posner, M. I., Friedrich, F. J., Inhoff, A. W. and Bernstein, E. (1988). Orienting of visual attention in progressive supranuclear palsy. *Brain*, 111: 267–280.

Recanzone, G. H. and Wurtz, R. H. (2000). Effects of attention on MT and MST neuronal activity during pursuit initiation. *J. Neurophysiol.*, 83: 777–790.

Remington, R. (1980). Attention and saccadic eye movements. *J. Exp. Psychol.: Hum. Percept. Perf.*, 6: 726–744.

Remington, R. W., Johnston, J. C. and Yantis, S. (1992). Involuntary attentional capture by abrupt onsets. *Percept. Psychophys.*, 51: 279–290.

Ress, D., Backus, B. T. and Heeger, D. J. (2000). Activity in primary visual cortex predicts performance in a visual detection task. *Nature Neurosci.*, 3: 940–945.

Reynolds, J. H., Chelazzi, L. and Desimone, R. (1999). Competitive mechanisms subserve attention in macaque areas V2 and V4. *J. Neurophysiol.*, 19: 1736–1753.

Richmond, B. J. and Sato, T. (1987). Enhancement of inferior temporal neurons during visual discrimination. *J. Neurophysiol.*, 58: 1292–1306.

Rivaud, S., Muri, R. M., Gaymard, B., Vermersch, A. I. and Pierrot-Deseilligny, C. (1994). Eye movement disorders after frontal eye field lesions in humans. *Exp. Brain Res.*, 102: 110–120.

Rizzolatti, G., Riggio, L., Dascola, I., and Umiltá, C. (1987). Reorienting attention across the horizontal and vertical meridians: evidence in favor of a premotor theory of attention. *Neuropsychologia.* 25: 31–40.

Rizzolatti, G., Camarda, R., Fogassi, L., Gentilucci, M., Luppino, G. and Matelli, M. (1988). Functional organization of inferior area 6 in the macaque monkey. II. Area F5 and the control of distal movements. *Exp. Brain Res.*, 71: 491–507.

Robinson, D. A. and Fuchs, A. F. (1969). Eye movements evoked by stimulation of frontal eye fields. *J. Neurophysiol.*, 32: 637–648.

Sapir, A., Soroker, N., Berger, A. and Henik, A. (1999). Inhibition of return in spatial attention: direct evidence for collicular generation. *Nature Neurosci.*, 2: 1053–1054.

Schiller, P. H., True, S. D. and Conway, J. L. (1979). Effects of frontal eye field and superior colliculus ablations on eye movements. *Science*, 206: 590–592.

Segraves, M. A. and Park, K. (1993). The relationship of monkey frontal eye field activity to saccade dynamics. *J. Neurophysiol.*, 69: 1880–1889.

Seidemann, E., and Newsome, W. T. (1999). Effect of spatial attention on the responses of area MT neurons. *J. Neurophysiol.*, 81: 1783–1794.

Sheliga, B. M., Riggio, L., Craighero, L. and Rizzolatti, G. (1995). Spatial attention-determined modifications in saccade trajectories. *NeuroReport*, 6: 585–588.

Sheliga, B. M., Riggio, L. and Rizzolatti, G. (1994). Orienting of attention and eye movements. *Exp. Brain Res.*, 98: 507–522.

Shepherd, M., Findlay, J. M. and Hockey, R. J. (1986). The relationship between eye movements and spatial attention. *Quart. J. Exp. Psychol. A: Hum. Exp. Psychol.*, 38: 475–491.

Snowden, R. J. and Hammett, S. T. (1998). The effects of surround contrast on contrast thresholds, perceived contrast and contrast discrimination. *Vision Res.*, 38:, 1935–1945.

Sommer, M. A. and Wurtz, R. H. (2000). Composition and topographic organization of signals sent from the frontal eye field to the superior colliculus. *J. Neurophysiol.*, 83: 1979–2001.

Spitzer, H., Desimone, R. and Moran, J. (1988). Increased attention enhances both behavioral and neuronal performance. *J. Neurophysiol.*, 240:, 338–340.

Tehovnik, E. J. (1996). Electrical stimulation of neural tissue to evoke behavioral responses. *J. Neurosci. Meth.*, 65: 1–17.

Tehovnik, E. J., Slocum, W. M. and Schiller, P. H. (1999). Behavioural conditions affecting saccadic eye movements elicited electrically from the frontal lobes of primates. *Eur. J. Neurosci.*, 11: 2431–2443.

Theeuwes, J., Kramer, A. F., Hahn, S., Irwin, D. E. and Zelinsky, G. J. (1999). Influence of attentional capture on oculomotor control. *J. Exp. Psychol.: Hum. Percept. Perf.*, 25: 1595–1608.

Treue, S. and Maunsell, J. H. R. (1996). Attentional modulation of visual motion processing in cortical areas MT and MST. *Nature*, 382: 539–541.

Treue, S. and Maunsell, J. H. R. (1999). Effects of attention on the processing of motion in macaque middle temporal and medial superior temporal visual cortical areas. *J. Neurosci.*, 19: 7591–7602.

Tu, T. A. and Keating, G. (2000). Electrical stimulation of the frontal eye field in a monkey produces combined eye and head movements. *J. Neurophysiol.*, 84: 1103–1106.

Vuilleumier, P. O. and Rafal, R. D. (2000). A systematic study of visual extinction: Between- and within-field deficits of attention in hemispatial neglect. *Brain*, 123: 1263–1279.

Weinstein, E. A. and Friedland, R. P. (1977). Behavioral disorders associated with hemi-inattention. *Adv. Neurol.*, 18: 51–62.

Witte, E. A., Davidson, M. C. and Marrocco, R. T. (1997). Effects of altering brain cholinergic activity on covert orienting of attention: comparison of monkey and human performance. *Psychopharmacol.*, 132: 324–334.

Yantis, S. and Jonides, J. (1984). Abrupt visual onsets and selective attention: evidence from visual search. *J. Exp. Psychol.: Hum. Percept. Perf.*, 10: 601–621.

Yeshurun, Y. and Carrasco, M. (2000). The locus of attentional effects in texture segmentation. *Nature Neurosci.*, 3: 622–627.

15 Neural mechanisms of attentional selection in visual search: evidence from electromagnetic recordings

J.-M. Hopf

Visual search – the operation of finding a particular object among many other objects – is involved in almost any situation of our daily life. In fact, being faced with isolated objects represents a rare exception, while most of the time we will have to select information among alternatives always involving some form of visual search. From introspection, searching for an object of interest may appear to be a simple unitary operation. This, however, turns out not to be the case, and most theories on visual search propose that a number of selection operations must be involved (Treisman and Gelade, 1980; Wolfe et al., 1989; Treisman and Sato, 1990; Wolfe, 1994; Cave, 1999). Take the simple situation where one aims to report the orientation of a red bar that is presented together with many other colored oriented bars. This will require the detection of the red color in the visual scene before the target's orientation can be determined. In other words it is logically necessary that the visual system first builds a neural representation of relevant features and then goes on to select potential target objects. Here, I will provide evidence from the electromagnetic brain response for a feature-based selection operation that may serve to build such initial representation in visual search. Based on the excellent temporal resolution of electromagnetic recordings (EEG, MEG), I will show that feature-based selection, indeed, appears prior to the onset of target selection, and that it operates in a location-independent manner – well suited to provide a location map of potentially relevant item locations.

Feature-based attentional selection thus represents a fast and effective mechanism to label potentially relevant locations in a visual scene. In a typical "real-word" scene this will include the location of many nontarget items whose feature sets happen to

Cortical Mechanisms of Vision, ed. M. Jenkin and L. R. Harris. Published by Cambridge University Press.
© Cambridge University Press 2009.

overlap with that of the target. Thus, feature-based selection will typically provide insufficient and ambiguous information about the target's location. How then does the visual system determine the actual location of the target? As will be outlined in the second part, solving this problem translates into resolving a principal coding problem inherent in the visual cortical processing hierarchy which arises because the visual system is massively convergent and receptive field (RF) size increases dramatically towards higher levels in the cortical hierarchy. Such a convergent architecture has been suggested to solve important coding problems like the computation of complex representations and transformational invariances (Sary et al., 1993; Riesenhuber and Poggio, 2000; Tanaka, 2003), but it has the consequence that precise location information is progressively lost and spatial resolution is inevitably reduced. Thus neural operations are needed that regain precise location information during visual processing. In the second section I will provide evidence from MEG and fMRI recordings suggesting a possible mechanism that may serve to resolve such ambiguities by adapting the spatial resolution of attention to the required perceptual scale. We will see that enhancing the spatial resolution of attention is accomplished by a coarse-to-fine selection in ventral extrastriate areas with progressively smaller receptive field size. In the last part, these observations will be discussed in the framework of the Selective Tuning Model (STM) (Tsotsos et al., 1995; Tsotsos, 2005) – a computational model that provides an explicit account for how spatial resolution and precise location information is (re)gained based on top-down selection in the visual hierarchy. It will turn out that the mechanism proposed by STM regarding the coarse-to-fine selection of spatial scale will receive direct support from our neuromagnetic and fMRI observations in extrastriate cortex areas. Importantly, top-down cross-hierarchical selection as formulated in STM leads to an important prediction regarding the spatial profile of the focus of attention. The latter may not be a simple monotonic gradient of enhanced neural processing, but rather a more complex shaped profile with a center enhancement surrounded by a zone of attenuation. In the last section, we will discuss neuromagnetic data that, indeed, demonstrate the existence of a center-surround profile of the spatial focus of attention in visual search (Hopf et al., 2006a).

15.1 Neural mechanisms of feature selection in visual search

Visual search will logically require some degree of decoding of relevant object features before the target object can be identified. Most theories on visual search (Treisman and Gelade, 1980; Wolfe et al., 1989; Treisman and Sato, 1990; Wolfe, 1994; Cave, 1999) propose some form of preliminary (preattentive) feature-based analysis of the visual scene that sets the stage for subsequent, and more elaborate operations of focal attention. According to an influential theory (feature integration theory, FIT) this preattentive decoding of relevant features may lead to instant target identification (and fast search) when the searched-for item feature is unique in the display. In this case the target's location will be unambiguously marked by the location of the relevant feature, no matter how many distractors are present. Searching for a combination of features (conjunction search) of which one or more is also present in the distractor set will, however, be slower because a simple determination of relevant feature locations will not identify the target's location unambiguously. FIT proposes that in the latter case focal attention comes into play forcing a decoding of features at each individual item's location in a serial item-by-item manner (serial search hypothesis). As a consequence, the time to find the target increases with the number of items in a given display.

However, under certain conditions, conjunction search was found to produce flatter slopes than expected (Egeth et al., 1984; Nakayama and Silverman, 1986; Wolfe et al., 1989). Wolfe et al. (1989) observed that triple-conjunctions (color, form, size) can produce flatter slopes than simple conjunctions when the target shares one feature with the distractors. These new observations contradicted the serial search hypothesis and turned out to be best accommodated by a modification of FIT, that proposed some form of parallel preattentive (top-down or bottom-up) feature-based analysis which parses the scene into candidate objects before focal attention comes into play (Wolfe et al., 1989; Treisman and Sato, 1990; Wolfe, 1994; Wolfe and Bennet, 1996). This initial "preattentive parse" is proposed to guide attentional focusing insofar as it reduces the search space requiring a serial operation (Duncan and Humphreys, 1989; Wolfe et al., 1989; Treisman and Sato, 1990; Wolfe, 1994; Wolfe and Bennet, 1996). Although feature-based guidance is referred to as a preattentive operation (Wolfe et al., 1989), guidance is not assumed to be preattentive in a strict sense (Wolfe, 2003). Guidance requires selectivity for relevant features or feature values, suggesting that it depends on some form of feature-based attentive operation to enhance their saliency. In fact attention to features has been shown to enhance feature saliency which biases the interpretation of an otherwise ambiguous percept (Lu and Sperling, 1995; Blaser et al., 1999). Thus, beyond the logical necessity to decode features before attention can be focused accordingly, there is firm psychophysical evidence for complex top-down driven feature-based segmentation processes that come into play before the serial operation of attentional focusing is involved in visual search.

It is thus important to ask whether there is neurophysiological evidence for such feature-based visual analysis prior to the processes mediating the spatial focusing of attention, and whether such feature-based operation would provide (location) information appropriate for guiding subsequent focusing.

Cell recordings in the monkey have reported candidate neural mechanisms that may underlie feature-based attentive selection (Motter, 1994; Treue and Martinez-Trujillo, 1999; McAdams and Maunsell, 2000; Mazer and Gallant, 2003; Martinez-Trujillo and Treue, 2004; Ogawa and Komatsu, 2004; Bichot et al., 2005; Maunsell and Treue, 2006). Motter (1994), for example, recorded from color-selective cells in macaque V4, and observed that presenting the cell's preferred color in its RF led to enhanced firing even when the monkey attended that color elsewhere in the visual field. Similarly, Treue and Martinez-Trujillo (1999) report that MT cells in the macaque enhance (reduce) firing when their preferred (anti-preferred) motion direction is attended outside their RF. Analogous feature-based attention effects (referred to as global feature-based attention) have been recently reported with fMRI in humans (Saenz et al., 2002, 2003). Addressing visual search more directly, Bichot et al. (2005) observed evidence for a parallel selection of relevant features (color or shape) in V4 neurons when monkeys performed a free-viewing visual search task.

As global feature-based attention operates in a location independent manner through-out the visual scene, it may serve to label item locations bearing relevant features inde-pendent of where attention is focused. It could, therefore, represent a potential neural mechanism that mediates feature guidance in visual search. At present, however, it is not clear whether these global feature-based attention effects are consistent with such operation, in particular because it is not clear whether they actually precede spatial focusing of attention in visual search.

We recently addressed this question explicitly using simultaneous recordings of event-related potential (ERP) and event-related magnetic fields (ERMF) in human ob-servers. Both methods provide very high temporal resolution in analyzing brain activity at the neural population level. They thus permit examination of the exact time course of neural activity underlying feature and location based selection.

To properly address the relative timing of these operations in visual search, it is necessary to dissociate processes of feature-based selection from processes of target selection proper; that is, from the actual operation of focusing attention onto the tar-get. To achieve this we asked subjects to search for a colored target item in multi-item displays, in which the spatial distribution of distractors sharing an orientation feature with the target (orientation-direction) was systematically varied with respect to the tar-get's location (Hopf et al., 2004). Specifically, on each search frame subjects had to discriminate the gap-orientation (left/right) of a red (or green) target C which randomly appeared in the left or right visual field (VF). Distractor Cs drawn in a different color (blue) were presented in both visual fields. Their gap-orientation could vary along the horizontal direction as the gap of the target (relevant orientation distractors) or they could vary along a vertical direction and differ from the target (irrelevant orientation distractors). The location of the relevant orientation feature (left/right) was varied rela-tive to the focus of attention by presenting relevant orientation distractors either in the target visual field only (Figure 15.1a (A)), in the nontarget visual field only (B), in both visual fields (C), or in neither visual field (D), with (D) serving as a control condition.

The neural activity reflecting the processing of the relevant orientation feature was then assessed by comparing the electromagnetic response elicited by condition A vs. D, B vs. D, and C vs. D. These comparisons were performed separately for targets pre-sented in the left and right VF. Figure 15.1b illustrates what was observed, for example, for target Cs presented in the left VF. Between 140 and 300 ms after search frame onset the electromagnetic response was enhanced at electrodes/sensor sites contralateral to the relevant orientation distractors (gray area between traces), no matter whether those distractors appeared in the target VF or the nontarget VF. For example, superimposing the ERP response of conditions A and D (upper row) reveals an enhancement of activ-ity between 140 and 300 ms after search frame onset at a right hemisphere electrode (PO8) contralateral to the relevant orientation distractors. A corresponding current source localization analysis on the magnetic difference wave (A-minus-D) between 140 and 200 ms confirmed this lateralization by showing a current maximum in the right inferior occipitotemporal cortex (Figure 15.1c). In contrast, when superimposing waveforms of conditions B and D (middle row in panel b) this relative enhancement appears at a left hemisphere electrode (PO7), while no effect is visible at PO8 con-tralateral to the target. Consistent with this lateralization, the current source maximum of the B-minus-D difference appears in the left inferior occipitotemporal cortex (panel

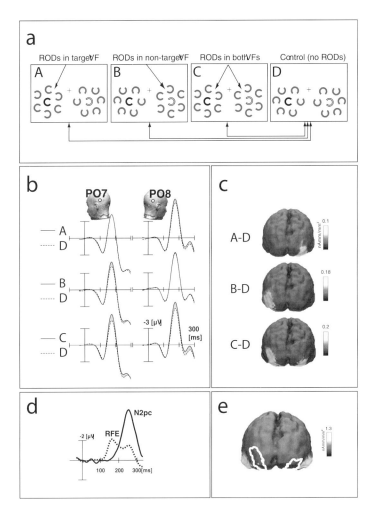

Figure 15.1. (a) Illustration of all possible distributions of relevant orientation distractors (ROD, gray Cs with horizontal gap-orientation) relative to a target item (black C) presented in the left visual field (VF). (b) Average ERP waveforms elicited by ROD distributions A-C (solid lines) for left VF targets superimposed onto waveforms elicited by the control condition (D, dashed line). Waveforms were recorded from a left (PO7) and a right (PO8) hemisphere parieto-occipital electrode site. The relevant feature effect (RFE) is highlighted by the gray area between traces. (c) Current source localization of the RFE based on average minimum norm least squares (MNLS) estimates of the waveform differences A-minus-D (A-D), B-minus-D (B-D), and C-minus-D (C-D) between 140 and 200 ms. (d) Time course of the RFE (from condition C in panel a) superimposed onto the time course of the N2pc effect. (e) Current density distribution of the RFE (white outlines) superimposed onto the current density estimates of the N2pc effect.

c), again contralateral to the relevant orientation distractors. Importantly, when relevant orientation distractors appear in both visual fields (C vs. D), this enhancement is seen at both the left and right hemisphere electrode sites, and current source maxima are seen in both the left and right inferior occipitotemporal cortex (panel c). An analogous, but mirror image modulation pattern was observed for targets in the right VF (Hopf et al., 2004). Apparently, the modulation highlighted in gray in panel (b) reflects the location of the relevant orientation feature value in a systematic way, while it is completely independent of where the target is located. It is important to see that target color (which is unique) would be sufficient to unambiguously pinpoint the target's location. This modulation therefore shows that orientation feature values were automatically registered at irrelevant item locations just by virtue of the fact that they were search-relevant (relevant feature effect, RFE).

The RFE shows obvious parallels to the global feature-based attention effects observed with single unit recordings in the monkey and with fMRI in humans. Like those effects the RFE signals a neural operation that is triggered in a retinotopically specific way from any location containing relevant feature values, no matter whether that location is consistent with the target or not. Accordingly, it could be a candidate neural mechanism that serves to transform the distribution of relevant feature values into a map of potentially relevant item locations that focal attention subsequently works on to bind features for target identification (Treisman and Gelade, 1980; Treisman and Gormican, 1988; Wolfe et al., 1989; Wolfe and Bennet, 1996; Cave, 1999). But, is the time course of the RFE consistent with this possibility? To answer this question, it would be critical to determine its time course relative to the time course of neural activity reflecting the actual focusing of attention onto the search target. Fortunately, this can easily be done by analyzing the so-called N2pc component (N2 posterior contralateral) in the present experiment. The N2pc – a relative negativity of the ERP response over the occipital cortex contralateral to the target – is a well characterized modulation of the event-related potential (Luck and Hillyard, 1994; Eimer, 1996; Luck et al., 1997b; Woodman and Luck, 1999) and the event-related magnetic field response (Hopf et al., 2000; Hopf et al., 2002).[1] The N2pc is known to reflect the operation of focusing attention onto the target item in visual search (Luck et al., 1997b), and has recently been shown to appear, although with different relative polarity, in the monkey ERP (Woodman et al., 2007). In typical search tasks, the N2pc arises between about 200 and 300 ms after the presentation of search items, and it has been demonstrated to permit rapid tracking of multiple shifts of the attentional focus during visual search (Woodman and Luck, 1999). Source localization analysis based on neuromagnetic data revealed that the N2pc originates from current sources in the parietal as well as inferior occipitotemporal cortex (Hopf et al., 2000) (see below).

Figure 15.1d illustrates the time course of the RFE (C–D difference wave, dotted trace) superimposed on the N2pc effect (solid trace). The N2pc is shown as the difference waveform attend left VF targets minus attend right VF targets and appears with an onset of ≈180 ms that is approximately 40 ms delayed relative to the onset of the RFE around 140 ms. Thus feature-based selection as reflected by the RFE, indeed,

---

[1]For simplicity I will refer to both the ERP effect as well as its analog in the neuromagnetic response as N2pc.

precedes the operation of focusing attention onto the target as reflected by the N2pc. In addition, as illustrated in Figure 15.1e the current source of the N2pc turns out to originate from inferior occipitotemporal cortex regions more anterior than the origin of the RFE (shown as white outlines), indicating that the neural generators of the RFE and the N2pc are also anatomically distinct. Notably, neural activity underlying the RFE appears to arise at earlier stages in the visual processing hierarchy, yet in a strategic cortical position that could feed forward the results of feature-based selection to subsequent higher levels of visual processing and thereby bias (guide) target selection based on prioritized feature representations.

Taken together, the reported differences in time course and cortical origin of the RFE and the N2pc provide support for the notion of a two-stage account of visual search as developed in FIT and related models. The RFE in particular suggests the existence of an initial parallel stage during which the processing of relevant features is biased in an automatic and location-independent manner. The RFE may therefore solve the general problem of detecting relevant features in a visual scene and thereby provide a distribution map of potentially relevant locations. However, as mentioned earlier, in conjunction search purely feature-based mechanisms will inevitably provide insufficient information to locate the target unambiguously. In fact, global feature-based selection as reflected by the RFE may obscure target-localization in many situations, as distractor locations sharing relevant feature values with the target will receive extra activation which increases their competitive weight. In other words, RFE will aggravate ambiguities of location coding under such conditions. Hence, there need to be mechanisms beyond feature-based selection that eliminate ambiguities of location coding in visual search. The next section will discuss evidence from neuromagnetic recordings and from fMRI suggesting a neural mechanism that may serve to solve such ambiguities of location coding.

15.2   Solving ambiguities of location coding in visual search

There is a principal neuroanatomical reason for ambiguities of location (and feature) coding to arise in the visual system. The visual system is massively convergent (Zeki, 1978; Felleman and Van Essen, 1991; Desimone, 1992), and receptive field (RF) size increases with increasing levels in the visual processing hierarchy. Items that fall in different RFs at lower levels of the hierarchy will fall into the same RF at higher levels. Accordingly, information about an item's location relative to other items is progressively lost upwards in the hierarchy. The size of RFs in higher level extrastriate visual areas is much larger than the spatial resolution of attention (Intriligator and Cavanagh, 2001). The visual system thus must be able to regain precise location information about individual items and their spatial relation in some way. One possible neural mechanism contributing to the solution of this problem has been suggested based on observations with cell recordings in macaque extrastriate cortex (Moran and Desimone, 1985; Chelazzi et al., 1993, 1998; Luck et al., 1997a; Reynolds et al., 1999). Moran and Desimone (1985) observed while recording from V4 neurons that attention modulated cell-firing, in particular when more than one item was simultaneously presented within the cell's RF. The effect of attention was to attenuate the influence of the unattended item onto its firing. For example, when two items appeared in a V4 RF, one being effective the other ineffective in driving that cell, firing rate depended on which item the monkey was attending. Attending the ineffective item reduced firing as if the cell responded to the ineffective item alone. Analogous observations were made in monkeys performing memory-guided visual search (Chelazzi et al., 1993, 1998). Chelazzi et al. (1993) trained monkeys to search for an effective or an ineffective item, both simultaneously presented within a cell's RF. The initial firing response (until 160 ms) to the search items did not differ when the monkey searched for the effective or the ineffective item, reflecting the initial response of the cell to the effective stimulus in the RF. After 160 ms, however, the firing rate depended on which item was searched for. The firing response was attenuated when the ineffective item was the target, but it remained at the initially increased level when the effective item was the target. Again, attention modulated the cell's firing as if it responded to the searched-for item in isolation, or in other words, as if the cell had eliminated the unattended item from its RF. These observations were taken to imply that attention shrinks the effective spatial extent of the RF around the target, thereby eliminating the influence of distractor items (Moran and Desimone, 1985). Evidence has been added showing that the spatial distribution of RFs can change dynamically with attention. RFs in macaque V4 were observed to shift and shrink towards the spatial focus of attention (Connor et al., 1996, 1997; Connor, 2001) or towards the saccade target (Tolias et al., 2001). Recently, similar effects of shifting and shrinking RFs have been reported to exist in dorsal-stream areas like area 7a (Quraishi et al., 2007) or MT (Womelsdorf et al., 2006). RF shape and size were even found to dynamically change with elementary brain-states like arousal (Wörgötter et al., 1998). Moreover, the particular timing and configuration of stimuli was found to change the shape of RFs (Fu et al., 2002). It appears that dynamic changes of RF properties like effective size, form and location represent a common feature of selection in the visual system. What is important here is that size change provides an efficient mechanism permitting the recovery of location information and enhancement of spatial resolution, both being inevitably lost with the initial feedforward sweep of processing upwards in the visual processing hierarchy.

A number of psychophysical observations provided indirect hints at RF dynamics being intrinsically tied to the change of attentional resolution (Tsal and Shalev, 1996; Morgan et al., 1998; Yeshurun and Carrasco, 1998, 1999; Carrasco et al., 2002; Talgar and Carrasco, 2002). Morgan et al. (1998), for example, observed that spatial cuing enhanced the acuity of orientation discrimination of a peripheral item among oriented distractors, even when distractors were crowded, suggesting that focal attention permits to restrict stimulus encoding to a small spatial range that excludes the interference from distractors. Without focal attention coarse-scale mechanisms dominate stimulus decoding. Likewise, Yeshurun and Carrasco (1999) report that focal attention improves performance on Vernier and gap resolution tasks indicating that attention truly enhances visual resolution. The authors suggest that attention does so by reducing the size of spatial filters at peripheral locations – an operation that is proposed to correspond with the shrinking of RFs. Finally, Tsal and Shalev (1996) report a particularly revealing phenomenon, namely that inattention enhances the perceived length of peripherally presented lines, while focal attention leads to more precise length judgments. According to Tsal and Shalev (1996), this phenomenon is best explained by assuming that under inattention the visual periphery undergoes a coarse spatial sampling by large attentional receptive fields. Focal attention, in contrast, is proposed to lead to smaller attentional receptive fields permitting spatial sampling at a higher resolution (attentional receptive field hypothesis).

Given that RF changes adapt the resolution of discrimination to the spatial scale of the relevant input, how is RF change brought about at the neural level? At present, firm experimental evidence on that point is rather sparse. Most theoretical proposals suggest some form of selective funneling of information upwards through the hierarchy, such that a restricted subset of afferent neurons is permitted to contribute to the next hierarchical level (Olshausen et al., 1993; Tsotsos et al., 1995; Salinas and Abbott, 1997; Mozer and Sitton, 1998; Reynolds and Desimone, 1999; Maunsell and McAdams, 2001; Spratling and Johnson, 2004). Increasing the resolution of attention will, thus, translate into a gating of afferent input at progressively lower levels in the hierarchy, with the particular level somehow reflecting the spatial scale of the attended input. Stimuli separated at a smaller spatial scale will produce ambiguities of location coding at lower levels in the visual hierarchy. The modulatory effects of attention mediating RF shrinking would, therefore, be predicted to appear with largest expression at lower levels of the hierarchy. We recently addressed this prediction with electromagnetic and fMRI recordings in human observers. To assess attention-driven modulatory activity in the magnetic response, we focused on the magnetic analog of the N2pc component. As already mentioned above, the N2pc is a well characterized modulation of the ERP/ERMF response, which reflects the operation of focusing attention onto the target item in visual search. MEG source localization revealed that the N2pc arises from a sequence of current sources in the parietal (180–200 ms) and ventral occipitotemporal cortex (200–350 ms), with the latter contributing most (Hopf et al., 2000). Notably, the N2pc amplitude was observed to reflect the degree distractors interfere with the target in visual search. It increases significantly when increasing the number of distractors, or the degree of feature-overlap with the target (Luck et al., 1997b; Hopf et al., 2002). These and a number of other properties led to the proposal that the N2pc reflects an attentional operation that serves to resolve ambiguities of coding in extrastriate visual cortex (ambiguity resolution theory) by filtering out distractor information (Luck and Hillyard, 1994; Luck et al., 1997b). In direct support of this notion, Luck and coworkers showed with a series of experiments (Luck et al., 1997b) that the N2pc parallels the suppressive firing effects in monkey extrastriate cortex reported by Chelazzi et al. (1993, 1998, 2001). Importantly, as outlined above, the latter firing effects are assumed to reflect the shrinking of RFs in extrastriate cortex. The N2pc is therefore a neurophysiological measure that permits to directly address the underlying mechanisms at the neural population level. We specifically predicted that the extrastriate current origin of the N2pc would change with the perceptual scale at which ambiguities of spatial coding arise.

To address this hypothesis, we aimed at changing the perceptual scale that would be attended without changing item spacing or the spatial layout of the stimulus (Hopf et al., 2006b). This is important as it is known from fMRI in humans that neural suppression in visual cortex due to multiple items scales with item distance (Kastner et al.,

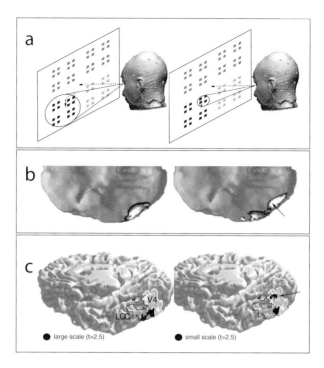

Figure 15.2. (a) Illustration of search frames requiring subjects to focus onto large-scale displacements (four dots displaced downwards, left) or small-scale displacements (one dot displaced upwards, right). (b) Current source density distribution (MNLS) of the N2pc effect between 250 and 300 ms after search frame onset for large scale trials (left) and small-scale trials (right). (c) fMRI activity for large-scale targets (left) and small-scale targets (right) overlaid onto the folded cortical surface of a single observer. Areas V4 and LOC are highlighted as regions with a white and a black outline, respectively.

1998, 1999, 2001), such that larger item distances cause a suppression in higher-level areas (with larger RFs) as compared with smaller item distances which lead to comparably larger BOLD reductions in lower level areas (Kastner et al., 2001). To avoid such stimulus-dependent scaling effect, we used self-similar stimuli (derived from a 2-dimensional Menger-sponge) as shown in Figure 15.2a. These stimuli were constructed by repeating a four-dot square pattern hierarchically at increasing spatial scale. Subjects were asked to discriminate a small displacement of a corner element, which could either be a single dot at the smallest spatial scale, or a four-dot corner at the next higher spatial scale. Identifying a small-scale displacement required a finer spatial resolution than a large-scale displacement, and thus entailed a narrower shrinking of RFs.

From trial to trial the scale of the displacement (large/small) varied unpredictably, forcing subjects to adjust the resolution of discrimination on each trial anew. Figure 15.2b shows the average current source distribution of the magnetic N2pc when subjects discriminated a large-scale displacement (left side). The current origin of the

N2pc was located in the ventral extrastriate cortex, confirming our previous observations. However, in trials where subjects were required to narrow the focus of attention to discriminate a small-scale displacement (right side), an additional current source maximum appeared in a more posterior ventral extrastriate region (arrow). This more posterior current maximum is clearly consistent with the prediction that attention to small-scale displacements modulated activity in an additional visual area that is lower in the visual hierarchy (and has smaller RFs) than the large-scale maximum. To confirm this observation with higher localizatory precision, we adapted the experiment as an fMRI version and combined it with a detailed retinotopic mapping of visual cortex areas in selected observers. Figure 15.2c shows BOLD maxima (black areas) reflecting the N2pc effect for large- (left) and small-scale (right) trials of one observer superimposed onto a 3D-surface segmentation of her right hemisphere. Notably, analogous to the MEG source localization results, large-scale trials are characterized by a BOLD maximum in ventral visual cortex which appears inside the so-called lateral occipital complex (LOC) shown with a black outline. Small-scale trials, on the other hand, show a BOLD maximum also in area V4 (region with a white outline) in addition to a maximum in LOC. While LOC and V4 are visual areas of the ventral stream, V4 represents a lower level than LOC in the visual hierarchy (Human LOC is suggested to be homolog to macaque TEO (Tootell et al., 2003)). Thus, attending to smaller separations produces an additional modulation of neural activity in a ventral stream visual area with smaller RFs. This suggests that attention resolves ambiguities of location coding by modulating visual areas at hierarchical levels where RF size matches the spatial scale of the attended input. Importantly, this observation hints at a possible mechanism for how RF shrinking is accomplished in the visual system. Shrinking of RF size may represent a consequence of modulatory effects at progressively lower levels in the processing hierarchy. But what do the MEG/fMRI observations just reported tell us about the nature of processing behind those modulations at different hierarchical levels? The reported data are clearly suggestive of a mechanism that involves input gating from afferent lower-level visual areas they do not, however, clarify this question completely. Narrowing RF size for higher spatial resolution may be achieved by changing the influence of projections converging from the level(s) below. This may, however, be mediated by different modulatory mechanisms. It is possible, for example, that RF shrinking at a given hierarchical level n is achieved by attenuating units at level $n - 1$ thereby eliminating their contribution to the next higher level. Alternatively, the projection of relevant units at level $n - 1$ may be strengthened by attention, producing a relative attenuation of irrelevant converging units at level n. Finally, it is possible that attenuation and enhancement combine in a selective manner in gating the contribution of level $n - 1$ input towards level n (Reynolds et al., 1999). A mechanism in line with a relative attenuation has been proposed based on computational considerations (Salinas and Abbott, 1997; Salinas and Thier, 2000) or on observations from single-unit recordings in the macaque (McAdams and Maunsell, 1999; Treue and Maunsell, 1999; Maunsell and McAdams, 2001). Maunsell and McAdams (2001) for example suggested that shrinking of RFs at a given hierarchical level may arise as a consequence of attention-driven multiplicative scaling of neural responses at a lower level in the hierarchy. With the reviewed evidence from MEG and fMRI recordings at hand, it is not possible to directly decide among those possibilities, not least because the link between these measures and the modulatory effects at the cellular level is still a debated issue that needs to be clarified by future research.

15.3   Recurrent processing and the center-surround profile of the spotlight of attention

Both MEG and fMRI data discussed above indicate that narrowing the focus of attention to discriminate small-scale displacements involved a modulation of extrastriate activity at more than one level in the processing hierarchy. Focusing onto small-scale displacements led to a modulation of activity not only in V4, but also in LOC, the region where large-scale displacements produced a maximum modulation by attention and where RFs are larger than in V4. This is a notable observation as sufficient spatial selectivity could be achieved by just modulating the lowest appropriate hierarchical level where RF size is small enough to permit item separation. An additional modulation at a higher level where the spatial resolution of RFs is coarser than required for item separation appears to be unnecessary, and in fact puzzling at a first glance. However, such a pattern would be reasonable to expect if spatial focusing proceeds as a top-down selection process in the visual system, where modulatory effects due to attention propagate from coarse to fine through the processing hierarchy. The latter notion has been suggested based on different experimental observations and theoretical considerations. (Tsotsos, 1993; Tsotsos et al., 1995; Lamme and Roelfsema, 2000; Hochstein and Ahissar, 2002; Lamme, 2003). Hochstein and Ahissar (2002), for example, review a large body of experimental data suggesting that explicit visual selection proceeds in reverse hierarchical direction. Their so-called Reverse Hierarchy Model proposes that visual selection starts with vision at a glance based on categorical discriminations in high-level areas with large generalizing RFs, and then proceeds by involving lower-level areas when vision with scrutiny is required.

A computationally more explicit theoretical framework for such top-down propagating selection mechanism has been proposed by Tsotsos and coworkers (Tsotsos, 1990; Tsotsos et al., 1995, 2001). This framework – referred to as the Selective Tuning Model (STM) – was developed to provide a computational solution to the formally intractable problem of coping with a combinatorial explosion of feature-coding possibilities in vision based on a complexity level analysis (Tsotsos, 1990). Importantly, STM proposes an explicit mechanism that explains how location information at any precision can be regained via top-down selection after it is lost with the feedforward sweep of processing the visual hierarchy. In keeping with the realistic neuroanatomical connectivity, STM assumes that the visual input first propagates upwards through the visual hierarchy to reach high-level visual areas (feedforward sweep of processing). This upward propagation produces a diverging sweep of activations with the biggest extension at the top level where RFs are largest. Here, attention comes into play in form of a winner-take-all (WTA) process at the global level. This WTA operates over its direct feedforward input by pruning away connections from the level below that do not contribute to the global winner. This pruning operation is then iteratively applied from level to level downwards through the hierarchy, thereby producing a pass zone of un-attenuated activity. Importantly, the spatial resolution of the pass zone increases with each step downwards the hierarchy, as its extension matches the RF size of the winner at the given hierarchical level. STM's coarse to fine multilevel selection process thus implements a mechanism capable of increasing spatial resolution directly in line with the observations reported in the previous section (Hopf et al., 2006b). Furthermore, it makes an important testable prediction regarding the spatial profile of the focus of attention. STM's top-down propagating WTA generates a pass zone of un-attenuated neural activity based on neural attenuation in the immediate surround. As the pruning operation reduces its spatial scope with each level downwards the visual hierarchy, surround attenuation will become strongest in a region adjacent to the un-attenuated center. As a consequence the spatial focus of attention will not be a simple gradient as traditionally envisioned, but rather show a center-surround structure that resembles a Mexican-hat profile. Several lines of psychophysical and neurophysiological evidence suggest that the spatial focus attention, in fact, has a center-surround structure instead of a simple gradient (Cave and Zimmerman, 1997; Caputo and Guerra, 1998; Bahcall and Kowler, 1999; Mounts, 2000; Slotnick et al., 2002; Cutzu and Tsotsos, 2003; Mounts and Gavett, 2004; Muller and Kleinschmidt, 2004; Muller et al., 2005; Carlson et al., 2007; McCarley and Mounts, 2007). Based on high-resolution MEG recordings, we recently provided direct neurophysiological evidence for the existence of such profile in visual search (Hopf et al., 2006a). Our general experimental approach was to probe the passive excitability of the visual cortex by flashing an irrelevant stimulus at varying distances from a popout target while subjects performed a visual search task. To avoid low-level stimulation confounds from changing the probe's location, the probe stimulus was flashed at a fixed spatial location while the location of the search target was varied relative to the probe from trial to trial. Specifically, subjects were required to discriminate the orientation of a red popout C (target) among eight randomly oriented blue Cs (distractors) presented at an iso-eccentric location in the right lower visual quadrant as shown in Figure 15.3a.

The search task involved a fine discrimination of the gap orientation, which guaranteed that subjects had to narrow their attentional focus onto the target. On 50% of the trials, a small irrelevant white ring (the probe) was flashed (50 ms) around the center item 250 ms after search frame onset (frame + probe trials (FP)), while on the remaining trials, no probe was presented (frame only trials (FO)). Whether a probe appeared or not on a given trial was not predictable. The location of the target item varied randomly from trial to trial, such that the focus of attention could be at the probe's location (probe distance 0 (PD0)), or one to four items away either towards the vertical or horizontal meridian (PD1–PD4). Figure 15.3a illustrates all possible probe distances towards the vertical meridian. The response elicited by the probe at the resulting nine possible probe distances (four towards either meridian and PD0) permitted to sample the spatial profile of cortical excitability at and around the focus of attention in a systematical way. Because we aimed at isolating the magnetic response to the probe proper, we subtracted activity elicited by FO-trials from that of FP-trials at each target location. This eliminated activity reflecting attentional focusing as well as activity reflecting stimulation differences due to the changing location of the color popout, but it left a clean measure of the magnitude of cortical excitability as a function of distance from the focus of attention. Figure 15.3b summarizes the probe related magnetic response (FP

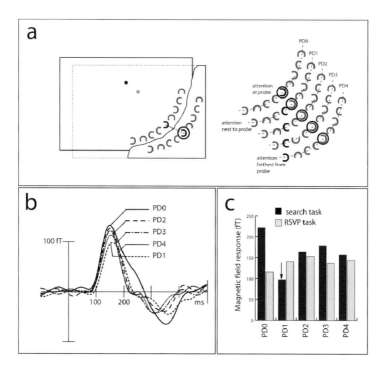

Figure 15.3. (a) Illustration of the passive probe paradigm. In 50% of the trials a white ring appeared 250 ms after search frame onset around the center item (left). The right side illustrates five possible target-to-probe distances (PD0–PD4). The target location also varied towards the horizontal meridian (not shown). (b) MEG waveforms elicited by the probe at different distances to the focus of attention. Shown are waveform differences frame-probe minus frame-only trials. (c) Average magnetic response elicited by the probe (average activity between 130 and 150 ms) when subjects performed the visual search task (black bars) or when attention was withdrawn from the search items by a demanding RSVP task at fixation (white bars).

minus-FO difference) over the occipital cortex for all probe distances averaged across 12 observers. Obviously, the probe response shows a relative enhancement when attention is focused onto the probe location (PD0). But when attention is focused onto the location next to the probe (PD1), a clear attenuation of the probe response is seen relative to PD0, and importantly, also relative to farther away probe distances (PD2–4). When attention was withdrawn from the search items by engaging subjects in a demanding RSVP task at fixation (experiment 2 in Hopf et al., 2006a) the Mexican-hat profile was eliminated (white bars in Figure 15.3c) indicating that the attenuation in the narrow surround of the search target is a true consequence of attentional focusing in visual search. Thus, the focus of attention – traditionally envisioned as a "spotlight" or "zoom-lens" – may not be a simple monotonic gradient that falls off gradually from its center. Instead, at least under conditions of visual search it may have a more complex profile with a center enhancement surrounded by a narrow zone of attenuation.

As outlined above, this center-surround profile is clearly in support of one key prediction of the STM. According to the STM the spatial focus of attention corresponds with a pass zone of unattenuated input resulting from a top-down pruning operation that propagates downwards the visual processing hierarchy from level to level. On its way downwards, feedforward connections from next lower-level RFs not contributing to the relevant subregion of the RF at a given level (i.e. the target's location) are eliminated. As a natural consequence of this iterative top-down pruning a narrow zone of surround attenuation arises. It should finally be emphasized that the observation of a center-surround profile of the focus of attention in visual search nicely dovetails with the results reported in the second section where we observed that enhancing the resolution of attention involves a modulation of neural activity at progressively lower levels in the visual hierarchy.

15.4   Conclusion

We have reviewed data from electromagnetic and fMRI recordings hinting at neural mechanisms that solve inevitable problems of stimulus coding in visual search. We have discussed modulations of the electromagnetic response reflecting the processing of relevant features prior to, and independent of, the operation of focusing attention onto the search target. This indicated that relevant features are initially registered in the visual system in a location-independent manner, which provided neurophysiological support for the notion of a so-called preattentional feature map – an intermediary state of stimulus representation proposed by many theories on visual search. We then focused on the problem of how attention accomplishes to change spatial resolution in a flexible way during visual search. We observed that enhancing spatial resolution involves modulations at progressively lower levels of the visual processing hierarchy where receptive field size matches the scale of the attended input. We finally discussed neuromagnetic evidence supporting the key notion of the Selective Tuning Model (Tsotsos et al., 1995, Tsotsos, 2005) that such coarse to fine selection across hierarchical levels gives rise to a spatial profile of the focus of attention that is not a simple monotonic gradient but a more complex profile with a center enhancement surrounded by a narrow zone of attenuation. The observations presented here, thus, emphasize the importance to consider the interplay of activity modulations across multiple levels of the cortical hierarchy for advancing our understanding of attentional selection in the visual system.

Acknowledgment

The research described here was supported by BMBF Grant 01G000202 (Center for Advanced Imaging), DFG Grant He 1531/3-5/9-1, and NIMH Grant (MH63001).

References

Bahcall D. O. and Kowler, E. (1999). Attentional interference at small spatial separations. *Vision Res.*, 39: 71–86.

Bichot, N. P., Rossi, A. F. and Desimone, R. (2005). Parallel and serial neural mechanisms for visual search in macaque area V4. *Science*, 308: 529–534.

Blaser, E., Sperling, G. and Lu, Z. L. (1999). Measuring the amplification of attention. *Proc. Nat. Acad. Sci. USA*, 96: 11681–11686.

Caputo. G. and Guerra, S. (1998). Attentional selection by distractor suppression. *Vision Res.*, 38: 669–689.

Carlson, T. A., Alvarez, G. A. and Cavanagh, P. (2007). Quadrantic deficit reveals anatomical constraints on selection. *Proc. Nat. Acad. Sci. USA*, 104: 13496–13500.

Carrasco, M., Williams, P. E. and Yeshurun, Y. (2002). Covert attention increases spatial resolution with or without masks: support for signal enhancement. *J. Vis.*, 2: 467–479.

Cave, K. R. (1999) The FeatureGate model of visual selection. *Psychological Res.*, 62:182–194.

Cave, K. R. and Zimmerman, J. M. (1997) Flexibility in spatial attention before and after practice. *Psychol. Sci.*, 8: 399–403.

Chelazzi, L., Duncan, J., Miller, E. K. and Desimone, R. (1998). Response of neurons in inferior temporal cortex during memory-guided visual search. *J. Neurophysiol.*, 80: 2918–2940.

Chelazzi, L., Miller, E. K., Duncan, J. and Desimone, R. (1993). A neural basis for visual search in inferior temporal cortex. *Nature*, 363: 345–347.

Chelazzi, L., Miller, E. K., Duncan, J. and Desimone, R. (2001). Responses of neurons in macaque area V4 during memory-guided visual search. *Cereb. Cortex*, 11: 761–772.

Connor, C. E. (2001). Shifting receptive fields. *Neuron*, 29: 548–549.

Connor, C. E., Gallant, J. L., Preddie, D. C. and Van Essen, D. C. (1996) Responses in area V4 depend on the spatial relationship between stimulus and attention. *J. Neurophysiol.*, 75: 1306–1308.

Connor, C. E., Preddie, D. C., Gallant, J. L. and Van Essen, D. C. (1997). Spatial attention effects in macaque area V4. *J. Neurosci.*, 19: 3201–3214.

Cutzu, F. and Tsotsos, J. K. (2003). The selective tuning model of attention: psychophysical evidence for a suppressive annulus around an attended item. *Vision Res.*, 43: 205–219.

Desimone, R. (1992). Neural substrates for visual attention in the primate brain. In G. A. Carpenter and S. Grossberg (eds.) *Neural Networks for Vision and Image Processing*. Cambridge, MA: MIT Press, pp. 343-364.

Duncan, J. and Humphreys, G. W. (1989). Visual search and stimulus similarity. *Psych. Rev.*, 96: 433–458.

Egeth, H. E., Virzi, R. A. and Garbat, H. (1984). Searching for conjunctively defined targets. *J. Exp. Psychol.: Hum. Percept. Perf.*, 10: 32–39.

Eimer, M. (1996). The N2pc component as an indicator of attentional selectivity. *Electroencephalogr. Clin. Neurophysiol.*, 99: 225–234.

Felleman, D. J. and Van Essen, D. C. (1991). Distributed hierarchical processing in the primate cerebral cortex. *Cereb. Cortex*, 1: 1–47.

Fu, Y. X., Djupsund, K., Gao, H., Hayden, B., Shen, K. and Dan, Y. (2002). Temporal specificity in the cortical plasticity of visual space representation. *Science*, 296: 1999–2003.

Hochstein, S. and Ahissar, M. (2002). View from the top: hierarchies and reverse hierarchies in the visual system. *Neuron*, 36: 791–804.

Hopf, J.-M., Boehler, N., Luck, S. J., Tsotsos, J. K., Heinze, H.-J. and Schoenfeld, M. A. (2006a). Direct neurophysiological evidence for spatial suppression surrounding the focus of attention in vision. *PNAS*, 103: 1053–1058.

Hopf, J.-M., Boelmans, K., Schoenfeld, A. M., Heinze, H.-J. and Luck, S. J. (2002). How does attention attenuate target-distractor interference in vision? Evidence from magnetoencephalographic recordings. *Cogn. Brain Res.*, 15: 17–29.

Hopf, J.-M., Boelmans, K., Schoenfeld, A., Luck, S. J. and Heinze, H.-J. (2004). Attention to features precedes attention to locations in visual search: evidence from electromagnetic brain responses in humans. *J. Neurosci.*, 24: 1822–1832.

Hopf, J.-M., Luck, S. J., Boelmans, K., Schoenfeld, A., Boehler, N., Rieger, J. W. and Heinze, H.-J. (2006b). The neural site of attention matches the spatial scale of perception. *J. Neurosci.*, 26: 3532–3540.

Hopf, J.-M., Luck, S. J., Girelli, M., Hagner, T., Mangun, G. R., Scheich, H. and Heinze, H.-J. (2000). Neural sources of focused attention in visual search. *Cereb. Cortex*, 10: 1233–1241.

Intriligator, J. and Cavanagh, P. (2001). The spatial resolution of visual attention. *Cogn. Psychol.*, 43: 171–216.

Kastner, S., De Weerd, P., Desimone, R. and Ungerleider, L. G. (1998). Mechanisms of directed attention in the human extrastriate cortex as revealed by functional MRI. *Science*, 282: 108–111.

Kastner, S., De Weerd, P., Pinsk, M. A., Elizondo, M. I., Desimone, R. and Ungerleider, L. G. (2001). Modulation of sensory suppression: implications for receptive field sizes in the human visual cortex. *J. Neurophysiol.*, 86: 1398–1411.

Kastner, S., Pinsk, M. A., De Weerd, P., Desimone, R. and Ungerleider, L. (1999). Increased activity in human visual cortex during directed attention in the absence of visual stimulation. *Neuron*, 22: 751–761.

Lamme, V. A. (2003). Why visual attention and awareness are different. *Trends Cogn. Sci.*, 7: 12 18.

Lamme, V. A. F. and Roelfsema, P. R. (2000). The distinct modes of vision offered by feedforward and recurrent processing. *Trends Neurosci.*, 23: 571–579.

Lu, Z. L. and Sperling, G. (1995). Attention-generated apparent motion. *Nature*, 377: 237–239.

Luck, S. J. and Hillyard, S. A. (1994). Spatial filtering during visual search: evidence from human electrophysiology. *J. Exp. Psychol.: Hum. Percept. Perf.*, 20: 1000–1014.

Luck, S. J., Chelazzi, L., Hillyard, S. A. and Desimone, R. (1997a). Neural mechanisms of spatial selective attention in areas V1, V2, and V4 of macaque visual cortex. *J. Neurophysiol.*, 77: 24–42.

Luck, S. J., Girelli, M., McDermott, M. T. and Ford, M. A. (1997b). Bridging the gap between monkey neurophysiology and human perception: an ambiguity resolution theory of visual selective attention. *Cogn. Psychol.*, 33: 64–87.

Martinez-Trujillo, J. C. and Treue, S. (2004). Feature-based attention increases the selectivity of population responses in primate visual cortex. *Curr. Biol.*, 14: 744–751.

Maunsell, J. H. and Treue, S. (2006). Feature-based attention in visual cortex. *Trends Neurosci.*, 29: 317–322.

Maunsell, J. H. R. and McAdams, C. J. (2001). Effects of attention on the responsiveness and selectivity of individual neurons in visual cerebral cortex. In J. Braun, C. Koch and J. L. Davis (eds.) *Visual Attention and Cortical Circuits*. Boston, MA: MIT Press, pp. 103–119.

Mazer, J. A. and Gallant, J. L. (2003). Goal-related activity in V4 during free viewing visual search. Evidence for a ventral stream visual salience map. *Neuron*, 40: 1241–1250.

McAdams, C. J. and Maunsell, J. H. (1999). Effects of attention on orientation-tuning functions of single neurons in macaque cortical area V4. *J. Neurosci.*, 19: 431–441.

McAdams, C. J. and Maunsell, J. H. (2000). Attention to both space and feature modulates neuronal responses in macaque area V4. *J. Neurophysiol.*, 83: 1751–1755.

McCarley, J. S. and Mounts, J. R. (2007). Localized attentional interference affects object individuation, not feature detection. *Perception*, 36: 17–32.

Moran, J. and Desimone, R. (1985). Selective attention gates visual processing in the extrastriate cortex. *Science*, 229: 782–784.

Morgan, M. J., Ward, R. M. and Castet, E. (1998). Visual search for a tilted target: tests of spatial uncertainty models. *Quat. J. Exp. Psychol. A*, 51: 347–370.

Motter, B. C. (1994). Neural correlates of attentive selection for color or luminance in extrastriate area V4. *J. Neurosci.*, 14: 2178–2189.

Mounts, J. R. (2000). Evidence for suppressive mechanisms in attentional selection: feature singletons produce inhibitory surrounds. *Percept. Psychophys.*, 62: 969–983.

Mounts, J. R. and Gavett, B. E. (2004). The role of salience in localized attentional interference. *Vision Res.*, 44: 1575–1588.

Mozer, M. C. and Sitton, M. (1998). Computational modelling of spatial attention. In H. Pashler (ed.) *Attention*. Hove, UK: Psychology Press, pp. 341–393.

Muller, N. G. and Kleinschmidt, A. (2004). The attentional 'spotlight's' penumbra: center-surround modulation in striate cortex. *NeuroReport*, 15: 977–980.

Muller, N. G., Mollenhauer, M., Rosler, A. and Kleinschmidt, A. (2005). The attentional field has a Mexican hat distribution. *Vision Res.*, 45: 1129–1137.

Nakayama, K. and Silverman, G. H. (1986). Serial and parallel processing of visual feature conjunctions. *Nature*, 320: 264–265.

Ogawa, T. and Komatsu, H. (2004). Target selection in area V4 during a multidimensional visual search task. *J. Neurosci.*, 24: 6371–6382.

Olshausen, B. A., Anderson, C. A. and Van Essen, D. C. (1993). A neurobiological model of visual attention and invariant pattern recognition based on dynamic routing of information. *J. Neurosci.*, 13: 4700–4719.

Quraishi, S., Heider, B. and Siegel, R. M. (2007). Attentional modulation of receptive field structure in area 7a of the behaving monkey. *Cereb. Cortex*, 17: 1841–1857.

Reynolds, J. H. and Desimone, R. (1999). The role of neural mechanisms of attention in solving the binding problem. *Neuron*, 24: 19–29.

Reynolds, J. H., Chelazzi, L. and Desimone, R. (1999). Competitive mechanisms subserve attention in macaque areas V2 and V4. *J. Neurosci.*, 19: 1736–1753.

Riesenhuber, M. and Poggio, T. (2000). Models of object recognition. *Nat. Neurosci.*, 3 Suppl: 1199–1204.

Saenz, M., Buracas, G. T. and Boynton, G. M. (2002). Global effects of feature-based attention in human visual cortex. *Nat. Neurosci.*, 5: 631–632.

Saenz, M., Buracas, G. T. and Boynton, G. M. (2003). Global feature-based attention for motion and color. *Vision Res.*, 43: 629–637.

Salinas, E. and Abbott, L. F. (1997). Invariant visual responses from attentional gain fields. *J. Neurophysiol.*, 77: 3267–3272.

Salinas, E. and Thier, P. (2000). Gain modulation: a major computational principle of the central nervous system. *Neuron*, 27: 15–21.

Sary, G., Vogels, R. and Orban, G. A. (1993). Cue-invariant shape selectivity of macaque inferior temporal neurons. *Science*, 260: 995–997.

Slotnick, S. D., Hopfinger, J. B., Klein, S. A. and Sutter, E. E. (2002). Darkness beyond the light: attentional inhibition surrounding the classic spotlight. *NeuroReport*, 13: 773–778.

Spratling, M. W. and Johnson, M. H. (2004). A feedback model of visual attention. *J. Cogn. Neurosci.*, 16: 219–237.

Talgar, C. P. and Carrasco, M. (2002). Vertical meridian asymmetry in spatial resolution: visual and attentional factors. *Psychon. Bull. Rev.*, 9: 714–722.

Tanaka, K. (2003). Columns for complex visual object features in the inferotemporal cortex: clustering of cells with similar but slightly different stimulus selectivities. *Cereb. Cortex*, 13: 90–99.

Tolias, A. S., Moore, T., Smirnakis, S. M., Tehovnik, E. J., Siapas, A. G. and Schiller, P. H. (2001). Eye movements modulate visual receptive fields of V4 neurons. *Neuron*, 29: 757–767.

Tootell, R. B., Tsao, D. and Vanduffel, W. (2003). Neuroimaging weighs in: humans meet macaques in "primate" visual cortex. *J. Neurosci.*, 23: 3981–3989.

Treisman, A. and Gelade, G. (1980). A feature-integration theory of attention. *Cogn. Psychol.*, 12: 97–136.

Treisman, A. and Gormican, S. (1988). Feature analysis in early vision: evidence from search asymmetries. *Psychol. Rev.*, 95: 15–48.

Treisman, A. and Sato, S. (1990). Conjunction search revisited. *J. Exp. Psychol.: Hum. Percept. Perf.*, 16: 459–478.

Treue, S. and Martinez-Trujillo, J. C. (1999). Feature-based attention influences motion processing gain in macaque visual cortex. *Nature*, 399: 575–579.

Treue, S. and Maunsell, J. H. (1999). Effects of attention on the processing of motion in macaque middle temporal and medial superior temporal visual cortical areas. *J. Neurosci.*, 19: 7591–7602.

Tsal, Y. and Shalev, L. (1996). Inattention magnifies perceived length: the attentional receptive field hypothesis. *J. Exp. Psychol.: Hum. Percept. Perform.*, 22: 233–243.

Tsotsos, J. K. (1990). Analyzing vision at the complexity level. *Behav. Brain Sci.*, 13: 423–469.

Tsotsos, J. K. (1993). An inhibitory beam for attentional selection. In L. Harris and M. Jenkin (eds.) *Spatial Vision in Humans and Robots*. Cambridge, UK: Cambridge University Press, pp. 313–331.

Tsotsos, J. K. (2005). The selective tuning model for visual attention. In L. Itti, G. Rees and J. K. Tsotsos (eds.) *Neurobiology of Attention*. San Diego, CA: Elsevier, pp. 562–569.

Tsotsos, J. K., Culhane, S. M. and Cutzu, F. (2001). From foundational principles to a hierarchical selection circuit for attention. In J. Braun, C. Koch and J. L. Davis (eds.) *Visual Attention and Cortical Circuits*. Cambridge, MA: MIT Press, pp. 285–306.

Tsotsos, J. K., Culhane, S. M., Wai, W. Y. K., Lai, Y., Davis, N. and Nuflo, F. (1995). Modeling visual attention via selective tuning. *Artif. Intell.*, 78: 507–545.

Wolfe, J. M. (1994). Guided search 2.0: a revised model of visual search. *Psychonomic Bull. Rev.*, 1: 202–238.

Wolfe, J. M. (2003). Moving towards solutions to some enduring controversies in visual search. *Trends Cogn. Sci.*, 7: 70–76.

Wolfe J. M. and Bennet, S. C. (1996). Preattentive object files: shapeless bundles of basic features. *Vision Res.*, 37: 25–43.

Wolfe, J. M., Cave, K. R., Franzel, S. L. (1989). Guided search: an alternative to the feature integration model for visual search. *J. Exp. Psychol.: Hum. Percept. Perf.*, 15: 419–433.

Womelsdorf, T., Anton-Erxleben, K., Pieper, F. and Treue, S. (2006). Dynamic shifts of visual receptive fields in cortical area MT by spatial attention. *Nat. Neurosci.*, 9: 1156–1160.

Woodman, G. F. and Luck, S. J. (1999). Electrophysiological measurement of rapid shifts of attention during visual search. *Nature*, 400: 867–869.

Woodman, G. F., Kang, M. S., Rossi, A. F. and Schall, J. D. (2007). Nonhuman primate event-related potentials indexing covert shifts of attention. *Proc. Natl. Acad. Sci. USA*, 104: 15111–15116.

Wörgötter, F., Suder, K., Zhao, Y., Kerscher, N., Eysel, U. T. and Funke, K. (1998). State-dependent receptive-field restructuring in the visual cortex. *Nature*, 396: 165–168.

Yeshurun, Y. and Carrasco, M. (1998). Attention improves or impairs visual performance by enhancing spatial resolution. *Nature*, 396: 72–75.

Yeshurun, Y. and Carrasco, M. (1999). Spatial attention improves performance in spatial resolution tasks. *Vision Res.*, 39: 293–306.

Zeki, S. M. (1978). Functional specialization in the visual cortex of the rhesus monkey. *Nature*, 274: 423–428.

Part IV

Attention and consciousness

16 Two visual systems: separate pathways for perception and action in the human cerebral cortex

M. A. Goodale and T. Ganel

Our appreciation of the world beyond our bodies owes more to vision than to any other sense. The perception of objects and events "out there" is so compelling that it is sometimes difficult to comprehend that this experience arises entirely from the activity of neurons inside our head. But the phenomenal intensity of visual consciousness makes us forget that this particular function of the visual system is a relative newcomer on the evolutionary landscape. Vision began, not as a system for "representing" the world, but as a system for the distal sensory control of movement. Primitive organisms, whose activity is modulated by light, do not "see" the world. Indeed, even when explaining the visually guided behavior of more complex organisms, there is no need to invoke representational vision; one can talk entirely in mechanistic terms without appealing to perception or experience. What is perhaps more difficult to accept is the idea that many of our own visually guided actions can be accounted for in exactly the same way. But to develop this idea will require a more detailed discussion of the origins of vision, first as a system for the control of movement, and then later, as a system for representing the world.

16.1 The origins of vision

As we have already emphasized, visual systems first evolved not to enable animals to perceive the world, but to provide distal sensory control of their movements. One clear example of this is phototaxis, a behavior exhibited by many simple organisms in which

Cortical Mechanisms of Vision, ed. M. Jenkin and L. R. Harris. Published by Cambridge University Press.
© Cambridge University Press 2009.

they move towards or away from light. Take the case of *Halobacterium salinarum*, a bacterium that lives in highly saline environments. *Halobacterium salinarum* uses orange light as energy source but ultraviolet light can damage its DNA. As a consequence, these halobacteria have developed differential phototaxis response, whereby the system measures light intensity at different wavelengths so that they end up moving towards orange light and away from UV light (Hildebrand and Schimz, 1985). To explain *Halobacterium salinarum's* light-sensitive behavior, it is not necessary to argue that this single-celled organism "perceives" the light or even that it has some sort of internal model of the outside world. One simply has to posit the existence of some sort of input-output device within *Halobacterium salinarum* that links the intensity of ambient orange and UV light to the pattern of locomotion. As we will see, even the visually guided behavior of more complex organisms, such as vertebrates, can be explained without reference to experiential perception or any "general-purpose" representation of the outside world.

In vertebrates, the visual control systems for different kinds of behavior have evolved as relatively independent neural systems. For example, in present-day amphibians, such as the frog, visually guided prey catching and visually guided obstacle avoidance are separately mediated by different neural pathways from the retina right through to the motor networks in the brain that produce the constituent movements (Ingle, 1973, 1980, 1982, 1991). The visual control of prey catching depends on circuitry involving retinal projections to a structure in the midbrain called the optic tectum, while the visual control of locomotion around barriers depends on circuitry involving retinal projections to a quite separate structure called the pretectum, which as the name implies is located immediately in front of the optic tectum. Each of these retinal targets in the brain projects in turn to different motor centers in the brainstem and spinal cord. In fact, evidence from several decades of work in both frog and toad suggests that there are at least five separate visuomotor modules, each responsible for a different kind of visually guided behavior and each having distinct neural pathways from input to output (Ingle, 1991; Ewert, 1987). The outputs of these different modules certainly have to be coordinated, but in no sense are they guided by a single general-purpose visual representation in the frog's brain.[1]

There is evidence that the same kind of visuomotor modularity found in the frog also exists in the mammalian and avian brain (for review, see Goodale, 1996 and Jäger, 1997). For example, lesions of the superior colliculus (the mammalian equivalent of the optic tectum in amphibians, reptiles, and birds) in a variety of mammals, including rats, hamsters, gerbils, cats, and monkeys, disrupt or dramatically reduce the animal's ability to orient to visual targets, particularly targets presented in the visual periphery (see review by Goodale and Milner, 1992). Conversely, stimulation of this structure, either electrically or pharmacologically, will often elicit contraversive movements of the eyes, head, limbs, and body that resemble normal orienting movements (see review by Dean et al., 1989). In contrast, lesions of the pretectum have been shown to interfere with barrier avoidance, leaving orienting movements relatively intact (Goodale and Milner, 1982). This striking parallel in the neural architecture of amphibians and mammals

---

[1]For a discussion of this issue, see Goodale (1996) and Milner and Goodale (2006).

suggests that modularity in visuomotor control is an ancient (and presumably efficient) characteristic of vertebrate brains.

But although there is considerable evidence for visuomotor modularity in all classes of vertebrates, the very complexity of the day-to-day living in many mammals, particularly in higher primates, demands much more flexible organization of the circuitry. In monkeys (and thus presumably in humans as well), many of the visuomotor circuits in the midbrain and brainstem that are shared with simpler vertebrates appear to be modulated by more recently evolved control systems in the cerebral cortex (for review, see Goodale and Milner, 2004a; Milner and Goodale, 2006). Having this layer of cortical control over the more ancient subcortical networks makes it possible for primates to have much more flexible visually guided behavior. But even so, the behavior of primates, particularly with their conspecifics, is so complicated and subtle, that direct sensory control of action is often not enough. To handle these complexities, representational systems have emerged in the primate brain (and presumably in other mammals as well), from which internal models of the external world can be constructed. These representational systems allow primates such as ourselves to perceive a world beyond our bodies, to share that experience with other members of our species, and to plan a vast range of different actions with respect to objects and events that we have identified. This constellation of abilities is often identified with consciousness, particularly those aspects of consciousness that have to do with decision-making and metacognition. It is important to emphasize that the perceptual machinery that has evolved to do this is not linked directly to specific motor outputs, but instead accesses these outputs via cognitive systems that rely on memory representations, semantics, spatial reasoning, planning, and communication. In other words, there are a lot of cognitive "buffers" between perceiving the world and acting on it, and the relationship between what is on the retina and the behavior of the organism cannot be understood without reference to other mental states, including those typically described as "conscious." But once a particular course of action has been chosen, the actual execution of the constituent movements of that action are typically carried out by dedicated visuomotor modules not dissimilar in principle from those found in frogs and toads.

To summarize: vision in humans and other primates (and perhaps other animals as well) has two distinct but interacting functions: (1) the perception of objects and their relations, which provides a foundation for the organism's cognitive life and its conscious experience of the world, and (2) the control of actions directed at (or with respect to) those objects, in which separate motor outputs are programmed and controlled online. These different demands on vision have shaped the organization of the visual pathways in the primate brain.

16.2   Two visual systems

More than a decade ago, Goodale and Milner (1992) proposed a model of cortical visual organization that reflected this division of labor between perception and action. According to their two-visual systems account, the ventral stream of projections from early visual areas to the inferotemporal cortex provides our perceptual representation of the world, whereas the dorsal stream of projections from early visual areas to the

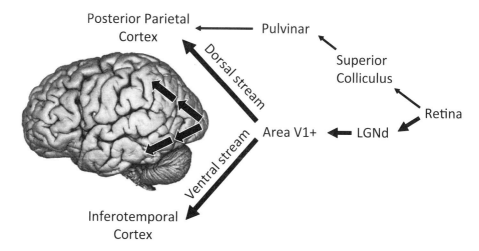

Figure 16.1. Schematic representation of the two streams of visual processing in human cerebral cortex. The retina sends projections to the dorsal part of the lateral geniculate nucleus in the thalamus (LGNd), which projects in turn to primary visual cortex (V1). Within the cerebral cortex, the ventral stream arises from early visual areas (V1+) and projects to regions in the occipito-temporal cortex. The dorsal stream also arises from early visual areas but projects instead to the posterior parietal cortex. The posterior parietal cortex also receives visual input from the superior colliculus via the pulvinar. On the left, the approximate locations of the pathways are shown on an image of the brain. The routes indicated by the arrows involve a series of complex interconnections.

posterior parietal cortex provides the visual control of actions (see Figure 16.1). Much of the evidence for this idea first came from work with neurological patients. The best known among these cases is the patient DF, who developed a profound visual form agnosia as a consequence of a hypoxic episode (Milner et al., 1991; Goodale et al., 1991). Even though DF shows no perceptual awareness of the form or dimensions of objects, she is able to scale her hand to the size, shape, and orientation of an object as she reaches out to pick it up. Furthermore, DF exhibits normal visuomotor control even in more complicated visuomotor tasks (Dijkerman et al., 1996), including stepping over obstacles during locomotion, despite the fact that her perceptual judgments about the height of these obstacles are far from normal (Patla and Goodale, 1996). As it turns out, even though DF shows some diffuse loss of tissue throughout her cerebral cortex (consistent with hypoxia), she also shows prominent focal lesions bilaterally in the lateral occipital cortex, a region of the human ventral stream that has been shown to be involved in the visual recognition of objects (James et al., 2003). It is presumably this selective damage to her ventral stream that has disrupted her ability to perceive the form of objects. But these lesions have not interfered with her ability to use visual information about form to shape her hand when she reaches out to grasp objects. The preservation of normal visually guided grasping in the face of ventral-stream damage, suggests that this ability is dependent on another visual pathway, probably one involving the dorsal stream. This conclusion was recently supported by neuroimaging evidence showing that, when DF grasps objects that vary in size and orientation, she shows relatively normal activation in the anterior intraparietal sulcus, an area in the dorsal stream that has been implicated in the visual control of grasping (James et al., 2003).

Consistent with these observations, neurological patients with damage to the dorsal stream, in the intraparietal sulcus and superior parietal cortex, often demonstrate impaired grasping movements, despite having relatively intact perception of object features (e.g. Perenin and Vighetto, 1988). As soon as their fingers make contact with the target, of course, they can use haptic information to adjust their hand to the correct posture. Many of these patients are also unable to avoid obstacles properly during reaching movements (Schindler et al., 2004) or even to reach in the correct direction to objects placed in different positions in the visual field contralateral to their lesion (Perenin and Vighetto, 1988). But despite exhibiting such clear deficits in the visual control of reaching and grasping (known clinically as "optic ataxia"), these same patients have little (if any) difficulties describing the orientation, size, shape, and even the relative spatial location of the very objects they are unable to grasp correctly (for review, see Milner and Goodale, 2006).

16.3 Different metrics and frames of reference for perception and action

But why did two separate streams of visual processing evolve in the primate brain? Or, to put it another way, why couldn't one "general-purpose" visual system handle both vision-for-perception and vision-for-action? The answer to this question lies in the computational requirements of vision-for-perception and vision-for-action. Simply put, perception and action require quite different transformations of the visual signals. To be able to grasp an object successfully, for example, it is essential that the brain compute the actual size of the object, and its orientation and position with respect to the grasping hand of the observer (i.e. in egocentric coordinates). The time at which these computations are performed is equally critical. Observers and goal objects rarely stay in a static relationship with one another and, as a consequence, the egocentric coordinates of a target object can often change radically from moment to moment. For these reasons, it is essential that the required coordinates for action be computed in an egocentric framework at the very moment the movements are to be performed.

Perceptual processing needs to proceed in a quite different way. Vision for perception does not require the absolute size of objects or their egocentric locations to be computed. In fact, such computations would be counterproductive because we almost never stay fixed in one place in the world. For this reason, it would be better to encode the size, orientation, and location of objects relative to each other. Such a scene-based frame of reference permits a perceptual representation of objects that transcends particular viewpoints, while preserving information about spatial relationships (as well as relative size and orientation) as the observer moves around. Indeed, if the perceptual machinery had to deliver the real size and distance of all the objects in the visual array, the computational load would be prohibitive (for discussion, see Goodale and Humphrey, 1998). The products of perception also need to be available over a much longer timescale than the visual information used in the control of action. We may need to recognize objects we have seen minutes, hours, days or even years before. To achieve this, the coding of the visual information has to be somewhat abstract, transcending particular viewpoint and viewing conditions. By working with perceptual representations that are object- or scene-based, we are able to maintain the constancies of size, shape, color, lightness, and relative location, over time and across different viewing conditions. Although there is much debate about the way in which this information is coded, it is clear that it is the identity of the object and its location within the scene, not its disposition with respect to the observer that is of primary concern to the perceptual system (see James et al., 2002). Thus current perception combined with stored information about previously encountered objects not only facilitates the object recognition but also contributes to the control of goal-directed movements when we are working in offline mode (i.e. on the basis of our memory of goal objects and their location in the world).

16.4   Perception, action and illusions

Although much of the evidence for the neural foundation for the two visual systems proposal comes from human neuropsychology and neuroimaging, as well as work with nonhuman primates,[2] evidence for fundamental differences in the metrics and frames of reference used by vision-for-perception and vision-for-action has largely come from studies in normal human observers. Because perception uses relative metrics and a scene-based reference frame, we tend to perceive the shape of objects in a configural or "holistic" manner, so that a given dimension cannot be perceptually isolated from the other dimensions of the object. This is why a tall tower can look thinner than a squat building, even though the building might be considerably wider. We simply cannot perceive the width of an object without also taking into account its overall shape. When we interact with objects, however, something different has to happen. Now it is important that our actions take into account only the most relevant dimension of an object without being influenced by its other dimensions. After all, if our visually guided movements were based on the relative rather than the absolute dimensions of objects, then many of our everyday actions, from driving a car to picking up wine glass, would be subject to critical errors.

   In two recent experiments, we tested people's ability to make perceptual judgments of the width of different rectangular objects or to grasp them across their width – while in both cases ignoring length (Ganel and Goodale, 2003). In both experiments, we used a modified version of a well-established psychophysical tool, Garner's speeded-classification task (Garner, 1974), which provides a reliable measure of how efficiently people can process one dimension of an object while ignoring dimensions of that

---

[2]For review, see Milner and Goodale (2006) and Goodale and Westwood (2003).

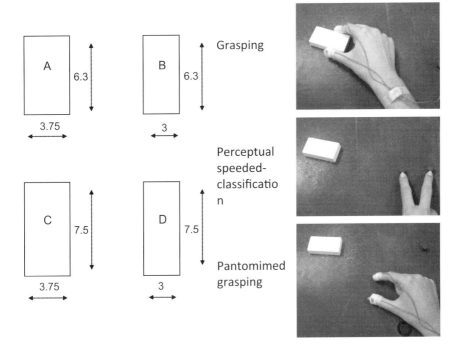

Figure 16.2. Objects and tasks that were used in Experiments 1 and 2 of the Ganel and Goodale (2003) study. The rectangles on the left-hand side of the figure depict the top view of the 3-dimensional objects that were used in both experiments. There were two different lengths and two different widths (the values shown are in cm). Objects A and B were presented in a random order in the first Baseline block; objects C and D were presented in the second Baseline block. Objects A, B, C, D were presented in the Filtering block. The right part of the figure illustrates the three tasks used in the experiments. From the top: Grasping and perceptual speeded-classification tasks (Experiment 1); Pantomimed grasping (perceptual estimates) (Experiment 2). (Adapted with permission from Ganel and Goodale, 2003.)

same object. In a typical Garner experiment, subjects are asked to classify objects on the basis of a single dimension (e.g. width) under two different conditions. In one condition (Baseline), the relevant dimension (width) varies but another, irrelevant, dimension (length) is kept constant. In the other condition (Filtering), both the relevant dimension (width) and the irrelevant dimension (length) vary. If participants are able to process the two dimensions independently, then the speed and accuracy should be identical for the Baseline and Filtering conditions. If participants cannot process the two dimensions independently and must instead treat them holistically, then speed and accuracy should be worse for the Filtering condition as compared with the Baseline condition (because participants cannot "filter out" the changes in the irrelevant dimension).

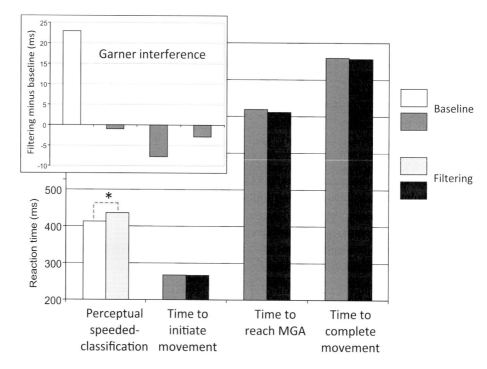

Figure 16.3. The effects of irrelevant variations in length on the perception of object width and on object-directed grasping (across the object's width). Reaction times (RTs) for speeded-classification of width were significantly slower in Filtering (right bar of pairs) than in Baseline (left bar of pairs). RTs for grasping were not different between Filtering and Baseline. Other kinematic measures of grasp also showed no differences between the conditions. The insert graph shows the Garner interference scores (Filtering minus Baseline), showing the magnitude of the effect on perceptual classification vs. grasping. (Adapted with permission from Ganel and Goodale, 2003.)

In the first of our initial experiments, we presented participants with rectangular objects and asked them either to classify the objects on the basis of their width or to reach out and grasp them across their width using a precision grip (see Figure 16.2 for more details). The objects were presented sequentially in either Baseline (different width but same length) or Filtering (different width and different length) conditions. We found that although subjects could not ignore length when making perceptual judgments of width, they could completely ignore length when grasping objects across their width. In other words, varying the length increased the time it took the subjects to classify objects according to their width, but had no effect on any kinematic variable (latency, movement time, grip aperture, and so on) when they reached out and picked up the object across its width (see Figure 16.3).

But when subjects were asked in a second experiment to pantomime the grasping movements without actually touching the target object, they showed Garner interference; that is, varying the length increased the response latency and the movement time

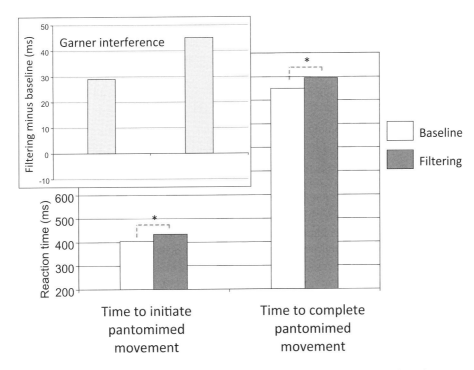

Figure 16.4. Effects of irrelevant variations in length on the reaction time for pantomimed grasping. The mean time to initiate the movement was slower in the Filtering condition (gray bars) than in the Baseline condition (open bars). The same was true for overall movement time. Garner-interference effects are shown in the inset graph. (Adapted with permission from Ganel and Goodale, 2003.)

(see Figure 16.4). This presumably reflects the fact that the production of a pantomimed movement utilizes perceptual rather than direct visuomotor processing (Goodale et al., 1994). Finally, as Figure 16.5 shows, although the amplitude of grip aperture was not affected by changes in length in the grasping task, it was affected by changes in length in the pantomime task (the longer the object, the narrower the pantomimed grasp). Taken together, these results lend support to the idea that in contrast to the configural and scene-based processing associated with perception, visuomotor systems are able to process the action-relevant dimension while at the same time ignoring changes in other, irrelevant, dimensions.

The differences in the metrics and frames of reference used by vision-for-perception and vision-for-action have also been demonstrated in experiments with pictorial illusions, particularly size-contrast illusions. Unlike the experiments described above, where the perception of one dimension of an object is affected by variations in another dimension of the same object, in size-contrast illusions, it is the context (scene) in which the object is embedded that affects the perception of its size. Aglioti et al. (1995), for example, showed that the scaling of grip aperture in flight was remarkably insensitive to the Ebbinghaus illusion, in which a target disk surrounded by smaller cir-

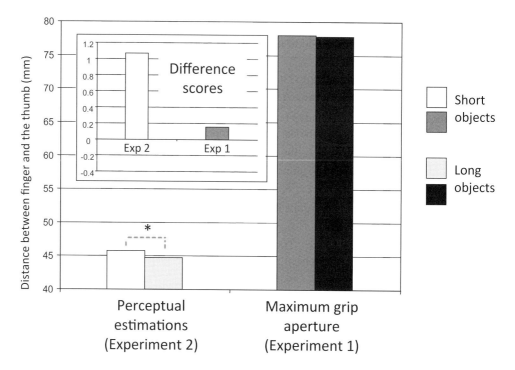

Figure 16.5. Effect of length on perceptual estimates (Experiment 2) and maximum grip aperture (Experiment 1). Note that with longer objects, the perceptual estimates of width were narrower but there was no effect of length of grip aperture. The inset shows the difference scores (short objects minus long objects). (Adapted with permission from Ganel and Goodale, 2003.)

cles appears to be larger than the same disk surrounded by larger circles. They found that maximum grip aperture was scaled to the real not the apparent size of the target disk. A similar dissociation between grip scaling and perceived size was reported by Haffenden and Goodale (1998), under conditions where participants had no visual feedback during the execution of grasping movements made to targets presented in the context of an Ebbinghaus illusion (see Figure 16.6). Although grip scaling escaped the influence of the illusion, the illusion did affect performance in a manual matching task, a kind of perceptual report, in which participants were asked to open their index finger and thumb to indicate the perceived size of a disk. Thus, the aperture between the finger and thumb was resistant to the illusion when the vision-for-action system was engaged (i.e. when the participant grasped the target) and sensitive to the illusion when the vision-for-perception system was engaged (i.e. when the participant estimated its size).

This dissociation between what people say they see and what they do underscores the differences between the vision-for-perception and vision-for-action. The obligatory size-contrast effects that give rise to the illusion (in which different elements of the array are compared) normally play a crucial role in scene interpretation, a cen-

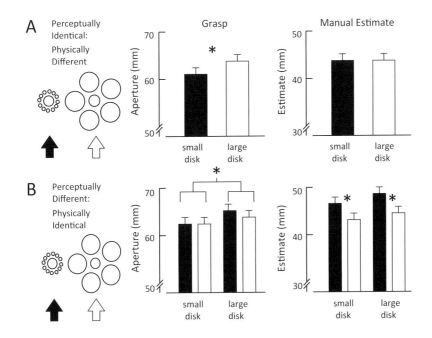

Figure 16.6. The effect of the Ebbinghaus illusion on maximum grip aperture and manual estimates of target size. Panel A shows the responses to targets in a display in which the two targets (one large and small) differed in their physical size but nevertheless appeared to be identical. In this case, participants opened their hand significantly wider when they picked up the larger of the two objects even though their manual estimates did not differ. Panel B shows the responses to targets in a display in which the two targets were physically identical but appeared to be different in size. On one set of trials, two identical large objects were presented whereas in another set of trials two identical small objects were presented. With these displays, participants' maximum grip aperture for the two targets in the two sets of trials (both large or both small) did not differ, whereas their manual estimates reflected the illusory differences in size. (Adapted with permission from Haffenden and Goodale, 1998.)

tral function of vision-for-perception. In contrast, the execution of a goal-directed act, such as manual prehension, requires metrical computations that are centered on the target itself, rather than on the relations between the target and other elements in the scene. Certainly, the true size of the target for calibrating the grip can be computed from the retinal-image size of the object coupled with an accurate estimate of distance. Such computations would be expected therefore to be quite insensitive to the kinds of pictorial cues that distort perception when familiar illusions are presented.

The initial demonstrations that grasping is refractory to pictorial illusions triggered a good deal of interest amongst researchers studying vision and motor control. Some investigators have replicated this dissociation between perception and action using different versions of the Ebbinghaus illusion (e.g. Fischer, 2001; Kwok and Braddick, 2003; Amazeen and DaSilva, 2005) as well as other illusions such as the Ponzo illusion (Brenner and Smeets, 1996; Jackson and Shaw, 2000), the horizontal-vertical illusion (Servos et al., 2000), the Müller-Lyer illusion (Dewar and Carey, 2006), the Diagonal illusion (Stöttinger and Perner, 2006), and the rod-and-frame illusion (Dyde and Milner, 2002). Some have reported that these illusions affect some aspects of motor control but not others (e.g. Gentilucci et al., 1996, Daprati and Gentilucci, 1997; van Donkelaar, 1999, Glazebrook et al. 2005; Biegstraaten et al., 2007). And a few investigators have found no dissociation whatsoever between the effects of pictorial illusions on perceptual judgments and the scaling of grip aperture (e.g. Franz et al. 2000, 2003).

But it is important to emphasize that the fact that actions such as grasping are sometimes sensitive to illusory displays is not by itself a refutation of the idea of two visual systems. Indeed, one should not be surprised that visual perception and visuomotor control can interact in the normal brain. After all, ultimately, perception has to affect our actions or the brain mechanisms mediating perception would never have evolved. The real surprise (at least for monolithic accounts of vision) is that there are instances where visually guided action is apparently unaffected by perception. But from the standpoint of our two-visual-systems proposal such instances are to be expected (Goodale and Milner, 1992). Nevertheless, the fact that action has been found to be affected by pictorial illusions in some experiments has led some authors to argue that the early studies demonstrating a dissociation had not adequately matched action and perception tasks for various input, attentional, and output demands (e.g. Smeets and Brenner, 2001; Vishton and Fabre, 2003) – and that when these factors were taken into account the apparent differences between perceptual judgments and motor control could be resolved without invoking the idea of two visual systems. Other authors, notably Glover (2004), have argued that action tasks involve multiple stages of processing from purely perceptual to more "automatic" visuomotor control. According to this so-called planning/control model, illusions would be expected to affect the early but not the late stages of a grasping movement (Glover and Dixon 2001a, b; Glover 2004).

Some of these competing accounts, particularly Glover's (2004) planning/control model, can simply be viewed as modifications of Goodale and Milner's original proposal. But even so, Glover's model fails to distinguish between planning in the sense of deciding upon one course of action rather than another, and planning in the sense of programming the actual constituent movements of an action (Goodale and Milner, 2004b). Goodale and Milner would not dispute that vision-for-perception (and thus, the ventral stream) is involved in the former kind of planning, but would argue that the other kind of planning (i.e. programming) is mediated by vision-for-action (and thus, the dorsal stream). In fact, Glover and Dixon's (2002) claim that perceptual processing intrudes into the early part of motor programming for grasping movements is based on findings that have been difficult to replicate (e.g. Danckert et al., 2002; Franz, 2003). Nevertheless, there are a number of other studies whose results cannot easily be reconciled with the two-visual-systems model, and it remains a real question as to why actions appear to be sensitive to illusions in some experiments but not in others.

As it turns out, there are several reasons why grip aperture might appear be sensitive to illusions under certain testing conditions. In some cases, notably the Ebbinghaus illusion, the flanker elements can be treated as obstacles, influencing the posture of the fingers during the execution of the grasp (Haffenden and Goodale, 2000; Haffenden et al., 2001; Plodowski and Jackson, 2001; de Grave et al., 2005). In other words, the apparent effect of the illusion on grip scaling in some experiments might simply reflect the operation of visuomotor mechanisms that treat the flanker elements of the visual arrays as obstacles to be avoided. Another critical variable is the timing of the grasp with respect to the presentation of the stimuli. When targets are visible during the programming of a grasping movement, maximum grip aperture is usually not affected by size-contrast illusions, whereas when vision is occluded before the command to initiate programming of the movement is presented, a reliable effect of the illusion on grip aperture is typically observed (Hu and Goodale, 2000; Westwood et al., 2000; Fischer, 2001; Westwood and Goodale, 2003). As discussed earlier, vision-for-action is designed to operate in real time and is not normally engaged unless the target object is visible during the programming phase, when (bottom-up) visual information can be immediately converted into the appropriate motor commands. The observation that (top-down) memory-guided grasping is affected by the illusory display reflects the fact that the stored information about the target's dimensions was originally derived from the earlier operation of vision-for-perception.[3]

Nevertheless, some have argued that if the perceptual and grasping tasks are appropriately matched, then grasping can be shown to be as sensitive to size-contrast illusions as psychophysical judgments (Franz et al., 2000; Franz, 2001). Although this explanation, at least on the face of it, is a compelling one, it cannot explain why Aglioti et al. (1995) and Haffenden and Goodale (1998) found that when the relative sizes of the two target objects in the Ebbinghaus display were adjusted so that they appeared to be perceptually identical, the grip aperture that participants used to pick up the two targets continued to reflect the physical difference in their size (see Figure 16.6). This explanation also cannot explain the results of a recent study we carried out using a version of the Ponzo (or railway track) illusion in which we pitted a real difference in size against a perceived difference in size (Ganel et al., 2008).

In the typical Ponzo illusion, when two objects of equal size are presented at the end of the display, the object placed at the converging end is usually perceived as longer than the one presented at the diverging end (see Figure 16.7a). In our experiments, however, the two target objects were always different in length. Critically, these different lengths were selected to create a situation in which, in a large subset of trials (incongruent trials), the target that was perceived to be the longer one was actually physically shorter than the other one (Figure 16.7b, c). In the first experiment, participants were shown the display and were then given an auditory instruction to pick up either the shorter or the longer target object. This meant that on many of the incongruent trials, when participants picked up the object they perceived to be shorter of the two, they were actually picking up the longer one (and vice versa). Thus, on these trials, we were able to assess whether the opening between the finger and thumb of the grasping hand followed this erroneous decision or was tuned instead to the real size differences between the objects.

---

[3]For a more detailed discussion of these and related issues, see Bruno et al., (2008); Goodale et al., (2004).

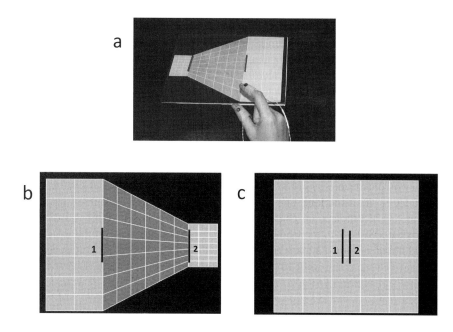

Figure 16.7. Stimuli and experimental design of Ganel et al.'s study (2008). (a) An overall illustration of the experimental paradigm and the version of the Ponzo illusion used. (b) A diagram of the arrangement of the objects on incongruent trials in which real size and the illusory size were pitted against one another. In this example, object 1 is perceived in most cases as shorter than object 2 (due to the illusory context), although it is actually longer. The real difference in size can be clearly seen in (c) where the two objects are placed next to one another (for illustrative purposes) on the nonillusory control display. (Adapted with permission from Ganel et al., 2008.)

As shown in Figure 16.8a (left-hand bars), the results were remarkably clear. Despite the fact that participants believed that the shorter object was the longer one (or vice versa), the in-flight aperture between the finger and thumb of their grasping hand reflected the real not the illusory size of the target objects. In other words, on the same trials in which participants erroneously decided that one object was the longer (or shorter) of the two, the anticipatory opening between their fingers reflected the real direction and magnitude of size differences between the two objects. Moreover, as can be seen by comparing Figure 16.8a and b, participants showed the same differential scaling to the real size of the objects whether the objects were shown on the illusory display or on the control display (Figure 16.7).

Still, it could be argued that these findings reflect the fact that, within a given trial, the overt decision about object size always preceded the grasp. To eliminate such an alternative account, we ran a second experiment using the same paradigm, in which participants first made overt size decisions but then, instead of actually grasping the

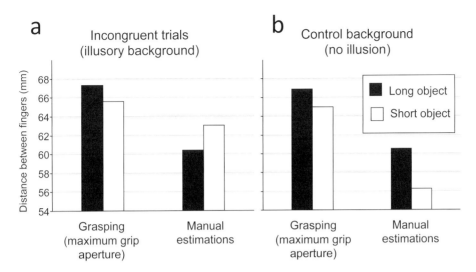

Figure 16.8. Maximum grip aperture and perceptual estimates of length for objects placed on illusory display (left-hand panel, a) and control display (right-hand panel, b). Only incongruent trials in which participants made erroneous decisions about real size are shown for the grip aperture and estimates with the illusory display. As the left-hand panel shows, despite the fact that participants erroneously perceived the physically longer object to be the shorter one (and vice versa), the opening between their finger and thumb during the grasping movements reflected the real difference in size between the objects. This pattern of results was completely reversed when they made perceptual estimates of the length of the objects. With the control display (right-hand panel), both grip aperture and manual estimates went in the same direction. (Adapted with permission from Ganel et al., 2008.)

object, they estimated its size by opening their finger and thumb a matching amount. This measure is akin to the typical magnitude estimation paradigms used in conventional psychophysics, but with the virtue that the manual estimation makes use of the same effector that is used in the grasping task. In the new experiment, the pattern of results was completely reversed and the manual estimates on incongruent trials now reflected the illusory, not the real, size of the objects (right-hand bars, Figure 16.8a). Note that with the control display (right-hand bars, Figure 16.8b), participant's estimates of the size of the two objects reversed direction from that seen with the illusory display. Across the two experiments then, the real and apparent differences in the size of the objects had opposite effects on action (grasping) and perception (manual estimations). Overall, these results underscore once more the profound difference in the way visual information is transformed for action and perception. Importantly too, the results are difficult to reconcile with any argument that suggests that grip aperture is sensitive to illusions, and that the absence of an effect found in many studies is simply a consequence of differences in the task demands (Franz et al., 2000, Franz, 2001).

Although the results presented so far are consistent with the idea that visually guided action and visual perception make use of different metrics and frames of reference, there is another account that can also handle the difference in sensitivity to size-contrast illusions, one that appeals to the idea that different visual information is used when we pick up an object versus when we make a judgment about its size. According to this explanation, which was put forward by Smeets and Brenner (1999, 2001), the trajectories of the two digits in a precision grasp are independently programmed with respect to the goal object. In other words, the visuomotor system does not compute the size of the object but instead computes the two locations on the surface of object where the digits will be placed. Thus, because size is irrelevant to the planning of these trajectories, the size-contrast illusion has no effect on grip aperture, the scaling of which is simply an epiphenomenon of the independent finger trajectories. Although Smeets and Brenner's account has been challenged (Mon-Williams and Tresilian, 2001), it has to be acknowledged that their digit-control model offers a convincing explanation for the lack of an effect of illusions on grasping. Nevertheless, there are some observations that cannot be accommodated by their model. For example, as discussed earlier, if a delay is introduced between viewing the target and initiating the grasp, the scaling of the anticipatory grip aperture is much more likely to be sensitive to size-contrast illusions (Hu and Goodale, 2000; Westwood et al., 2000; Fischer, 2001; Westwood and Goodale, 2003). These results cannot be explained by the Smeets and Brenner model without conceding that – with delay – grip-scaling is no longer a consequence of programming individual digit trajectories, but instead reflects the perceived size of the target object. Nor can the Smeets and Brenner model explain what happens when unpracticed finger postures (e.g. the thumb and ring finger) are used to pick up objects in the context of a size-contrast illusion. In contrast to skilled grasping movements, grip-scaling with unpracticed awkward grasping is quite sensitive to the illusory difference in size between the objects (Gonzalez et al., 2008). Only with practice does grip aperture begin to reflect the real size of the target objects. Smeets and Brenner's model cannot account for this result without positing that individual control over the digits occurs only after practice. Finally, recent neuropsychological findings with patient DF suggest that she could use action-related information about object size (presumably from her intact dorsal stream) to make explicit perceptual judgments regarding the length of an object that she was about to pick up (Schenk and Milner, 2006). At this point, the difference between the Goodale and Milner account and the (modified) Smeets and Brenner account begins to blur. Both accounts posit that real-time control of skilled grasping depends on visuomotor transformations that are quite distinct from those involved in the control of delayed or unpracticed grasping movements. The difference in the two accounts turns on the nature of the control exercised over skilled movements performed in real time. But note that even if Smeets and Brenner are correct that the trajectories of the individual digits are programmed individually on the basis of spatial information that ignores the size of the object, this would not obviate the idea of two visual systems, one for perceiving the world and one for controlling our actions in that world. Indeed, the virtue of Goodale and Milner's proposal is that it accounts not only for the dissociations outlined above between the control of action and psychophysical report in normal observers in a number of different settings, but it also accounts for a broad range of neuropsychological, neurophysiological, and neuroimaging data.

16.5   Interactions between the two streams

Although there is a good deal of evidence to suggest that vision-for-perception and vision-for-action can be separately mapped onto the ventral and dorsal visual streams, the two pathways clearly must work together in providing us with a seamless visual life. It has been suggested that there is a close analogy between the interaction of the two visual streams and "tele-assistance", one of the most efficient schemes that has been devised for the remote control of robots working in hostile environments (Pook and Ballard 1996; Goodale and Humphrey, 1998; Goodale and Milner, 2004a). Consider the case of a human operator on earth communicating with a semi-autonomous robot operating on the surface of Mars. In the tele-assistance mode, the human operator can identify potential goal objects, such as an interesting rock formation, by viewing the Martian surface via a videocam mounted on the robot. Once the goal has been identified, the operator can then send an instruction to the robot to approach the rock formation and take a sample. Notice that in tele-assistance, the human operator simply identifies or "flags" a target object and specifies what kind of action is to be performed, in general terms, to achieve the desired goal. Once this information is communicated to the semi-autonomous robot, the robot can use its on-board rangefinders and other sensing devices to program and control the required movements for achieving the specified goal.

The interaction between the ventral and dorsal stream is an example of "biological tele-assistance." The perceptual systems in the ventral stream, in association with memory and other cognitive systems in the brain, perform the role of the human operator in recognizing a potentially important target. These systems parse the visual array and identify different objects in the scene, using a representational system that is rich and detailed but not metrically precise. When a particular goal object has been flagged, dedicated visuomotor networks in the dorsal stream, in conjunction with output systems elsewhere in the brain (such as the premotor cortex, motor cortex, basal ganglia, and brainstem) are activated to perform the desired motor act. In other words, dorsal stream networks, with their precise egocentric coding of the location and orientation of the goal object along with accurate metric coding of its size and shape, could be viewed as the robotic component of tele-assistance. Thus, the ventral and dorsal streams work together in the production of purposive behavior – one system selects the goal object from the visual array while the other carries out the required metrical computations for the goal-directed action. In a very real sense, the strengths and weaknesses of the two streams complement each other in the production of adaptive behavior.

Of course, the tele-assistance analogy is far too simplified. For one thing, the ventral stream by itself does not constitute an intelligent operator that can make assessments and plans. In fact the ventral and dorsal streams are merely two players in a highly complex and recursive system that involves a lot of other brain areas. Clearly, there has to be some sort of top-down executive control – almost certainly engaging prefrontal mechanisms – that can initiate the operation of attentional search and thus set the whole process of planning and goal selection in motion (for review, see Goodale and Haffenden, 2003). Reciprocal interactions between prefrontal/premotor areas and the areas in the posterior parietal cortex undoubtedly play a critical role in recruiting specialized dorsal-stream structures, such as the lateral intraparietal area (LIP), which appear to control both voluntary eye movements and covert shifts of spatial attention (without eye movements) in monkeys and humans (Corbetta et al., 2002; Bisley and Goldberg, 2003). In terms of the tele-assistance analogy, area LIP can be seen as acting like the videocam scanning the visual scene, and thereby providing new inputs that the ventral stream can process and pass on to frontal systems that assess their potential importance. In practice, of course, the videocam/LIP system does not scan the environment randomly: it is constrained to a greater or lesser degree by top-down information about the nature of the potential targets and where those targets might be located, information that reflects the priorities of the operator/organism that are presumably elaborated in prefrontal systems.

What happens next goes beyond even these speculations. Before instructions can be transmitted to the visuomotor control systems in the dorsal stream (the semi-autonomous robot), the nature of the action required needs to be determined. This means that praxis systems, perhaps located in the left hemisphere, need to "instruct" the relevant visuomotor systems. After all, objects such as tools demand a particular kind of hand posture. Achieving this not only requires that the tool be identified (presumably using ventral-stream mechanisms) but also that the required actions to achieve that posture be selected as well (via a link to these praxis systems). At the same time, the ventral stream (and its related cognitive apparatus) has to communicate the locus of the goal object to these visuomotor systems in the dorsal stream. One way that this ventral-dorsal transmission could happen is via recurrent projections from foci of activity in the ventral stream back downstream to primary visual cortex and other adjacent visual areas. Once a target has been "highlighted" on these retinotopic maps, its location could then finally be forwarded to the dorsal stream for action (for a version of this idea, see Lamme and Roelfsema, 2000). Moreover, LIP itself, by virtue of the fact that it would be "pointing" at the goal object, could also provide the requisite coordinates, once it has been cued by recognition systems in the ventral stream. Again, it must be emphasized that all of this is highly speculative. Nevertheless, whatever complex interactions might be involved, it is clear that goal-directed action is unlikely to be mediated by a simple serial processing system. Multiple iterative processing is almost certainly required, involving a constant interplay among different control systems at different levels of processing (for a discussion of these and related issues, see Milner and Goodale, 2006).

16.6 Conclusion

We began this chapter by arguing that Goodale and Milner's (1992) proposed division of labor between vision-for-perception and vision-for-action in the ventral and dorsal streams provides a powerful theoretical framework for understanding how vision works. According to this duplex model, both visual pathways transform visual information into motor output. In the dorsal stream, the transformation is quite direct: visual input and motor output are essentially "isomorphic" with one another. In the ventral stream, however, the transformation is quite indirect: and the construction of a perceptual representation of the world permits a "propositional" relationship between input and output, taking into account previous knowledge and experience. Although both streams process information about the structure of objects and about their spatial locations, they use quite different frames of reference and metrics to deal with this information. The operations carried out by the ventral stream use scene-based frames of reference and relational metrics; those carried out by the dorsal stream use egocentric frames of reference and absolute metrics. Both streams work together in the production of goal-directed behavior. The ventral stream (together with associated cognitive machinery) identifies goals and plans appropriate actions; the dorsal stream (in conjunction with related circuits in premotor cortex, basal ganglia, and brainstem) programs and controls those actions. Thus, a full understanding of the integrated nature of visually guided behavior will require that we specify the nature of the interactions and information exchange that take place between the two streams of visual processing.

References

Aglioti, S., DeSouza, J. F. X. and Goodale, M. A. (1995). Size-contrast illusions deceive the eye but not the hand. *Curr. Biol.*, 5: 679–685.

Amazeen, E. L. and DaSilva, F. (2005). Psychophysical test for the independence of perception and action. *J. Exp. Psychol.: Hum. Percept. Perf.*, 31: 170–182.

Biegstraaten, M., de Grave, D. D., Brenner, E. and Smeets, J. B. (2007). Grasping the Müller-Lyer illusion: not a change in perceived length. *Exp. Brain Res.*, 176: 497–503.

Bisley, J. W. and Goldberg, M. E. (2003). Neuronal activity in the lateral intraparietal area and spatial attention. *Science*, 299: 81–86.

Brenner, E. and Smeets, J. B. (1996). Size illusion influences how we lift but not how we grasp an object. *Exp. Brain Res.*, 111: 473–476.

Bruno, N., Bernardis, P. and Gentilucci, M. (2008). Visually guided pointing, the Müller-Lyer illusion, and the functional interpretation of the dorsal-ventral split: Conclusions from 33 independent studies. *Neurosci. Biobehav. Rev.*, 32: 423–437.

Corbetta, M., Kincade, J. M. and Shulman, G. L. (2002). Two neural systems for visual orienting and the pathophysiology of unilateral spatial neglect. In H.-O. Karnath, A. D. Milner and G. Vallar (eds.) *The Cognitive and Neural Bases of Spatial Neglect*. Oxford, UK: Oxford University Press, pp. 259–273.

Danckert, J., Sharif, N., Haffenden, A. M., Schiff, K. C. and Goodale, M. A. (2002). A temporal analysis of grasping in the Ebbinghaus illusion: planning versus on-line control. *Exp. Brain Res.*, 144: 275–280.

Daprati, E. and Gentilucci, M. (1997). Grasping an illusion. *Neuropsychologia*, 35: 1577–1582.

Dean, P., Redgrave, P. and Westby, G. W. M. (1989). Event or emergency? Two response systems in the mammalian superior colliculus. *Trends Neurosci.*, 12: 137–147.

de Grave, D. D., Biegstraaten, M., Smeets, J. B. and Brenner, E. (2005). Effects of the Ebbinghaus figure on grasping are not only due to misjudged size. *Exp. Brain Res.*, 163: 58–64.

Dewar, M. T. and Carey, D. P. (2006). Visuomotor "immunity" to perceptual illusion: a mismatch of attentional demands cannot explain the perception-action dissoci- ation. *Neuropsychologia*, 44: 1501–1508.

Dijkerman, H. C., Milner, A. D. and Carey, D. P. (1996). The perception and prehen- sion of objects oriented in the depth plane. I. Effects of visual form agnosia. *Exp. Brain Res.*, 112: 442–451.

Dyde, R. T. and Milner, A. D. (2002). Two illusions of perceived orientation: one fools all of the people some of the time; the other fools all of the people all of the time. *Exp. Brain Res.*, 144: 518–527.

Ewert, J.-P. (1987). Neuroethology of releasing mechanisms: prey-catching in toads. *Beh. Brain Sci.*, 10: 337–405.

Fischer, M. H. (2001). How sensitive is hand transport to illusory context effects? *Exp. Brain Res.*, 136: 224–230.

Franz, V. H. (2001). Action does not resist visual illusions. *Trend. Cogn. Sci.*, 5: 457–459.

Franz, V. H. (2003). Planning versus online control: dynamic illusion effects in grasp- ing? *Spatial Vis.*, 16: 211–223.

Franz, V. H., Bülthoff, H. H. and Fahle, M. (2003). Grasp effects of the Ebbinghaus illusion: obstacle avoidance is not the explanation. *Exp. Brain Res.*, 149: 470– 477.

Franz, V. H., Gegenfurtner, K. R., Bülthoff, H. H. and Fahle, M. (2000). Grasping visual illusions: no evidence for a dissociation between perception and action. *Psychol. Sci.*, 11: 20–25.

Ganel, T. and Goodale, M. A. (2003). Visual control of action but not perception requires analytical processing of object shape. *Nature*, 426: 664–667.

Ganel, T., Tanzer, M. and Goodale, M. A. (2008). A double dissociation between action and perception in the context of visual illusions: Opposite effects of real and illusory size. *Psychol. Sci.*, 19: 221–225.

Garner, W. R. (1974). *The Processing of Information and Structure*. Potomac, MA: Lawrence Erlbaum.

Gentilucci, M., Chieffi, S., Daprati, E., Saetti, M. C. and Toni, I. (1996). Visual illusion and action. *Neuropsychologia*, 34: 369–376.

Glazebrook, C. M., Dhillon, V. P., Keetch, K. M., Lyons, J., Amazeen, E., Weeks, D. J. and Elliott, D. (2005). Perception-action and the Muller-Lyer illusion: amplitude or endpoint bias? *Exp. Brain Res.*, 160: 71–78.

Glover, S. (2004). Separate visual representations in the planning and control of action. *Behav. Brain Sci.*, 27: 3–24; discussion 24–78.

Glover, S. and Dixon, P. (2001a). Motor adaptation to an optical illusion. *Exp. Brain Res.*, 137: 254–258.

Glover, S. and Dixon, P. (2001b). The role of vision in the on-line correction of illusion effects on action. *Can. J. Exp. Psychol.*, 55: 96–103.

Gonzalez, C. L., Ganel, T., Whitwell, R. L., Morrissey, B. and Goodale, M. A. (2008). Practice makes perfect, but only with the right hand: Sensitivity to perceptual illusions with awkward grasps decreases with practice in the right but not the left hand. *Neuropsychologia*, 46: 624–631.

Goodale, M. A. (1996). Visuomotor modules in the vertebrate brain. *Can. J. Physiol. Pharmacol.*, 74: 390–400.

Goodale, M. A. and Haffenden, A. M. (2003). Interactions between dorsal and ventral streams of visual processing. In A. Siegel, R. Andersen, H.-J. Freund, and D. Spencer (Eds.) *Advances in Neurology (Vol. 93): The Parietal Lobe.* Philadelphia: Lippincott-Raven, pp. 249–267.

Goodale, M. A. and Humphrey, G. K. (1998). The objects of action and perception. *Cognition*, 67: 179–205.

Goodale, M. A. and Milner, A. D. (1984). Fractionating orientation behavior in rodents. In D. J. Ingle, M. A. Goodale and R. J. W. Mansfield (Eds.) *Analysis of Visual Behavior*, Cambridge, MA: MIT Press, pp. 267–299.

Goodale, M. A. and Milner, A. D. (1992). Separate visual pathways for perception and action. *Trends Neurosci.*, 15: 20–25.

Goodale, M. A. and Milner, A. D. (2004a). *Sight Unseen: An Exploration of Conscious and Unconscious Vision.* Oxford: Oxford University Press.

Goodale, M. A. and Milner, A. D. (2004b). Plans for action. *Behav. Brain Sci.*, 2: 37–40.

Goodale, M. A. and Westwood, D. A. (2004). An evolving view of duplex vision: separate but interacting cortical pathways for perception and action. *Curr. Opin. Neurobiol.*, 14: 203–211.

Goodale, M. A., Jakobson, L. S. and Keillor, J. M. (1994). Differences in the visual control of pantomimed and natural grasping movements. *Neuropsychologia*, 32: 1159–1178.

Goodale, M. A., Milner, A. D., Jakobson, L. S. and Carey, D. P. (1991). A neurological dissociation between perceiving objects and grasping them. *Nature*, 349: 154–156.

Goodale, M. A., Westwood, D. A. and Milner, A. D. (2004). Two distinct modes of control for object-directed action. *Prog. Brain Res.*, 144: 131–144.

Haffenden, A. M. and Goodale, M. A. (1998). The effect of pictorial illusion on prehension and perception. *J. Cogn. Neurosci.*, 10: 122–136.

Haffenden, A. M. and Goodale, M. A. (2000). Independent effects of pictorial displays on perception and action. *Vis. Res.*, 40. 1597–1607.

Haffenden, A. M. and Goodale, M. A. (2001). The dissociation between perception and action in the Ebbingaus Illusion: nonilusory effects of pictorial cues on grasp. *Curr. Biol.*, 11: 177–181.

Hildebrand, E. and Schimz, A. (1985). Behavioral pattern and its sensory control in *Halobacterium halobium*. In M. Eisenbach and M. Balaban (eds.) *Sensing and Response in Microorganisms*. Amsterdam: Elsevier, pp. 129–142.

Hu, Y. and Goodale, M. A. (2000). Grasping after a delay shifts size-scaling from absolute to relative metrics. *J. Cogn. Neurosci.*, 12: 856–868.

Humphrey, G. K. and Goodale, M. (1998). Probing unconcious visual processing with the McCullogh effect. *Conscious Cogn.*, 7: 494–519.

Ingle, D. J. (1973). Two visual systems in the frog. *Science* 181: 1053–1055.

Ingle, D. J. (1980). Some effects of pretectum lesions on the frog's detection of stationary objects. *Behav. Brain Res.*, 1: 139–163.

Ingle, D. J. (1982). Organization of visuomotor behaviors in vertebrates. In D. J. Ingle, M. A. Goodale and R. J. W. Mansfield (eds.) *Analysis of Visual Behavior*. Cambridge, MA: MIT Press, pp. 67–109.

Ingle, D. J. (1991). Functions of subcortical visual systems in vertebrates and the evolution of higher visual mechanisms. In R. L. Gregory and J. Cronly-Dillon (eds.) *Vision and Visual Dysfunction, Volume 2: Evolution of the Eye and Visual System*. London: Macmillan, pp. 152–164.

Jackson, S. R. and Shaw, A. (2000). The Ponzo illusion affects grip-force but not grip-aperture scaling during prehension movements. *J. Exp. Psych.: Hum. Percept. Perf.*, 26: 418–423.

Jäger, R. (1997) Separate channels for visuomotor transformation in the pigeon. *Eur. J. Morphol.*, 35: 277–289.

James, T. W., Culham, J., Humphrey, G. K., Milner, A. D. and Goodale, M. A. (2003). Ventral occipital lesions impair object recognition but not object-directed grasping: an fMRI study. *Brain*, 126: 2463–2475.

James, T. W., Humphrey, G. K., Gati, J. S., Menon, R. S. and Goodale, M. A. (2002). Differential effects of viewpoint on object-driven activation in dorsal and ventral streams. *Neuron*, 35: 793–801.

Kwok, R. M. and Braddick, O. J. (2003). When does the Titchener Circles illusion exert an effect on grasping? Two- and three-dimensional targets. *Neuropsychologia*, 41: 932–940.

Lamme, V. A. F. and Roelfsema, P. R. (2000). The distinct modes of vision offered by feedforward and recurrent processing. *Trends Neurosci.*, 23: 571–579.

Milner, A. D. and Goodale, M. A. (2006). *The Visual Brain in Action*. 2nd Edition, Oxford, UK: Oxford University Press.

Milner, A. D., Perrett, D. I., Johnston, R. S., Benson, P. J., Jordan, T. R., Heeley, D. W., Bettucci, D., Mortara, F., Mutani, R., Terazzi, E. and Davidson, D. L. W. (1991). Perception and action in visual form agnosia. *Brain*, 114: 405–428.

Mon-Williams, M. and Tresilian, J. R. (2001). A simple rule of thumb for elegant prehension. *Curr. Biol.*, 11: 1058–1061.

Patla, A. E. and Goodale, M. A. (1996). Obstacle avoidance during locomotion is unaffected in a patient with visual form agnosia. *NeuroReport*, 8: 165–168.

Perenin, M. T. and Vighetto, A. (1988). Optic ataxia: a specific disruption in visuomotor mechanisms. I. Different aspects of the deficit in reaching for objects. *Brain*, 111: 643–674.

Plodowski, A. and Jackson, S. R. (2001). Vision: getting to grips with the Ebbinghaus illusion. *Curr. Biol.*, 11: 304–306.

Pook, P. K. and Ballard, D. H. (1996). Deictic human/robot interaction. *Robot. Aut. Sys.*, 18: 259–269.

Schenk, T. and Milner, A. D. (2006). Concurrent visuomotor behaviour improves form discrimination in a patient with visual form agnosia. *Eur. J. Neurosci.*, 24: 1495–1503.

Schindler, I., Rice, N. J., McIntosh, R. D., Rossetti, Y., Vighetto, A. and Milner, A. D. (2004). Automatic avoidance of obstacles is a dorsal stream function: evidence from optic ataxia. *Nat. Neurosci.*, 7: 779–784.

Servos, P., Carnahan, H. and Fedwick, J. (2000). The visuomotor system resists the horizontal-vertical illusion. *J. Motor Behav.*, 32: 400–404.

Smeets, J. B. and Brenner, E. (1999). A new view on grasping. *Motor Control*, 3: 237–271.

Smeets, J. B. and Brenner, E. (2001). Independent movements of the digits in grasping. *Exp. Brain Res.*, 139: 92–100.

Stöttinger, E. and Perner, J. (2006). Dissociating size representation for action and for conscious judgment: grasping visual illusions without apparent obstacles. *Conscious. Cogn.*, 15: 269–284.

van Donkelaar, P. (1999). Pointing movements are affected by size-contrast illusions. *Exp. Brain Res.*, 125: 517–520.

Vishton, P. M. and Fabre, E. (2003). Effects of the Ebbinghaus illusion on different behaviors: one- and two-handed grasping; one- and two-handed manual estimation; metric and comparative judgment. *Spatial Vis.*, 16: 377–392.

Westwood, D. A. and Goodale, M. A. (2003). Perceptual illusion and the real-time control of action. *Spatial Vis.*, 16: 243–254.

Westwood, D. A., Heath, M. and Roy, E. A. (2000). The effect of a pictorial illusion on closed-loop and open-loop prehension. *Exp. Brain Res.*, 134: 456–463.

17 Requirements for conscious visual processing

H. R. Wilson

Conscious brain processes likely evolved because they increase survival by enabling animals to better evaluate alternative plans of action in order to attain goals driven by primitive emotions such as hunger, thirst, and sex. To achieve this, it is argued that prefrontal cortex must be activated and must reciprocally interact with brain areas devoted to emotion, episodic memory, and the higher levels of cortical vision in inferior temporal and posterior parietal cortex. Furthermore, recurrent excitatory and inhibitory interactions within prefrontal and other cortical areas are critical to the emergence of conscious vision. These ideas are illustrated by the dynamics of very simple neural networks that represent generalizations of networks implicated in binocular rivalry and prefrontal control of eye movements. Finally, it is argued that feedback within and among cortical areas avoids the infinite regress engendered in the concept of the homunculus.

17.1 Introduction

I shall begin this chapter with the assertion that all mammals are conscious of some of their actions and deliberations at least some of the time. By this I mean that they are capable of initiating conscious reflection analogous to that engaged in by humans when they evaluate alternative courses of action under relatively complex circumstances. This, of course, does not imply that all mammals are conscious to the same degree or in precisely the same manner as humans. In particular, it is obvious that conscious human reflection frequently, but by no means always, involves language. Such linguistic aspects of conscious processes do not appear to be present in other mammals, except possibly the great apes. Furthermore, it is very probable that highly social mammals, such as primates, dogs, and wolves, have more highly developed conscious faculties than their more solitary counterparts. Social interactions clearly put a premium on be-

Cortical Mechanisms of Vision, ed. M. Jenkin and L. R. Harris. Published by Cambridge University Press.
© Cambridge University Press 2009.

ing able to predict the responses of other individuals to one's contemplated course of action. Finally, it may well be that many nonmammalian vertebrates (e.g. birds) are also capable of conscious processing, but I shall remain agnostic on this issue, as it is not germane to my argument.

Before going further, I must emphasize that "conscious" is an adjective that is only misleadingly nominalized into "consciousness." This is because conscious is descriptive of a variety of brain or cognitive processes rather than being an entity itself. This is presumably what William James was emphasizing in his stream of consciousness metaphor. Once the adjectival nature of conscious attribution is accepted, one is perhaps less likely to feel the need to associate it with a specific set of neurons in a particular brain area. For conciseness in this essay, I shall therefore refer to a conscious brain process as CBP.

The argument for CBPs in mammals derives from the observation that humans are capable of conscious deliberation, and humans have evolved from ancestors common to many other mammals. Given the evolution of CBPs, it is overwhelmingly likely that they confer some survival advantage. I shall postulate that at least one such advantage is the planning of action, the ability to decide among several mutually exclusive alternatives that all have pros and cons. A corollary of this is that CBPs also provide the evolutionary advantage of enhancing learning from mistakes. This follows because a mistake in an action plan throws the individual back into the previous realm of possible actions minus the failure.

Granted these points, two questions arise. First, why should CBPs be related to action plans? Second, as plans for action invariably have goals, what basic goals did CBPs evolve to achieve? The first question is quite easy to answer. Action requires brain guided motion, even in the case where the actor is human and the motion is of larynx and vocal cords (i.e. speech). In addition, achievement of goals almost always requires body locomotion. Thus, it appears that the evolution of brain guided movement is essential to the evolution of CBPs. A consequence of this is that plants have not evolved any form of conscious processing, as tropisms are essentially reflexive growth responses to the local environment.

The second question has been answered elegantly by Denton (2006). He argues that a range of primordial survival requirements drove the evolution of CBPs. Among these were hunger, thirst, need to maintain internal salt balance, and sex. A synopsis of his argument is that demands for food, water, and various salts periodically arise and must be satisfied if the individual is to survive. Interestingly, the range of homeostatic internal salt balances across mammalian species is almost constant (Denton, 2006), thus supporting their emergence early in evolution. In short, homeostasis must be maintained. Similarly, sexual contact must occur if the species is to survive. Denton's argument is that these drives constitute the primordial basis of emotions, and I find this general argument compelling.

Thus, we have arrived at the hypothesis that primordial survival requirements have facilitated the evolution of CBPs. The role of CBPs would therefore be to enhance the probability that a course of action would temporarily lead to satisfaction of such a primordial emotion. Given this, it seems apparent that a primary advantage of CBPs will be to enhance decision-making under conditions where the optimal decision, given the initial evidence, is less than obvious. The focus of this essay will therefore be on two issues. First, can we conjecture what assemblage of brain regions must necessarily be activated during any visual CBP? Second, can we formulate any requirements or constraints on the nature of neural interactions within and between these brain regions? To answer this, I shall discuss decision making networks in prefrontal cortex and their similarity to the visual circuits involved in binocular rivalry. This represents a very different conception of the relevance of rivalry to elucidating CBPs than that espoused by others (Leopold and Logothetis, 1996; Logothetis et al., 1996). It leads naturally to a generalization of rivalry circuits that will be argued to form a dynamical basis for arriving at difficult decisions. These networks also embody aspects of several previous discussions of CBPs: coalitions of neurons (Crick and Koch, 2003), a dynamic core of neurons (Tononi and Edelman, 1998), and neural network implementations of a global work space (Dehaene et al., 1998, 2003). Feedback, both excitatory and inhibitory, will emerge as necessary constitutive elements of CBPs.

As a scientist, I should emphasize that I shall propose and argue that certain conditions are requirements for CBPs. I shall not provide nor claim to provide logically definitive arguments that any of these must certainly be the case. The quest for elucidation of CBPs will involve an interaction between plausible hypotheses, logic, and empirical observation in the best scientific tradition.

17.2   Cortical networks for conscious vision

There have been several synopses of the plethora of visual cortical areas and their interconnections (Van Essen et al., 1992; Young, 1992). The most extensive data are almost entirely from macaques, but brain imaging (fMRI) studies have revealed many homologous areas in humans (Van Essen et al., 1998). For the purposes of this essay I shall make the assumption that the cortical visual systems of humans and macaques map quite accurately onto one another. This will doubtless turn out to be false in detail, although further data in both species will be required to decide the issue. The only key assumption here is that differences in the details are not relevant to the elucidation of basic visual CBPs. This assumption obviously does not preclude the likelihood that human cortical vision instantiates more and perhaps higher CBPs than those in other primates. In the following, therefore, I shall largely base my arguments on macaque data with appropriate references to human fMRI.

Given these caveats, it is convenient to focus on the schematic of cortical brain areas in Figure 17.1, which is derived from macaque data. This diagram is schematic in the sense that a number of visual areas have been ignored (e.g. V2, V3, MST), while others have been condensed (e.g. retina and LGN represented as input, IT representing TEO and TE). The area labeled Emotion represents the amygdala and other areas of the limbic system, while Episodic Memory incorporates the hippocampus and associated structures. Despite these simplifications, this abbreviated representation of cortical anatomy will suffice to instantiate the core areas requisite for conscious visual processing.

Each area in Figure 17.1 is shown as providing feedback connections to all areas that provide it with input by double-headed arrows. This serves to emphasize the anatomical fact that there are feedback loops between all interconnected cortical ar-

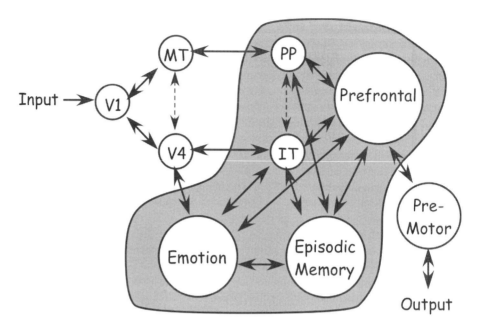

Figure 17.1. Simplified diagram of visual brain areas and associated brain areas critical for conscious vision. Beginning with Input (retina, LGN), V1 provides input to the dorsal visual pathway, approximated by MT (middle temporal cortex) and PP (posterior parietal cortex). In parallel with this, V1 provides input to the ventral visual pathway that includes V4 and IT (inferior temporal cortex). Dorsal and ventral pathways are weakly interconnected (dashed arrows) and converge in prefrontal cortex. These pathways also interact with brain areas related to emotion (e.g. amygdala and limbic system) and with areas critical for episodic memory (hippocampus, parahippocampal gyrus). Prefrontal cortex activity activates premotor areas, which ultimately lead to motor activity. Double-headed arrows indicate major interconnections among areas and highlight the fact that all involve both feedforward and feedback interactions. The areas and interconnections within the gray region are argued to be the essential substrate for conscious visual processes.

eas. The only exception to this feedback rule known in mammals is the lack of neural feedback from the LGN to retinal neurons (although such feedback is present in birds). The diagram represents the dorsal visual pathway by MT and posterior parietal cortex (PP) and the ventral pathway by V4 and inferior temporal cortex (IT). Although dorsal and ventral pathways are frequently treated as though they are virtually independent, it is known that there are at least modest feedback interconnections between them, which are illustrated by the dashed arrows between MT-V4 and IT-PP (Van Essen et al., 1992). Finally, dorsal and ventral pathways both activate adjacent regions of prefrontal cortex, which interact via feedback (Wilson et al., 1993; Courtney et al., 1996; Goldman-Rakic, 1998). In addition, there is fMRI evidence that areas of human medial frontal cortex are involved in social cognition (Amodio and Frith, 2006), and it is reasonable to suppose a similar role of medial frontal cortex in other social mammals (primates, wolves, dogs) on evolutionary grounds.

Both the dorsal and ventral visual hierarchies thus remain largely distinct but partially reciprocally interconnected as far as prefrontal cortex. Furthermore, prefrontal cortex incorporates circuits known to be involved in visual short-term memory (Fuster, 1995; Goldman-Rakic, 1998). Beyond prefrontal cortex one encounters premotor cortex and ultimately motor cortex mediating control of behavior. Thus, the various areas of prefrontal cortex can be regarded as the apex of the visual sensory system before the transformation into motor output. This leads naturally to my first hypothesis: activation of visual prefrontal areas is necessary *for any visual CBP*. For visual areas of prefrontal cortex to be activated, it follows that feedback loops between prefrontal areas, IT, and PP will be activated.

It may be noted here that Milner and Goodale have argued that only the ventral pathway via IT is involved in visual CBPs and that the dorsal pathway via IPS does not provide input into conscious vision (Milner and Goodale, 1995). As they state it (p. 200): "Attentional modulation of ventral-stream processing leads to conscious perception; attention modulation of the dorsal stream leads to action." However, this view of the dorsal pathway as being exclusively a nonconscious visual action pathway is no longer tenable. In humans we now know that parietal areas such as PP are critical for arithmetic (Abdullaev and Melnichuk, 1996), which clearly has claim to being a CBP. In addition, recent recordings from monkey parietal cortex demonstrate that neurons there can compute conditional probabilities implicitly represented in sequences of visual images (Yang and Shadlen, 2007). Conditional probabilities are obviously relevant to conscious visual decisions, so it seems clear that parietal areas such as PP must be involved in at least some aspects of conscious vision. In light of this, the dorsal pathway may be best construed not as a nonconscious visual action pathway but rather as a visual measurement pathway. Visual measurement may indeed be nonconscious for highly overlearned actions such as visually guided grasping, but it will be a part of CBPs in more unique visual situations. It is worth noting that the concept of a visual measurement pathway subsumes both the vision for action concept (Milner and Goodale, 1995) and the original concept of the dorsal pathway as the "where" pathway (Mishkin et al., 1983).

The presence of CBPs involving the dorsal visual pathway may also be related to the distinction between action in peripersonal as opposed to extrapersonal space. Peripersonal space is essentially the space within arm's reach and research related to the lack of conscious processing in the dorsal stream has been restricted to peripersonal space (Milner and Goodale, 1995). However, there is a double dissociation from lesion studies showing that different parietal areas are involved in peripersonal as opposed to extrapersonal space processing (Halligan and Marshall, 1991; Cowey et al., 1994). In light of this, a plausible hypothesis is that the importance of CBPs in action planning increases as a function of distance from the viewer. Thus, grasping an object within arm's reach is highly overlearned and may seldom or never require conscious processing (Milner and Goodale, 1995). However, a wolf pack stalking an antelope at a distance of several hundred meters must generally plan a course of action contingent upon wind direction, intervening obstacles, etc. Indeed, there is video footage of a pack of gray wolves planning an attack of two deer they had discovered in an upwind clearing (Coren, 2000, pp. 158–161). The alpha male used pointing to indicate to each of several other wolves where to go in order to surround the deer. Such spatial planning must surely have involved CBPs in the wolf analog of the dorsal visual stream. In fact, Coren (2000) compares this planning directly to maneuvers he engaged in during military training exercises. Clearly such planning in both species must involve conscious visuospatial planning that would occur in the dorsal pathway.

The foregoing clearly implies that visual CBPs entail concurrent neural activity in prefrontal cortex as well as in its major visual input areas IT and PP. To the extent that prefrontal activation is prolonged beyond about 200 ms, feedback circuits between prefrontal cortex and both IT and PP will be activated. (The time delay here is simply because feedback, of necessity, entails time beyond the feedforward sweep.) Furthermore, excitatory feedback within prefrontal cortex is generally held to provide the substrate for short-term memory (Fuster, 1995; González-Burgos et al., 2000). It is therefore reasonable to hypothesize that *recurrent activity between and within prefrontal cortex, IT and PP is essential for visual CBPs.* This is supported by Lamme and Roelfsema (2000) who conclude from a review of research on feedforward and feedback processing that (p. 577): "the feedforward sweep of information processing is mainly involved in pre-attentive, unconscious vision, whereas recurrent processing is required for attentive vision and visual awareness."

It should also be noted from Figure 17.1 that both emotional areas and episodic memory areas have recurrent feedback connections with prefrontal cortex. The argument that CBPs arose to facilitate the satisfaction of primordial emotions has already been made (Denton, 2006) and Damasio has extended the argument to much of human reason (Damasio, 1994). The amygdala, a key emotional area, has reciprocal connections with the ventral visual pathway (V4 and IT in Figure 17.1), but not with the dorsal pathway (Barton and Aggleton, 2000). This is consistent with the notion that object recognition, but not visual measurement, plays a dominant role in driving emotional learning and recall, and the amygdala is known to play a major role in these emotional processes (LaBar and Cabeza, 2006). In addition, decisions related to the planning of actions to fulfill emotional needs are frequently conscious and clearly require access to episodic memory. Thus, we can extend the argument above to include feedback interactions between prefrontal cortex, emotional areas, and episodic memory areas as necessary ingredients in visual CBPs.

All of the visual areas deemed necessary for CBPs are encompassed by the gray field in Figure 17.1. They represent the higher levels of the visual hierarchy along with their interactions. But what of activity in lower visual areas such as V1, MT, and V4, or areas like premotor cortex? Others have argued that V1 activity is not necessary for visual CBPs (Crick and Koch, 1995), and recent research on binocular rivalry has substantiated this conclusion. In this work, the effects of selective attention on traveling rivalry dominance waves (Wilson et al., 2001) was assessed using fMRI (Lee et al., 2007). It was shown that dominance waves were present in V1 whether or not the subject was attending to them. When the subjects attended to a task at fixation and ignored the waves, they reported that they were not perceptually aware of the waves. This switch due to attention was signaled in V2 and V3, where evidence of wave activity was directly correlated with visual awareness. Thus, V1 activity is not necessary or sufficient for visual awareness. Further evidence supporting the lack of V1 input to CBPs has been reported from studies of chromatic flicker in which perceptually invisible flicker rates are nevertheless evident in the V1 BOLD signal (Jiang et al., 2007). The situation for V2, V3, V4, and MT is not yet clear and awaits further research. Similarly, it may well be that feedback between prefrontal cortex and premotor areas is necessary for CBPs underlying some aspects of complex action planning, but it suffices for present purposes to remain agnostic.

17.3 Neural decisions and generalized rivalry

Binocular rivalry has frequently been touted in the consciousness literature as an ideal candidate for isolating the neural correlates of consciousness (NCC) (Leopold and Logothetis, 1996; Logothetis et al., 1996). As indicated above, fMRI exploration of traveling waves in rivalry provides strong evidence that V1 activity is neither necessary nor sufficient for CBPs (Lee et al., 2007). In fact, rivalry in V1 may or may not propagate up the visual hierarchy contingent on the top-down state of visual attention. Thus, neither fMRI studies of rivalry in humans nor single unit rivalry recordings in monkeys are likely to elucidate CBPs. Rather, my argument shall be that rivalry provides a paradigm of our most fully explored example of a neural circuit involved in decision making, albeit at preconscious levels. This, in turn, suggests that generalizations of rivalry will provide insights into CBPs. This argument rests on three observations. First, rivalry entails competitive inhibitory interactions between neural populations signaling different and mutually incompatible interpretations of the available visual input data (Wilson, 2005, 2007). Second, studies of decisions related to eye movements in the primate prefrontal cortex implicate neural networks with reciprocal competitive inhibition comparable to that in rivalry networks (Schall, 2003). Finally, there is evidence that rivalrous competition occurs at several levels of the visual hierarchy and therefore may represent a general principle of decision making throughout the visual system (Wilson, 2003). Thus, it is predicted that analogous networks will explain decision making at the highest levels of the visual hierarchy in prefrontal cortex. Consonant with this conclusion, Dennett argues that CBPs become conscious in consequence of winning competitions with alternative possibilities (Dennett, 1996).

Support for these arguments is buttressed by a comparison of V1 rivalry networks with prefrontal decision networks. Binocular rivalry requires reciprocal inhibition between two distinct groups of monocular neurons driven by stimuli to the left and right eyes (Wilson, 2005, 2007). Within each monocular group there is evidence for excitatory feedback, in this case due to contour collinearity (Alais and Blake, 1999; Wilson et al., 2001). To generalize, rivalry networks may be described as embodying recurrent excitation among mutually compatible responses (collinearity in V1) and strong competitive inhibition between incompatible (extremely different monocular) representations. Experiments carried out in prefrontal cortex by Schall have investigated primate decisions regarding the initiation of eye movements (Schall, 2003). Remarkably, the neural networks producing such decisions have the same recurrent inhibitory structure as rivalry networks! This lends credence to the hypothesis that rivalry networks can be generalized to elucidate higher level visual decision making.

A very simple neural network that instantiates these ideas is depicted in Figure 17.2. The network comprises 15 neurons arranged in five columns of three neurons each. Each of the five columns may be regarded as representing a different generalized attribute or component relevant to the situation. In face areas of IT, for example, the five columns might represent face elongation, eye separation, nose length, mouth width, and chin shape. The three neurons within each column would then represent above average, average, and below average values for each component. As a more speculative example, in prefrontal cortex, the five columns might represent emotional valance (positive, neutral, and negative), similarity to previous experience (high, medium, and low), familiarity of visual object (known, uncertain, unknown), location relative to observer, and direction of attention or gaze of visual object (if another human or other mammal). Although these are very small examples, the important point is that multiplication of each dimension by perhaps 10^6 begins to incorporate a richness and complexity that is truly germane to understanding CBPs.

Given the simple network in Figure 17.2, the next task is to specify the neural interactions. It should be emphasized at the outset that the precise details of these connections are not critical to the argument, although the general pattern is. In this example, I have assumed that the three neurons in each column are reciprocally connected by powerful inhibitory connections, thus precluding more than one of these cells from firing at the same time. This is consistent with the notion that a particular attribute must be either above average, average, or below average. As the five attributes represented by the different columns are not mutually exclusive, it will be assumed that previous episodic experiences have generated excitatory interconnections among them via some form of Hebbian learning. This is depicted in Figure 17.2A for a pattern represented by the gray neurons in a / shape. All pairwise connections, represented by double headed arrows, have been assigned a value of 0.5, thus providing positive feedback within this subset of neurons. The same network of 15 neurons has also been trained on the patterns depicted by the gray neurons in Figure 17.2B and C. For clarity, the recurrent excitatory connections within these patterns, although present in the model, are not illustrated. It is important to recognize that each of these three patterns represents a population code, and the elements of these codes overlap. For example, activation of neurons in the rightmost two columns of patterns A and B are identical; these patterns differ only in the remaining three neurons. Similarly, patterns A and C are identical regarding activation of neurons in the leftmost two columns.

This network has been simulated using an extension of the differential equations recently described for rivalry (Wilson, 2007). Briefly, the firing rate of the ith neuron, E_i, is given by:

$$\tau \frac{dE_i}{dt} = -E_i + \frac{[S_i + g \cdot H_i]_+}{1 + [S_i - g \cdot H_i]_+^{0.8}}$$
$$\tau_H \frac{dH_i}{dt} = -H_i + E_i \tag{17.1}$$

The variable H_i governed by the second equation represents a slow self-hyperpolarizing variable generally associated with Ca^{2+} modulated K^+ currents known to be present in human and other mammalian cortical excitatory neurons (McCormick and Williamson, 1989). These currents, which have time constants on the order of a second or more, have been proposed as a key factor in the alternations present in binocular rivalry (Wilson, 2005, 2007). In the current simulations, $\tau = 15$ ms, and $\tau_H = 700$ ms, although

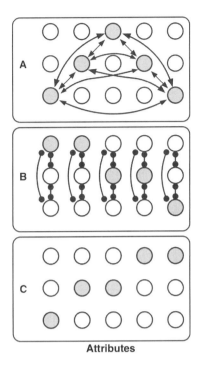

Attributes

Figure 17.2. Schematic of a simple neural network that supports a generalized rivalry competition. The network comprises 15 neurons organized in five columns and three rows. Each column represents a different attribute, while each row represents a different level of that attribute (see text for details). (A) One of three learned patterns of attributes (represented by a / shape) is highlighted in gray with all pairwise feedback excitatory connections represented by double-headed arrows. (B) This shows the same network with the inhibitory feedback within each column represented by the connections terminating in filled circles. Although only illustrated within one column, the same connection pattern is present in all columns. A second learned pattern is depicted by the gray neurons, although the excitatory feedback interconnections analogous to those in (A), although present, are not shown. (C) A third pattern learned by the network is illustrated by the gray neurons (excitatory interconnections not shown). Note that (A)–(C) all represent the same 15 neuron network and simply highlight different aspects of the neural connectivity.

neither value is critical so long as the latter is much greater than the former. The function in brackets, $[X]_+$, is a simple threshold function with a threshold value that valuates to zero for subthreshold stimulation levels X_i:

$$[X_i]_+ = \max \left\{ \begin{array}{c} X_i - \theta \\ 0 \end{array} \right\} \qquad (17.2)$$

The net stimulus is given by:

$$S_i = \text{Input} + 0.5 \sum_{\text{columns}} E_j - 3 \sum_{\text{row}} E_k \qquad (17.3)$$

where the first term on the right is the external input to the neuron, the first summation represents recurrent excitation from neurons in other columns to which the ith neuron has been connected via Hebbian facilitation and the final subtracted summation term represents inhibition from the other neurons within the same row. As illustrated in Figure 17.1, there is neither direct self-excitation nor direct self-inhibition in the network. The coefficients values 0.5 for excitation and -3 for inhibition are not critical so long as the inhibition is much stronger than the excitation.

The ratio $[S_i]_+/(1 + [S_i]_+^{0.8})$ in Equation (17.1) simply generates a compressive nonlinearity at higher Si levels, which agrees with firing rates of human neurons and has been shown to explain certain aspects of binocular rivalry (Wilson, 2007). Thus, Equation (17.1) is a spike rate description of neural firing and adaptation with the same general type of response nonlinearity as the Wilson-Cowan equations (Wilson and Cowan, 1973).

The network just described represents a generalization of binocular rivalry networks (Wilson, 2007) and is a plausible candidate for a generalized decision network. Suppose that the network is stimulated by a weighted sum of the three input patterns depicted in Figure 17.2A–C. Each of these input patterns can be considered as evidence in favor of a particular interpretation of sensory information or as evidence in favor of a particular course of action. Therefore, one might expect that when evidence for one pattern is significantly stronger than evidence for the others, the network response should simply represent the dominant evidence and suppress the other patterns. Simulations show that this indeed occurs whenever stimulation by one of the patterns is at least 40% stronger than stimulation by either of the other patterns. Thus, the network immediately makes easy decisions and suppresses other possibilities by settling into a "winner take all" mode.

The situation becomes quite different when the evidence for each of the three patterns is quite similar. In this case, one might say that the information available to the prefrontal cortex is closely balanced among several alternatives. To simulate this, the three patterns in Figure 17.2 were given the relative weights of 1.0, 0.95, and 0.90 respectively. The network response, as illustrated in Figure 17.3, is now quite striking. Instead of settling into a winner take all mode reflecting the strongest input, the network goes into an oscillation in which first the pattern with the strongest evidence is dominant and temporarily suppresses the other patterns. Next, the pattern with the second strongest input becomes dominant and suppresses the others, and finally the pattern with the least evidence becomes dominant. This sequence then repeats itself in the same order again and again. Two aspects of this response are significant. First, the network automatically rank orders its responses in the order of the available evidence. Second, it exhibits what is known as "inhibition of return" in the selective attention literature (Klein, 2000) as it does not return to its first excitatory state until it has sequenced through the other available states. I submit that this network behavior is suggestive of CBPs in cases where a decision among alternatives is difficult because of ambiguities in the evidence. It reminds me of my own experience at gourmet restau-

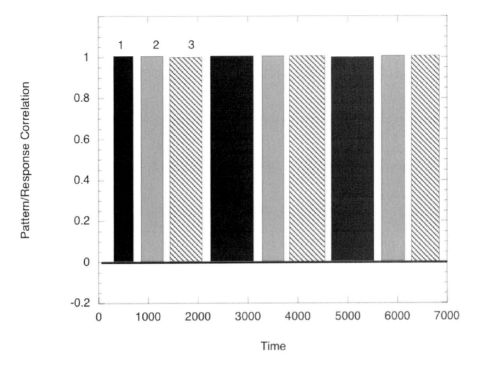

Figure 17.3. A sequence of patterns that the network in Figure 17.2 cycles through in response to appropriate stimulation. The patterns are the three shown in Figure 17.2. Network activity in simulations was assigned to a particular pattern if the correlation with that pattern was > 0.99. The times between response to one pattern and its sequel represent transition periods when no single pattern was dominant. Note that the patterns repeat in the same order shown by the numerals 1–3.

rants, where I have difficulty deciding among several tempting entrees (e.g. venison, duck, or lobster) and consciously revisit the appeal of each one in turn before my final choice.

It should be obvious that this network represents a generalization of a rivalry network in that it cycles among three global states rather than just two binocular inputs. Cycling among more patterns is also possible in larger networks. Furthermore, rather than incorporating positive feedback due to collinear facilitation, the positive feedback here is due to a learned pattern of correlations among diverse attributes.

This network needs to be placed within the context of the anatomy sketched in Figure 17.1. If this network were situated in prefrontal cortex, then each of the three activity states would send a different neural feedback signal to PP, IT, and emotional and episodic memory centers. Presumably such feedback has evolved to facilitate transmission of any further supportive evidence back to prefrontal cortex. This feedback (or reentrance for those enamored of neologisms (Tononi and Edelman, 1998)) would thus play a role related to (and perhaps constitutive of) selective attention in roughly the manner espoused by Tsotsos (1993). If this resulted in augmentation of positive

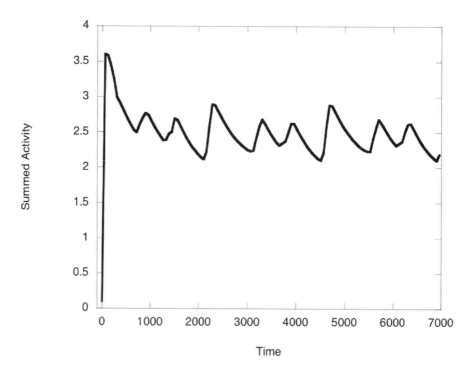

Figure 17.4. Summed network activity as a function of time. The summed activity shows an oscillation driven by the pattern transitions shown in Figure 17.3. This oscillation would be reflected in the electroencephalogram (EEG) under appropriate conditions.

evidence at some stage in the prefrontal network oscillation, this could terminate the oscillation and lead to a decision via bifurcation to a winner-take-all mode. If not, the oscillation would continue until feedback from some state generated sufficiently enhanced information to win the competition.

A final point about this simple network is illustrated by the graph in Figure 17.4. This plots the sum of all neural activity in the network as a function of time under the conditions producing the state alternations in Figure 17.3. The summed neural activity generates a brain wave oscillation of the sort frequently present in the electroencephalogram (EEG). No attempt has been made here to tune the oscillation frequency to any particular value, although this could easily be done by scaling τ and τ_H appropriately. The salient point is that any decision network in the brain that is alternating among several possible outcomes will ipso facto generate an EEG type oscillation. In this instance the oscillation is not performing binding of attributes; that is being done by the positive feedback connections. Rather, the oscillation is an emergent property or epiphenomenon of the cycling among competing neural groups in decision making.

17.4 Significance of feedback

The simple model just described depends critically on feedback, both excitatory and inhibitory. The excitatory feedback is essential for pattern completion and to stabilize each of the learned input patterns. Similarly, inhibitory feedback is critical to the selection of patterns one at a time in sequence instead of generating a sum of all patterns. Self-adaptation via the feedback variable H_i in Equation 17.1 is likewise critical for switching between patterns. Without feedback, oscillations among patterns are not possible. Similarly, feedback is crucial to stabilization of one pattern with very strong supporting evidence at the expense of other patterns for which there is weaker evidence via a network bifurcation to a winner take all regime.

Without pattern completion and competition generated by positive and negative feedback, it is hard to imagine how a brain could make any decisions at all. The alternative is a feedforward system in which visual information flows through just once to generate each action without any possible neural activation representing alternative possibilities. This certainly does occur in many extremely simple decision situations but not in all. In fact, any action planning that precedes execution must necessarily involve feedback in order for the first planning step to be recalled for use in planning further steps. There has been some discussion of zombies among those studying CBPs (Koch and Crick, 2001). Here I offer the hypothesis that it is impaired feedback that is responsible for zombie-like behavior. In the extreme case this would generate a purely feedforward neural system that would produce a sequence of actions without any conscious, competitive evaluation of alternatives.

The crucial role of feedback in CBPs leads to an important point regarding processing speed. Feedback such as that in the generalized rivalry network above ipso facto results in slower processing than simple feedforward processing. This is simply because passage through feedback loops several times accumulates processing time. To this may be added the observation that prolonged neural activity entails a metabolic cost, especially as active neurons are the cells most demanding of energy in the body. The fact that CBPs are inherently slow therefore implies that only some aspects of visual experience will be conscious, while rapid responses will not be. For example, a back in Canadian football running downfield and suddenly cutting to one side to avoid tacklers will be best served by rapid feedforward processing within his brain. In short, it would be a waste of valuable time and metabolic resources for all visual brain processes to be conscious.

This emphasis on feedback as an essential ingredient in CBPs has been argued forcefully by several others. Edelman and colleagues have emphasized the importance of "reentrant" processing in understanding CBPs (Sporns et al., 1991; Tononi and Edelman, 1998). As is evident from examination of their work, reentrance is just a neologism for feedback. Dehaene and his coworkers have gone even farther and have developed explicit neural networks for various visual CBPs (Dehaene et al., 1998, 2003). These are more complex networks but otherwise similar in spirit to the network discussed above, and feedback is ubiquitous in their simulations.

17.5   The homunculus and the Cartesian Theater

One of the major critiques by those opposing explanations of CBPs in purely neural terms is couched in the form of an infinite regress. This is exemplified by two metaphors. In the homunculus metaphor, it is assumed that a miniscule humanoid in the brain is required to explain the perception of CBPs. In the Cartesian Theater metaphor CBPs are conceptualized as a play upon a stage. However, this raises the question of what audience is present to be conscious of the play. Either metaphor, if true, would imply an infinite regress of the homunculus within the homunculus or the theater within the minds of the audience, and so forth. Thus, any proposed theory of CBPs that is open to the criticism of implicitly requiring an infinite regress cannot be correct.

Feedback provides a natural resolution of the infinite regress problem. In the feedback network depicted in Figure 17.2 different subsets of neurons respond in an ongoing sequence. As the same neurons are involved in each case, no problem of an infinite regress can arise. Depending on changes in the stimulation of the network triggered by feedback to its inputs (IT, PP, emotional, and memory areas in Figure 17.1), it is possible for the network to reach a decision by settling into a winner take all state driven by the strongest available evidence. Note further that no particular neuron is involved in all of the network responses, so no neuron or unique group of neurons is necessary for the occurrence of a CBP. In short, there is no homunculus within the network. A preferable metaphor would be to say that networks underlying CBPs function as a committee that arrives at decisions through evaluation of evidence germane to the issue. The committee does not arrive at its decisions through consensus, however, but rather by having a subset of members silence the opposition due to a preponderance of evidence, that is, winner take all. This committee metaphor answers the question "who is conscious of all the conscious processes within the entire committee?," the answer being nobody!

17.6   Discussion

The essential requirements for any visual CBP may now be summarized. They are:

(1) Activation of prefrontal visual networks. This may happen either through their inputs from the dorsal and ventral visual pathways or else through emotional centers activated by primordial emotions.

(2) Activation of feedback to highest areas of dorsal and ventral pathways.

(3) Input from and activation of feedback to emotional areas (e.g. amygdala)

(4) Activation of feedback to episodic memory areas.

(5) Activation of both positive (cooperative) and negative (competitive) feedback circuits within prefrontal cortex and the areas to which it is connected.

All of these requirements are entirely consistent with the known anatomy and physiology of the visual system (Van Essen et al., 1992; Young, 1992). Furthermore, feedback excitation in prefrontal cortex appears to be the key component of neural short-term memory (Fuster, 1995; Goldman-Rakic, 1998), and short term memory is clearly an essential ingredient of CBPs. Also, feedback inhibition, which is crucial in the generalized rivalry network described above, exists in prefrontal circuits that control the decision to make a saccadic eye movement (Schall, 2003).

The generalized rivalry network developed above is most similar in spirit to the detailed network simulations by Dehaene and colleagues (Dehaene et al., 1998). Their networks contain recurrent feedback among several levels as sketched in Figure 17.1 above. Their recent network includes the interesting additional feature that feedforward activation is mediated by AMPA receptors, whereas feedback projections are represented by NMDA receptors (Dehaene et al., 2003). Due to the properties of NMDA synapses, this gives the feedback a primarily modulatory function and may represent an important further insight into neural networks supporting CBPs.

The importance of feedback in the guise of reentrance has also been emphasized by Edelman's group (Tononi and Edelman, 1998). Varela has also argued for the importance of both feedforward and feedback activation in any understanding of CBPs (Varela, 2002). Crick and Koch (2003) have acknowledged that their qualitative ideas concerning "coalitions of neurons" and CBPs, are very similar to those of the Dehaene group and also to Edleman's "dynamic core" hypothesis. The key to all these models as well as to the generalized rivalry network described above is that a combination of positive and negative feedback can combine to activate one population of neurons and suppress others in a manner contingent on the details of stimulation. The additional contribution of the generalized rivalry network is to show how the network can cycle through several different population responses in a manner indicative of conscious decision making under difficult or ambiguous circumstances.

A natural criticism of this network would be that it is too repetitive in its responses. There are three rejoinders to this. First, feedback from this network to its high-level cortical inputs (albeit not simulated) will ultimately shift the sequence and result in a winner of the decision competition. Second, addition of noise in the H_i equation in Equation (17.1) will result in a much more varied repetition sequence (Wilson, 2007). Most interesting, however, is the possible onset of mathematical chaos. In significantly larger networks with feedback excitation and inhibition it has been observed that chaotic dynamics frequently ensue (Van Vreeswijk and Sompolinsky, 1996; Wilson and Wilkinson, 2000). Although chaos is deterministic, it is unpredictable except on very short timescales. Thus, a chaotic decision network, although deterministic, would appear to be making quasi-random jumps among possible states. It is plausible that networks in such a chaotic state provide the neural substrate for novelty and creativity, an idea whose possible evolutionary basis has been discussed elsewhere in the context of "Machiavellian Intelligence" (Miller, 1997).

It has been emphasized that CBPs are inherently subjective (Searle, 1992) and this is fully consistent with the current model. Given the requirements above, any visual CBP will encompass idiosyncratic memory recall, emotional valance, etc. that is perforce unique to the individual brain. No other brain could be privy to all of the idiosyncratic details unless that other brain had exactly the same neural connectivity patterns driven by a lifetime of exactly the same learning and experience. This does not happen even in the case of identical twins who unavoidably view the world from different locations in space throughout their lives. This seems to me a definition of subjective: idiosyncratic emotional and memory recall within a particular brain that cannot in principle (due to the presence of a finite number of neurons in every brain) be known or experienced in complete detail by any other brain. This, I think, also provides a basis for the resolution of the "qualia" problem.

In closing, it is worth quoting Searle:

> Consciousness is a higher-level or emergent property of the brain in the utterly harmless sense – in which solidity is a higher-level emergent property of H_2O molecules when they are in a lattice structure (ice), and liquidity is similarly a higher-level emergent property of H_2O molecules when they are, roughly speaking, rolling around on each other (water). (p. 14)

In other words, CBPs are simply the global or macroscopic ramifications of dynamical interactions in large populations of microscopic neurons. This is precisely the sense in which the generalized rivalry network above generates simulations of conscious deliberation and decisions. The list above of five necessary requirements for conscious visual processing is doubtless incomplete and therefore not sufficient. Refining and expanding the list are thus tasks for future research and simulations.

References

Abdullaev, Y. G. and Melnichuk, K. V. (1996). Counting and arithmetic functions of neurons in the human parietal cortex. *NeuroImage*, 3: S216.

Alais, D. and Blake, R. (1999). Grouping visual features during binocular rivalry. *Vision Res.*, 39: 4341–4353.

Amodio, D. M. and Frith, C. D. (2006). Meeting of minds: the medial frontal cortex and social cognition. *Nat. Rev. Neurosci.*, 7: 268–277.

Barton, R. A. and Aggleton, J. P. (2000). Primate evolution and the amygdala. In J. P. Aggleton (ed.) *The Amygdala: A Functional Analysis*. New York: Oxford University Press, pp. 479–508.

Coren, S. (2000). *How to Speak Dog: Mastering the Art of Dog–Human Communication*. New York: Free Press.

Courtney, S. M., Ungerleider, L. G., Keil, K. and Haxby, J. V. (1996). Object and spatial visual working memory activate separate neural systems in human cortex. *Cereb. Cortex*, 6: 39–49.

Cowey, A., Small, M. and Ellis, S. (1994). Left visuo-spatial neglect can be worse in far than in near space. *Neuropsychologia*, 32: 1059–1066.

Crick, F. and Koch, C. (1995). Are we aware of neural activity in primary visual cortex? *Nature*, 375: 121–123.

Crick, F. and Koch, C. (2003). A framework for consciousness. *Nat. Neurosci.*, 6: 119–126.

Damasio, A. R. (1994). *Descartes' Error: Emotion, Reason, and the Human Brain.* New York: G. P. Putnam.

Dehaene, S., Kerszberg, M. and Changeux, J. P. (1998). A neuronal model of a global workspace in effortful cognitive tasks. *Proc. Nat. Acad. Sci.,* 95: 14529–14534.

Dehaene, S., Sergent, C. and Changeux, J. P. (2003). A neuronal network model linking subjective reports and objective physiological data during conscious perception. *Proc. Nat. Acad. Sci.,* 100: 8520–8525.

Dennett, D. C. (1996). *Kinds of Minds: Toward an Understanding of Consciousness.* New York: Basic Books.

Denton, D. (2006). *The Primordial Emotions: The Dawning of Consciousness.* Oxford, UK: Oxford University Press.

Fuster, J. M. (1995). *Memory in the Cerebral Cortex.* Cambridge, MA: MIT Press.

Goldman-Rakic, P. S. (1998). The prefrontal landscape: implications of functional architecture for understanding human mentation and the central executive. In A. C. Roberts, T. W. Robbins and L. Weiskrantz (eds.) *The Prefrontal Cortex: Executive and Cognitive Functions.* Oxford, UK: Oxford University Press, pp. 87–102).

González-Burgos, G., Barrionuevo, G. and Lewis, D. A. (2000). Horizontal synaptic connections in monkey prefrontal cortex: an in vitro electrophysiological study. *Cereb. Cortex,* 10: 82–92.

Halligan, P. W. and Marshall, J. C. (1991). Left neglect for near but not far space in man. *Nature,* 350: 498–500.

Jiang, Y., Zhou, K. and He, S. (2007). Human visual cortex responds to invisible chromatic flicker. *Nat. Neurosci.,* 10: 657–662.

Klein, R. M. (2000). Inhibition of return. *Trends Cogn. Sci.,* 4: 138–147.

Koch, C. and Crick, F. (2001). On the zombie within. *Nature,* 411: 893.

LaBar, K. S., and Cabeza, R. (2006). Cognitive neuroscience of emotional memory. *Nat. Rev. Neurosci.,* 7: 54–64.

Lamme, V. A. F. and Roelfsema, P. R. (2000). The distinct modes of vision offered by feedforward and recurrent processing. *Trends Neurosci.,* 23: 571–557.

Lee, S. H., Blake, R. and Heeger, D. J. (2007). Hierarchy of cortical responses underlying binocular rivalry. *Nat. Neurosci.,* 10: 1048–1054.

Leopold, D. A. and Logothetis, N. K. (1996). Activity changes in early visual cortex reflect monkeys' percepts during binocular rivalry. *Nature,* 379: 549–553.

Logothetis, N. K., Leopold, D. A. and Scheinberg, D. L. (1996). What is rivaling during binocular rivalry? *Nature,* 380: 621–624.

McCormick, D. A. and Williamson, A. (1989). Convergence and divergence of neurotransmitter action in human cerebral cortex. *Proc. Nat. Acad. Sci.,* 86: 8098–8102.

Miller, G. F. (1997). Protean primates: the evolution of adaptive unpredictability in competition and courtship. In A. Whiten and R. W. Byrne (eds.) *Machiavellian Intelligence II: Extensions and Evaluations*. Cambridge, UK: Cambridge University Press, pp. 312–340.

Milner, A. D. and Goodale, M. A. (1995). *The Visual Brain in Action*. Oxford, UK: Oxford University Press.

Mishkin, M., Ungerleider, L. G. and Macko, K. A. (1983). Object vision and spatial vision: two cortical pathways. *Trends Neurosci.*, 6: 414–417.

Schall, J. D. (2003). On building a bridge between brain and behavior. *Ann. Rev. Psychol.*, 55: 1–28.

Searle, J. R. (1992). *The Rediscovery of the Mind*, Cambridge, MA: MIT Press.

Sporns, O., Tononi, G. and Edelman, G. M. (1991). Modeling perceptual grouping and figure-ground segregation by means of active reentrant connections. *Proc. Nat. Acad. Sci.*, 88: 129–133.

Tononi, G. and Edelman, G.M. (1998). Consciousness and complexity. *Science*, 282: 1846–1851.

Tsotsos, J. K. (1993). An inhibitory beam for attentional selection. In L. Harris and M. Jenkin (eds.) *Spatial Vision in Humans and Robots*, New York: Cambridge University Press, pp. 313–331.

Van Essen, D. C., Anderson, C. H. and Felleman, D. J. (1992). Information processing in the primate visual system: an integrated systems perspective. *Science*, 255: 419–423.

Van Essen, D. C., Drury, H. A. Joshi, S. and Miller, M. I. (1998). Functional and structural mapping of human cerebral cortex: solutions are in the surfaces. *Proc. Nat. Acad. Sci.*, 95: 788–795.

Van Vreeswijk, C. and Sompolinsky, H. (1996). Chaos in neuronal networks with balanced excitatory and inhibitory activity. *Science*, 274: 1724–1726.

Varela, F. J. (2002). Upwards and downwards causation in the brain. In K. Yasue, M. Jibu and T. Della Senta (eds.) *No Matter, Never Mind*. Amsterdam: John Benjamins, pp. 95–107.

Wilson, F. A. W., Scalaidhe, S. P. O. and Goldman-Rakic, P. S. (1993). Dissociation of object and spatial processing domains in primate prefrontal cortex. *Science*, 260: 1955–1958.

Wilson, H. R. (2003). Computational evidence for a rivalry hierarchy in vision. *Proc. Nat. Acad. Sci. USA*, 100: 14499–14503.

Wilson, H. R. (2005). Rivalry and perceptual oscillations: a dynamical synthesis. In D. Alais and R. Blake (eds.) *Binocular Rivalry*. Cambridge, MA: MIT Press, pp. 317–335.

Wilson, H. R. (2007). Minimal physiological conditions for binocular rivalry and rivalry memory. *Vision Res.*, 47: 2741–2750.

Wilson, H. R., Blake, R. and Lee, S. H. (2001). Dynamics of travelling waves in visual perception. *Nature*, 412: 907–910.

Wilson, H. R. and Cowan, J. D. (1973). A mathematical theory of the functional dynamics of cortical and thalamic nervous tissue. *Kybernetik*, 13: 55–80.

Wilson, H. R. and Wilkinson, F. (2000). Dynamics of perceptual oscillations in form vision. *Nat. Neurosci.*, 3: 170–176.

Yang, T. and Shadlen, M. N. (2007). Probabilistic reasoning by neurons. *Nature*, 447: 1075–1080.

Young, M. P. (1992). Objective analysis of the topological organization of the primate cortical visual system. *Nature*, 358: 152–155.

Author index

Subject index